Quality Assurance in the Era of Individualized Medicine

Anastasius S. Moumtzoglou
P. & A. Kyriakou Children's Hospital, Greece

A volume in the Advances in
Medical Diagnosis, Treatment, and
Care (AMDTC) Book Series

IGI Global
DISSEMINATOR OF KNOWLEDGE

Published in the United States of America by
IGI Global
Medical Information Science Reference (an imprint of IGI Global)
701 E. Chocolate Avenue
Hershey PA, USA 17033
Tel: 717-533-8845
Fax: 717-533-8661
E-mail: cust@igi-global.com
Web site: http://www.igi-global.com

Library of Congress Cataloging-in-Publication Data

Names: Moumtzoglou, Anastasius S., 1959- editor.
Title: Quality assurance in the era of individualized medicine / Anastasius S. Moumtzoglou, editor.
Description: Hershey, PA : Medical Information Science Reference, [2020] | Includes bibliographical references and index. | Summary: "This book explores the science of individuality in the practice of health care quality and health services management"-- Provided by publisher.
Identifiers: LCCN 2019039494 (print) | LCCN 2019039495 (ebook) | ISBN 9781799823902 (hardcover) | ISBN 9781799823919 (ebook)
Subjects: MESH: Quality Assurance, Health Care | Precision Medicine--methods
Classification: LCC RA418 (print) | LCC RA418 (ebook) | NLM W 84.41 | DDC 362.1--dc23
LC record available at https://lccn.loc.gov/2019039494
LC ebook record available at https://lccn.loc.gov/2019039495

This book is published in the IGI Global book series Advances in Medical Diagnosis, Treatment, and Care (AMDTC) (ISSN: 2475-6628; eISSN: 2475-6636)

British Cataloguing in Publication Data
A Cataloguing in Publication record for this book is available from the British Library.

Advances in Medical Diagnosis, Treatment, and Care (AMDTC) Book Series

ISSN:2475-6628
EISSN:2475-6636

MISSION

Advancements in medicine have prolonged the life expectancy of individuals all over the world. Once life-threatening conditions have become significantly easier to treat and even cure in many cases. Continued research in the medical field will further improve the quality of life, longevity, and wellbeing of individuals.

The **Advances in Medical Diagnosis, Treatment, and Care (AMDTC)** book series seeks to highlight publications on innovative treatment methodologies, diagnosis tools and techniques, and best practices for patient care. Comprised of comprehensive resources aimed to assist professionals in the medical field apply the latest innovations in the identification and management of medical conditions as well as patient care and interaction, the books within the AMDTC series are relevant to the research and practical needs of medical practitioners, researchers, students, and hospital administrators.

COVERAGE

- Medical Testing
- Disease Prevention
- Disease Management
- Medical Procedures
- Critical Care
- Experimental Medicine
- Patient-Centered Care
- Patient Interaction
- Emergency Medicine
- Internal Medicine

The Advances in Medical Diagnosis, Treatment, and Care (AMDTC) Book Series (ISSN 2475-6628) is published by IGI Global, 701 E. Chocolate Avenue, Hershey, PA 17033-1240, USA, www.igi-global.com. This series is composed of titles available for purchase individually; each title is edited to be contextually exclusive from any other title within the series. For pricing and ordering information please visit http://www.igi-global.com/book-series/advances-medical-diagnosis-treatment-care/129618. Postmaster: Send all address changes to above address.

Titles in this Series

For a list of additional titles in this series, please visit:
https://www.igi-global.com/book-series/advances-medical-diagnosis-treatment-care/129618

Strategies to Overcome Superbug Invasions Emerging Research and Opportunities
Dimple Sethi Chopra (Punjabi University, India)
Medical Information Science Reference • © 2020 • 284pp • H/C (ISBN: 9781799803072) • US $225.00 (our price)

Advanced Applications of Nanotechnology in Cancer Detection and Therapy
Alireza Heidari (Faculty of Chemistry, California South University, USA)
Medical Information Science Reference • © 2020 • 280pp • H/C (ISBN: 9781799801399) • US $275.00 (our price)

Developmental Challenges and Societal Issues for Individuals With Intellectual Disabilities
Rejani Thudalikunnil Gopalan (Mahatma Gandhi Medical College and Hospital, India)
Medical Information Science Reference • © 2020 • 416pp • H/C (ISBN: 9781799812234) • US $265.00 (our price)

Global Applications of One Health Practice and Care
Sandul Yasobant (Center for Development Research (ZEF), Germany) and Deepak Saxena (Indian Institute of Public Health Gandhinagar, India)
Medical Information Science Reference • © 2019 • 306pp • H/C (ISBN: 9781522563044) • US $245.00 (our price)

Pre-Screening Systems for Early Disease Prediction, Detection, and Prevention
Thierry Edoh (Technical University of Munich, Germany) Pravin Pawar (Philips Research, India) and Sagar Mohammad (Philips Research, India)
Medical Information Science Reference • © 2019 • 395pp • H/C (ISBN: 9781522571315) • US $245.00 (our price)

Advanced Methodologies and Technologies in Medicine and Healthcare
Mehdi Khosrow-Pour, D.B.A. (Information Resources Management Association, USA)
Medical Information Science Reference • © 2019 • 591pp • H/C (ISBN: 9781522574897) • US $325.00 (our price)

IGI Global
DISSEMINATOR OF KNOWLEDGE

701 East Chocolate Avenue, Hershey, PA 17033, USA
Tel: 717-533-8845 x100 • Fax: 717-533-8661
E-Mail: cust@igi-global.com • www.igi-global.com

To my cousins, Costas & Dimitrios Birtachas

Table of Contents

Detailed Table of Contents

Anastasius S. Moumtzoglou argues that the application of linear models to human systems and healthcare management and quality has improved our understanding of their system structure and function. However, such models often fall short of explaining experimental results or predicting future abnormalities in complex nonlinear systems which help in dissecting and analyzing individual system components. Nonlinear models may better explain how the individual components collectively act and interact to produce a dynamic system in constant flux. They also assist in filling in some of the results which are not adequately explained by linear models. In this context, we should consider the integration of linear and non-linear theories in healthcare quality and management, drawing the initial conditions of chaotic behavior from the standardization of the linear theory, and distinguishing between desirable and undesirable variation relegating statistical process control only to issues of high certainty regarding the outcome.

Anastasius S. Moumtzoglou and Abraham Pouliakis contend that population health management (PHM) has been a discipline which studies and facilitates care delivery across a group of individuals or the general population. In the context of PHM, the life science industry has had no motivation to design drugs or devices and even offer treatment of patient management that is only effective for a distinct population segment. The primary outgrowth of the science of individuality, as well as the rising 'wiki medicine', fully recognizes the uniqueness of the individual. Cloud computing, Big Data, M-Health and recently Internet of Things can nowadays offer the resources to deal with numerous shortcomings such as data collection and processing, of the PHM approach, as they facilitate the propagation of the science of individuality.

Dimitrios G. Katehakis and Angelina Kouroubali analyze the digital transformation challenges related to the implementation of quality electronic medical record systems in Greece, within the broader frame of the European digital single market. The authors explore characteristics of quality, interoperable and secure electronic medical records, and provide an overview of the challenges and factors affecting their adoption, implementation, and operation. Key challenges relate to linking electronic medical records with the workflow, building trust and acceptance by making the best use of champions and key stakeholders, and financing the digital transformation transition and sustainability. The foreseen benefits include better support of medical decisions across all stages of the patient pathway, patients empowered to carry with them clinically relevant information, fostering research and unlocking the full potential of vendors to implement innovative tools to support continuity of care.

Stavros Pitoglou cites evidence that Machine Learning, closely related to Artificial Intelligence and standing at the intersection of Computer Science and Mathematical Statistical Theory, comes in handy when the truth is hiding in a place that the human brain has no access to. Given any prediction or assessment problem, the more complicated this issue is, based on the difficulty of the human mind to understand

Abraham Pouliakis et al. compare Machine Learning Algorithms (MLAs) in the discrimination between benign and malignant endometrial nuclei and lesions. Nuclei characteristics are obtained via image analysis and were measured from liquid-based cytology slides. 416 histologically confirmed patients were involved, 168 healthy, and the remaining with pathological endometrium. 50% of the cases were used to three MLAs: a feedforward artificial neural network (ANN) trained by the backpropagation algorithm, a learning vector quantization (LVQ) and a competitive learning ANN. The outcome of this process was the classification of cell nuclei as benign or malignant. Based on the nuclei classification, an algorithm to classify individual patients was constructed. The sensitivity of the MLAs in training set for nuclei classification was in the range of 77%-84%. Patients' classification had sensitivity in the range of 90%-98%. These findings indicate that MLAs have good performance for the classification of endometrial nuclei and lesions.

Katerina Giazitzi, Vaios T. Karathanos, and George Boskou declare that the nutritional information on food services could be part of a public health policy against the increasing rate of obesity. The aim of their work is to present the state of the art for the nutritional information on food services and the mHealth application usage, worldwide. A particular case study is presented that refers to an Electronic Intelligent System of Personalized Dietary Advice ("DISYS") for tablets and smart-phones. This application provides nutritional analysis of menu items and personalized suggestions according to the nutritional demands of each customer. The application was characterized as an easy-to-use, comprehensive and useful tool. Volunteers considered that this application contributes to overall health by enabling the modulation of body weight throughout healthier choices, reduction of calorie intake and self-monitoring. MHealth applications designed to provide nutritional information, seem to be useful for customers as they recommend appropriate nutritional options. They are an effective tool for caterers and nutritionists, who can provide value-added services.

Yannis Koumpouros asserts that the ageing of the population is one of the major societal and financial problems. The prevalence of disability increases dramatically by age. The loss of mobility can be devastating to the elderly, while falls belong to the main geriatric syndromes. Mobility aids are a one-way street to maintain independent mobility. The performance of daily activities is restrained by a series of factors related to the assistive device limitations, or the ones emerged from environmental causes. A literature review reveals minimal tools for assessing assistive mobility devices able to capture users' satisfaction. The chapter presents an assessment methodology in order to investigate mobility assistive devices' limitations, dissatisfaction reasons and identify the most appropriate tools to study such limitations and conclude in valid outcomes. One of the valuable characteristics of the study presented in its generalizability since it is not disease-oriented. A summary of the results from both the literature review and the real case study on a mixed group of end-users are presented in the chapter.

Marilena Stamouli and Antonia Mourtzikou state that role that clinical laboratories play in the detection, diagnosis and treatment of diseases is evident. Clinical laboratories need to sustain a commitment to quality and demonstrate a certifiable level of compliance. Many strategies are used to reduce laboratory errors, including internal QC procedures, external quality assessment programs, implementation of QIs and six-sigma methodology. All strategies should be consistent with the requirements of the International Standard for medical laboratory accreditation and suitable for promoting corrective/preventive actions. They must promote total quality and patient safety and be consistent with the definition of a laboratory error. Harmonization process is in progress; however, further efforts must be made. Total quality management must be evaluated periodically. For a patient-centered approach, there is the need to assure that every step of the whole testing process is correctly performed, that weaknesses are recognized and that corrective and preventive actions are designed and implemented.

Pranil Vijay Sawalakhe asserts that ensuring the quality of testing laboratory services plays an essential role in the field of service sector. Acknowledging the revolution occurred by Six Sigma (SS) in corporate world, and service sector, testing laboratories can also be benefited by the application of the same. SS focuses on process improvement that is a major determinant of customer satisfaction. CTQs (Critical to Quality) is a quality characteristic of a product or a service which is required to be improved from a customer's point of view. CTQs are the vital measurable indicators of a product or process whose performance standards or specification limits must be met in order to satisfy the customer. The aim of this research is to develop a model for establishing CTQ for testing laboratories. The focus is on establishing process-wise CTQ characteristics from the voice of customer taken from direct and indirect customers associated with testing laboratories. The list of established CTQs will be a useful guide for both practitioners and academics willing to evaluate performance of testing laboratories.

Dimitrios G. Katehakis, George Pangalos, and Andriana Prentza claim that preserving patient safety, patient rights, and safeguarding trust are crucial components for the provision of high-quality medical treatments across borders. This chapter focuses on required technological improvements to address quality challenges through the adoption of generic building blocks (BBs), towards enabling seamless care between European healthcare systems. The authors present essential considerations that are relevant to incremental, cross-sectorial advancements for the enhancement of the technology used for the implementation of the directive on the application of patients' rights in cross-border healthcare. These include cross-domain technical BBs to support non-repudiation, capability lookup, dynamic service location, and electronic identification. The authors use cross-border electronic prescription and patient summary, as a case to discuss the use of related international interoperability standards, together with recommendations for future work relevant to the introduction of better quality, trustworthy, cross-border, electronic health services in Europe.

Preface

There is a significant deficiency of contemporary medicine which is reflected by the use of experts to make recommendations or guidelines for a large proportion of decisions for which no or minimal data exists. Fortunately, our capacity to get just that information is rapidly arising. An era which is characterized by the right drug and dose, at the right cost and timing has begun (Topol, 2012). Medicine for the common good is not sufficient. A rebooted life science, instead of a mass-population-directed strategy, would leverage the science of individuality, getting the relevant digital readout from an individual to shape a therapy. We now have the tools to do this on a broad basis throughout medicine and for the first time, promote a level of prescription precision we have never seen before.

The era of individualized medicine ultimately promises to do away with terms like 'cryptogenic' and 'essential,' fully recognizing the uniqueness of the individual who needs to be seen and treated with utter respect for his or her individuality. It will not be long until digitizing a person unlocks the cause for what is wrong, creating valuable knowledge that can save a life or markedly improve the quality of life. That is a significant outgrowth of the science of individuality.

In this context, the entire classification system of medical conditions and diagnoses is about to be rewritten. Instead of our current reductionist model for which individuals are unwisely assigned to such categories as one of two types of diabetes or cancer of a particular organ, the science of individuality will promote a new molecular taxonomy that invokes the primary biologic basis, regarding genes or pathways.

The implementation of health IT is among the essential components. However, the adoption of electronic health records is just the first step toward the creation of the requisite infrastructure, although direct access to a health record of a patient is not seen as entirely positive. In the current debate, a discrepancy is noted between the legislation, policies and decision ambitions versus the care professionals' preferences and knowledge regarding the issue. Many healthcare professionals are concerned about how the information will be understood by patients when reading without any medical support. Patients, on the other hand, want to communicate and interact more with healthcare which can be facilitated and streamlined by information technology.

Moreover, as beneficial as data interoperability is to healthcare, at present, it is mostly an unreached goal. That is chiefly because electronic health information systems have been developed independently. As a result, they include a large number of heterogeneous and distributed proprietary models for representing and recording patients' information. Consequently, the seamless, productive and meaningful exchange of patients' information is yet to be achieved across healthcare systems.

Consequently, an appraisal of the concepts of interoperability in the context of healthcare, its benefits and its attendant challenges is vital. In this context, we have to take into account that achieving complete interoperability of health information systems requires:

- The adoption of standardized healthcare terminology.
- An education strategy.
- The design of useable interfaces for ICT tools.
- Consideration of privacy and security issues.

On the other hand, Artificial Intelligence (AI) techniques and numerous applications have been reported which include the use of classical statistical models, as well as more advanced techniques, such as neural networks.

Furthermore, Machine Learning is the subfield of computer science that gives computers the ability to learn without being explicitly programmed. That is a description of the significant paradigm shift Machine Learning brings to the world of solving problems, answering questions and making decisions with the use of information technologies. It implies that we can delegate to a computer the task to make sense out of a dataset without needing humans to define the exact course of calculations and actions.

At the micro-level, it is well known that the clinical laboratory plays an essential role in the treatment of diseases. Patient management, treatment, detection of complications, hospital admission and discharge, are based on laboratory test results. Thus, the laboratory is accountable in providing reliable, analytic measurements to clinicians facilitating the prevention, diagnosis, treatment and management of the disease.

Quality assurance programs in cytology constitute the most critical methods to maintain and improve the diagnostic acumen of cytotechnologists and cytopathologists, although there are difficulties in carrying out such programs. However, a long turnaround time of the glass slides is a significant drawback. In this context, the use of photographed slides has been a partial and unsatisfactory solution due to cost and delay in preparation.

Finally, the lack of all European citizens' confidence in the protection of their data has become more than obvious. As a result, a comprehensive, initial proposal was submitted in 2012. After several years of deliberations, the new General Data Privacy Regulation (GDPR), was voted by the EU parliament in April 2015. Its primary objective was to homogenize the legal frameworks of all EU members on data privacy protection. By the 25th of May 2018, all the EU members were obliged to fully apply the General Data Protection Regulation ensuring that all data are protected appropriately.

THE CHALLENGES

Long-term thinking is necessary for the health and social care systems because significant changes in the population, society, technology and other areas are likely to shape social and health care in the future.

As an illustration, economic growth and its distribution will shape future standards of living. National governments' policies are one set of factors that will impact the economy and living standards in the future. However, being unemployed, in insecure work, or working in impoverished conditions contributes to poor health, as work and health are inextricably linked. In this context, the future of work is widely debated, and the implications for health are complex and uncertain as there is significant uncertainty around macroeconomic forecasts for earnings and employment (Lovell & Bibby, 2018).

Furthermore, much has been written about the likely impact of automation and particularly the potential for job displacement, but predictions for the future vary widely (Office for National Statistics, 2019).

On the flip side, there is also optimism about opportunities technology could bring. As some roles are replaced, others will be adapted and integrated with technology, and new ones will be created. As automation replaces routine tasks, people could be freed to undertake more rewarding work (Willis et al., 2019).

Nonetheless, there are limits to the tasks that technology can perform, especially where human intelligence and perception are still essential (Frey & Osborne, 2017). As a result, social skills, intelligence and perception, are likely to be of enduring value, and the caring roles and skills that depend on human interaction could become sought after.

How well industries and governments prepare the current workforce with the knowledge, skills and flexibility needed to adapt to new types of work will also influence the impact of new technologies. As work changes, it is likely that social attitudes and expectations of working will change too. Accordingly, alternatives to traditional employment models have been proposed as policy responses to promote people's economic security and wellbeing within a shifting labor market.

The economic, societal and technological shifts are likely to alter the way that people connect, as well as their communities and broader institutions (Pantel et al., 2013; Holt-Lunstad et al., 2015; Laugesen, et al., 2018). Still, social networks are essential for our health. People who are socially isolated have a higher risk of early mortality, comparable with other well-established risk factors.

Furthermore, the older population, which is particularly vulnerable to isolation, is growing while young people grow up in a time when technology has fundamentally changed the way that people interact. In digital terms, people are more connected than ever, although it is now recognized that technology use also has the potential to harm young people's psychological health.

On the other hand, the world population is ageing and growing, as the proportion of older people increases due to improved life expectancy, which is projected to continue to rise over the coming years. As people live longer, they are spending more years in poor health and are increasingly likely to live with multiple conditions. Moreover, the burden of disease is shaped by the prevalence of the major health risk factors, but it is hard to predict how the prevalence of health risk factors will change over time.

Additionally, recent analysis has suggested that over the next years, health spending will need to rise to maintain current service levels, while the picture is starker for social care (Evans, 2018).

Moreover, even with additional funding, the health and social care system risk not having enough staff to deliver services in the future as there are no simple solutions to the workforce challenge. Increasing the pipeline of professionals and creating the working cultures and conditions that encourage retention takes time and investment.

There is also a consensus that health and social care services need to change in future to respond to the population's changing health needs and new models of team-based primary care are being developed that aim to better respond to people's changing health needs while also helping address health professionals' shortages.

Similarly, medical and technological advances shape the future supply of health services while personalized medicine and quantum technology, also bring new questions for policymakers (Willis et al., 2019). Advances in precision medicine are intersecting with the understanding of the social determinants of health. However, some researchers worry about the potential for medical approaches to reducing health inequalities (Bayer & Galea, 2015).

Correspondingly, a growing body of research demonstrates the biological consequences of adverse social circumstances and their impact on health (Notterman & Mitchell, 2015; Wolfe, Evans & Seeman, 2012; Mitchell et al., 2014). That includes how social deprivation changes gene expression, shifting people's susceptibility to a variety of physical and mental health conditions. One future scenario involves better prevention and treatment efforts through the health system. However, even if social factors were incorporated into precision medicine efforts, population health benefits would still be limited given that medicalizing social issues could lead to a misdiagnosis of the causes of ill health and a misallocation of resources. Finally, precision medicine targeting individuals will not replace the need for social policy to reduce health inequalities across populations.

Besides, the climate is warming globally, with severe consequences for health (Watts et al., 2018). As the earth warms, weather extremes occur with more frequency, and the risk of disease increases and access to clean air, water and food could be compromised.

Currently, there is no regulatory framework to prevent overheating in hospitals and care homes. Moreover, the workforce will need to develop new capabilities relating to the climate-related changing illness patterns. At the same time, as the sector adapts to changing environmental conditions, its role in mitigating environmental impact will become critical.

By the same token, advancement in artificial intelligence, nanotechnology and genomics are driving rapid technological change in the public and private health sector (Topol, 2019). There are several technological trends related to health and health care that seem likely to continue or accelerate:

- People are embracing technology to monitor and manage their health.
- The expansion of remote care models.
- Genomics and precision medicine.
- Data held by the health system.
- The application of artificial intelligence and machine learning techniques.

Overall, digital and data-driven technologies have the potential to improve care quality and outcomes. However, excitement about the potential benefits of new technology often outpaces evidence of impact. A more comprehensive review of the evidence on bringing Artificial Intelligence into health care found that the field is undoubtedly high on promise but relatively low on data and proof.

Data and technology are instrumental goods; they do not, in themselves, lead to better health or health care. As a result, the challenge for policymakers is in ensuring data and technologies are used maximally for public benefit, with minimum adverse impact.

There are also ethical challenges in applying Artificial Intelligence and other technologies in the health system (Wellcome Trust, 2019). These include algorithmic bias in tools used for decision making, as well as the lack of transparency in how Artificial Intelligence aided decisions are reached.

However, the emergence of new technologies does not necessarily mean that health and social care systems will be able to implement and benefit from them in the future. The health systems are currently not well equipped to use data they already have to monitor and improve the quality and efficiency of services (Bardsley, 2016). Moreover, there is the question of who is accountable for technology-led decisions if something goes wrong while the potential of data-driven technologies (such as machine learning) is also limited by the current quality of health and social care data, collected in disjointed and inconsistent ways.

Lastly, implementing and spreading new technologies in the health systems is as much about people as technology (Greenhalgh et al., 2017). As a result, those seeking to embed new digital innovations must take into account the complex social and organizational contexts in which new technologies are being introduced. Moreover, they should consider that all areas of outlined changes and uncertainty are affected, to varying degrees, by political choices, which are also shaped by the public's attitudes and engagement.

However, changes in the population, society, technology and other areas are only one side of the coin. On the flip side, people using healthcare services, to be treated as an individual is an essential component of their whole experience while each patient experiences healthcare in a unique and individual way. For many, healthcare forms a small but essential part of their wider life. Being recognized and treated as an individual remains essential to a person when they become a patient. Nevertheless, healthcare is based on the average.

SEARCHING FOR A SOLUTION

The application of linear models to human systems and healthcare management and quality has improved our understanding of their system structure and function. However, such models often fall short of explaining experimental results or predicting future abnormalities in complex nonlinear systems which help in dissecting and analyzing individual system components. Nonlinear models may better explain how the individual components collectively act and interact to produce a dynamic system in constant flux. They also assist in filling in some of the results which are not adequately explained by linear models.

However, as not all medicine is nonlinear, linear modeling should not be abandoned, as the use of both models is complementary and leads to a complete understanding of system behavior.

Chaos theory also provides new insights in standard as well as abnormal behavior within systems. Applications of chaos, especially fractals, may detect disease in its early stages and proves valuable in managing illness while the pursue of complexity theory provides new insights regarding the genetic encryption of the environment in the context of biological evolution, cellular automata, and modulation of protein production using biological pulse signals (Lewin, 1999).

In this context, we could easily consider the integration of linear and non-linear theories in healthcare quality and management, as we can draw the initial conditions of chaotic behavior from the standardization of the linear theory. Moreover, we can distinguish between desirable and undesirable variation relegating statistical process control only to issues of high certainty regarding the outcome.

The book intends to:

- Support students understand the science of Individuality.
- Help healthcare professionals better understand the needs of their patients.
- Act as an assistant for patients to derive more benefits from their healthcare.
- Encourage e-health systems' designers and managers to ground everyday practice on the science of individuality.

The prospective audience includes undergraduate and extended degree programs students, graduate students of health care quality and health services management, executive education and continuing education, health care managers and health professionals.

ORGANIZATION OF THE BOOK

In Chapter 1, Anastasius S. Moumtzoglou argues that the application of linear models to human systems and healthcare management and quality has improved our understanding of their system structure and function. However, such models often fall short of explaining experimental results or predicting future abnormalities in complex nonlinear systems which help in dissecting and analyzing individual system components. Nonlinear models may better explain how the individual components collectively act and interact to produce a dynamic system in constant flux. They also assist in filling in some of the results which are not adequately explained by linear models. In this context, we should consider the integration of linear and non-linear theories in healthcare quality and management, drawing the initial conditions of chaotic behavior from the standardization of the linear theory, and distinguishing between desirable and undesirable variation relegating statistical process control only to issues of high certainty regarding the outcome.

In Chapter 2, Anastasius S. Moumtzoglou and Abraham Pouliakis contend that population health management (PHM) has been a discipline which studies and facilitates care delivery across a group of individuals or the general population. In the context of PHM, the life science industry has had no motivation to design drugs or devices and even offer treatment of patient management that is only effective for a distinct population segment. The primary outgrowth of the science of individuality, as well as the rising 'wiki medicine', fully recognizes the uniqueness of the individual. Cloud computing, Big Data, M-Health and recently Internet of Things can nowadays offer the resources to deal with numerous shortcomings such as data collection and processing, of the PHM approach, as they facilitate the propagation of the science of individuality.

In Chapter 3, Dimitrios G. Katehakis and Angelina Kouroubali analyze the digital transformation challenges related to the implementation of quality electronic medical record systems in Greece, within the broader frame of the European digital single market. The authors explore characteristics of quality, interoperable and secure electronic medical records, and provide an overview of the challenges and factors affecting their adoption, implementation, and operation. Key challenges relate to linking electronic medical records with the workflow, building trust and acceptance by making the best use of champions and key stakeholders, and financing the digital transformation transition and sustainability. The foreseen benefits include better support of medical decisions across all stages of the patient pathway, patients empowered to carry with them clinically relevant information, fostering research and unlocking the full potential of vendors to implement innovative tools to support continuity of care

In Chapter 4, Stavros Pitoglou cites evidence that Machine Learning, closely related to Artificial Intelligence and standing at the intersection of Computer Science and Mathematical Statistical Theory, comes in handy when the truth is hiding in a place that the human brain has no access to. Given any prediction or assessment problem, the more complicated this issue is, based on the difficulty of the human mind to understand the inherent causalities/patterns and apply conventional methods towards an acceptable solution, Machine Learning can find a fertile field of application. This article's purpose is to give a general non-technical definition of Machine Learning, provide a review of its latest implementations in the Healthcare domain and add to the ongoing discussion on this subject. It suggests the active involvement of entities beyond the already active academic community in the quest for solutions that "exploit" existing datasets and can be applied in the daily practice, embedded inside the software processes that are already in use.

In Chapter 5, Abraham Pouliakis et al. compare Machine Learning Algorithms (MLAs) in the discrimination between benign and malignant endometrial nuclei and lesions. Nuclei characteristics are obtained via image analysis and were measured from liquid-based cytology slides. 416 histologically confirmed patients were involved, 168 healthy, and the remaining with pathological endometrium. 50% of the cases were used to three MLAs: a feedforward artificial neural network (ANN) trained by the backpropagation algorithm, a learning vector quantization (LVQ) and a competitive learning ANN. The outcome of this process was the classification of cell nuclei as benign or malignant. Based on the nuclei classification, an algorithm to classify individual patients was constructed. The sensitivity of the MLAs in training set for nuclei classification was in the range of 77%-84%. Patients' classification had sensitivity in the range of 90%-98%. These findings indicate that MLAs have good performance for the classification of endometrial nuclei and lesions.

In Chapter 6, Katerina Giazitzi, Vaios T. Karathanos, and George Boskou declare that the nutritional information on food services could be part of a public health policy against the increasing rate of obesity. The aim of their work is to present the state of the art for the nutritional information on food services and the mHealth application usage, worldwide. A particular case study is presented that refers to an Electronic Intelligent System of Personalized Dietary Advice ("DISYS") for tablets and smart-phones. This application provides nutritional analysis of menu items and personalized suggestions according to the nutritional demands of each customer. The application was characterized as an easy-to-use, comprehensive and useful tool. Volunteers considered that this application contributes to overall health by enabling the modulation of body weight throughout healthier choices, reduction of calorie intake and self-monitoring. MHealth applications designed to provide nutritional information, seem to be useful for customers as they recommend appropriate nutritional options. They are an effective tool for caterers and nutritionists, who can provide value-added services.

In Chapter 7, Yannis Koumpouros asserts that the ageing of the population is one of the major societal and financial problems. The prevalence of disability increases dramatically by age. The loss of mobility can be devastating to the elderly, while falls belong to the main geriatric syndromes. Mobility aids are a one-way street to maintain independent mobility. The performance of daily activities is restrained by a series of factors related to the assistive device limitations, or the ones emerged from environmental causes. A literature review reveals minimal tools for assessing assistive mobility devices able to capture users' satisfaction. The chapter presents an assessment methodology in order to investigate mobility assistive devices' limitations, dissatisfaction reasons and identify the most appropriate tools to study such limitations and conclude in valid outcomes. One of the valuable characteristics of the study presented in its generalizability since it is not disease-oriented. A summary of the results from both the literature review and the real case study on a mixed group of end-users are presented in the chapter.

In Chapter 8, Marilena Stamouli and Antonia Mourtzikou state that role that clinical laboratories play in the detection, diagnosis and treatment of diseases is evident. Clinical laboratories need to sustain a commitment to quality and demonstrate a certifiable level of compliance. Many strategies are used to reduce laboratory errors, including internal QC procedures, external quality assessment programs, implementation of QIs and six-sigma methodology. All strategies should be consistent with the requirements of the International Standard for medical laboratory accreditation and suitable for promoting corrective/preventive actions. They must promote total quality and patient safety and be consistent with the definition of a laboratory error. Harmonization process is in progress; however, further efforts must be made. Total quality management must be evaluated periodically. For a patient-centered approach, there is the need to assure that every step of the whole testing process is correctly performed, that weaknesses are recognized and that corrective and preventive actions are designed and implemented.

In Chapter 9, Pranil Vijay Sawalakhe asserts that ensuring the quality of testing laboratory services plays an essential role in the field of service sector. Acknowledging the revolution occurred by Six Sigma (SS) in corporate world, and service sector, testing laboratories can also be benefited by the application of the same. SS focuses on process improvement that is a major determinant of customer satisfaction. CTQs (Critical to Quality) is a quality characteristic of a product or a service which is required to be improved from a customer's point of view. CTQs are the vital measurable indicators of a product or process whose performance standards or specification limits must be met in order to satisfy the customer. The aim of this research is to develop a model for establishing CTQ for testing laboratories. The focus is on establishing process-wise CTQ characteristics from the voice of customer taken from direct and indirect customers associated with testing laboratories. The list of established CTQs will be a useful guide for both practitioners and academics willing to evaluate performance of testing laboratories.

In Chapter 10, Dimitrios G. Katehakis, George Pangalos, and Andriana Prentza claim that preserving patient safety, patient rights, and safeguarding trust are crucial components for the provision of high-quality medical treatments across borders. This chapter focuses on required technological improvements to address quality challenges through the adoption of generic building blocks (BBs), towards enabling seamless care between European healthcare systems. The authors present essential considerations that are relevant to incremental, cross-sectorial advancements for the enhancement of the technology used for the implementation of the directive on the application of patients' rights in cross-border healthcare. These include cross-domain technical BBs to support non-repudiation, capability lookup, dynamic service location, and electronic identification. The authors use cross-border electronic prescription and patient summary, as a case to discuss the use of related international interoperability standards, together with recommendations for future work relevant to the introduction of better quality, trustworthy, cross-border, electronic health services in Europe.

REFERENCES

Bardsley, M. (2016). *Understanding analytical capability in health care: Do we have more data than insight?* The Health Foundation.

Evans, H. (2018). *Does the public see tax rises as the answer to NHS funding pressures?* London: The King's Fund.

Frey, C. B., & Osborne, M. A. (2017). The Future of Employment: How susceptible are jobs to computerisation? *Technological Forecasting and Social Change, 114*, 254–280. doi:10.1016/j.techfore.2016.08.019

Greenhalgh, T., Wherton, J., Papoutsi, C., Lynch, J., Hughes, J., A'Court, C., ... Shaw, S. (2017). Beyond Adoption: A New Framework for Theorizing and Evaluating Nonadoption, Abandonment, and Challenges to the Scale-Up, Spread, and Sustainability of Health and Care Technologies. *Journal of Medical Internet Research, 19*(11), e367. doi:10.2196/jmir.8775 PMID:29092808

Holt-Lunstad, J., Smith, T. B., Baker, M., Harris, T., & Stephenson, J. (2015). Loneliness and Social Isolation as Risk Factors for Mortality: A Meta-Analytic Review. *Perspectives on Psychological Science, 10*(2), 227–237. doi:10.1177/1745691614568352 PMID:25910392

Laugesen, K., Baggesen, L. M., Schmidt, S. L. J., Glymour, M. M., Mathias, L., Arnold, M., & .... (2018). Social isolation and all-cause mortality:a population-based cohort study in Denmark. *Scientific Reports, 8*(1), 4731. doi:10.103841598-018-22963-w PMID:29549355

Lewin, R. (1999). *Complexity: Life at the Edge of Chaos*. Chicago: The University of Chicago Press.

Lovell, N., & Bibby, J. (2018). *What makes us healthy? An introduction to the social determinants of health*. London: The Health Foundation.

Mitchell, C., Hobcraft, J., McLanahan, S. S., Siegel, S. R., Berg, A., Brooks-Gunn, J., ... Notterman, D. (2014). Social disadvantage, genetic sensitivity,and children's telomere length. *Proceedings of the National Academy of Sciences of the United States of America, 111*(16), 5944–5949. doi:10.1073/pnas.1404293111 PMID:24711381

Notterman, D. A., & Mitchell, C. (2015). Epigenetics and understanding the impact of social determinants of health. *Pediatric Clinics of North America, 62*(5), 1227–1240. doi:10.1016/j.pcl.2015.05.012 PMID:26318949

Office for National Statistics. (n.d.). *Which occupations are at highest risk of being automated?* Retrieved June 3, 2019, from www.ons.gov.uk/employmentandlabourmarket/peopleinwork/employmentandemployeetypes/articles/whichoccupationsareathighestriskofbeingautomated/2019-03-25

Pantell, M., Rehkopf, D., Jutte, D., Syme, S. L., Balmes, J., & Adler, N. (2013). Social isolation: A predictor of mortality comparable to traditional clinical risk factors. *American Journal of Public Health*, *103*(11), 2056–2062. doi:10.2105/AJPH.2013.301261 PMID:24028260

Topol, E. (2019). High-performance medicine: The convergence of human and artificial intelligence. *Nature Medicine*, *25*(1), 44–56. doi:10.103841591-018-0300-7 PMID:30617339

Topol, E. J. (2012). *The creative destruction of medicine: how the digital revolution will create better health care*. New York: Basic Books.

Wellcome Trust. (2019). *The ethical, social and political challenges of using artificial intelligence in healthcare*. Retrieved June 3, 2019 from https://wellcomeac.uk/funding/ethical-social-and-political-challenges-using-artificial-intelligence-healthcare

Willis, M., Duckworth, P., Coulter, A., Meyer, E. T., & Osborne, M. (2019). The Future of Health Care: Protocol for Measuring the Potential of Task Automation Grounded in the National Health Service Primary Care System. *JMIR Research Protocols*, *8*(4), e11232. doi:10.2196/11232 PMID:30964437

Wolfe, B., Evans, W., & Seeman, T. E. (Eds.). (2012). The Biological Consequences of Socioeconomic Inequalities. Russell Sage Foundation.

Acknowledgment

I would like to thank the reviewers for the care with which they reviewed the manuscripts and all the authors for their diverse and outstanding contributions to this book.

Chapter 1
The Science of Individuality and Healthcare Quality

Anastasius S. Moumtzoglou
https://orcid.org/0000-0002-5899-1033
P. & A. Kyriakou Children's Hospital, Greece

ABSTRACT

The application of linear models to human systems and healthcare management and quality has improved our understanding of their system structure and function. However, such models often fall short of explaining experimental results or predicting future abnormalities in complex nonlinear systems which help in dissecting and analyzing individual system components. Nonlinear models may better explain how the individual components collectively act and interact to produce a dynamic system in constant flux. They also assist in filling in some of the results that are not adequately explained by linear models. In this context, we should consider the integration of linear and non-linear theories in healthcare quality and management, drawing the initial conditions of chaotic behavior from the standardization of the linear theory, and distinguishing between desirable and undesirable variation relegating statistical process control only to issues of high certainty regarding the outcome.

INTRODUCTION

Long-term thinking is necessary for the health and social care systems because significant changes in the population, society, technology and other areas are likely to shape social and health care in the future.

DOI: 10.4018/978-1-7998-2390-2.ch001

As an illustration, economic growth and its distribution will shape future standards of living. National governments' policies are one set of factors that will impact the economy and living standards in the future. However, being unemployed, in insecure work, or working in impoverished conditions contributes to poor health, as work and health are inextricably linked. In this context, the future of work is widely debated, and the implications for health are complex and uncertain as there is significant uncertainty around macroeconomic forecasts for earnings and employment (Lovell & Bibby, 2018).

Furthermore, much has been written about the likely impact of automation and particularly the potential for job displacement, but predictions for the future vary widely (Office for National Statistics, 2019).

On the flip side, there is also optimism about opportunities technology could bring. As some roles are replaced, others will be adapted and integrated with technology, and new ones will be created. As automation replaces routine tasks, people could be freed to undertake more rewarding work (Willis et al., 2019).

Nonetheless, there are limits to the tasks that technology can perform, especially where human intelligence and perception are still essential (Frey & Osborne, 2017). As a result, social skills, intelligence and perception, are likely to be of enduring value, and the caring roles and skills that depend on human interaction could become sought after.

How well industries and governments prepare the current workforce with the knowledge, skills and flexibility needed to adapt to new types of work will also influence the impact of new technologies. As work changes, it is likely that social attitudes and expectations of working will change too. Accordingly, alternatives to traditional employment models have been proposed as policy responses to promote people's economic security and wellbeing within a shifting labor market.

The economic, societal and technological shifts are likely to alter the way that people connect, as well as their communities and broader institutions (Pantel et al., 2013; Holt-Lunstad et al., 2015; Laugesen, et al., 2018). Still, social networks are essential for our health. People who are socially isolated have a higher risk of early mortality, comparable with other well-established risk factors.

Furthermore, the older population, which is particularly vulnerable to isolation, is growing while young people grow up in a time when technology has fundamentally changed the way that people interact. In digital terms, people are more connected than ever, although it is now recognized that technology use also has the potential to harm young people's psychological health.

On the other hand, the world population is ageing and growing, as the proportion of older people increases due to improved life expectancy, which is projected to continue to rise over the coming years. As people live longer, they are spending more years in poor health and are increasingly likely to live with multiple conditions.

Moreover, the burden of disease is shaped by the prevalence of the major health risk factors, but it is hard to predict how the prevalence of health risk factors will change over time.

Additionally, recent analysis has suggested that over the next years, health spending will need to rise to maintain current service levels, while the picture is starker for social care (Evans, 2018).

Moreover, even with additional funding, the health and social care system risk not having enough staff to deliver services in the future as there are no simple solutions to the workforce challenge. Increasing the pipeline of professionals and creating the working cultures and conditions that encourage retention takes time and investment.

There is also a consensus that health and social care services need to change in future to respond to the population's changing health needs and new models of team-based primary care are being developed that aim to better respond to people's changing health needs while also helping address health professionals' shortages.

Similarly, medical and technological advances shape the future supply of health services while personalized medicine and quantum technology, also bring new questions for policymakers (Willis et al., 2019). Advances in precision medicine are intersecting with the understanding of the social determinants of health. However, some researchers worry about the potential for medical approaches to reducing health inequalities (Bayer & Galea, 2015).

Correspondingly, a growing body of research demonstrates the biological consequences of adverse social circumstances and their impact on health (Notterman & Mitchell, 2015; Wolfe, Evans & Seeman, 2012; Mitchell et al., 2014). That includes how social deprivation changes gene expression, shifting people's susceptibility to a variety of physical and mental health conditions. One future scenario involves better prevention and treatment efforts through the health system. However, even if social factors were incorporated into precision medicine efforts, population health benefits would still be limited given that medicalizing social issues could lead to a misdiagnosis of the causes of ill health and a misallocation of resources. Finally, precision medicine targeting individuals will not replace the need for social policy to reduce health inequalities across populations.

Besides, the climate is warming globally, with severe consequences for health (Watts et al., 2018). As the earth warms, weather extremes occur with more frequency, and the risk of disease increases and access to clean air, water and food could be compromised.

Currently, there is no regulatory framework to prevent overheating in hospitals and care homes. Moreover, the workforce will need to develop new capabilities relating to the climate-related changing illness patterns. At the same time, as the sector adapts to changing environmental conditions, its role in mitigating environmental impact will become critical.

By the same token, advancement in artificial intelligence, nanotechnology and genomics are driving rapid technological change in the public and private health sector (Topol, 2019). There are several technological trends related to health and health care that seem likely to continue or accelerate:

- People are embracing technology to monitor and manage their health.
- The expansion of remote care models.
- Genomics and precision medicine.
- Data held by the health system.
- The application of artificial intelligence and machine learning techniques

Overall, digital and data-driven technologies have the potential to improve care quality and outcomes. However, excitement about the potential benefits of new technology often outpaces evidence of impact. A more comprehensive review of the evidence on bringing Artificial Intelligence into health care found that the field is undoubtedly high on promise but relatively low on data and proof.

Data and technology are instrumental goods; they do not in themselves lead to better health or health care. As a result, the challenge for policymakers is in ensuring data and technologies are used maximally for public benefit, with minimum adverse impact.

There are also ethical challenges in applying Artificial Intelligence and other technologies in the health system (Wellcome Trust, 2019). These include algorithmic bias in tools used for decision making, as well as the lack of transparency in how Artificial Intelligence aided decisions are reached.

However, the emergence of new technologies does not necessarily mean that health and social care systems will be able to implement and benefit from them in the future. The health systems are currently not well equipped to use data they already have to monitor and improve the quality and efficiency of services (Bardsley, 2016). Moreover, there is the question of who is accountable for technology-led decisions if something goes wrong while the potential of data-driven technologies (such as machine learning) is also limited by the current quality of health and social care data, collected in disjointed and inconsistent ways.

Lastly, implementing and spreading new technologies in the health systems is as much about people as technology (Greenhalgh et al., 2017). As a result, those seeking to embed new digital innovations must take into account the complex social and organizational contexts in which new technologies are being introduced. Moreover, they should consider that all areas of outlined changes and uncertainty are affected, to varying degrees, by political choices, which are also shaped by the public's attitudes and engagement.

However, changes in the population, society, technology and other areas are only one side of the coin. On the flip side, people using healthcare services, to be treated as an individual is an essential component of their whole experience while each patient experiences healthcare in a unique and individual way. For many, healthcare forms a small but essential part of their wider life. Being recognized and treated as an individual remains essential to a person when they become a patient. Nevertheless, healthcare is based on the average.

As a result, the objective of the chapter is to examine the idea of 'average', its evolution, ways of overthrowing it and the impact on healthcare quality and patient safety.

THE INVENTION OF THE AVERAGE

The societal average relates to Lambert Adolphe Jacques Quetelet (1796-1874), a Belgian mathematician dealing with astronomy, contemplated that the Belgian revolution of 1830 against the Dutch would put an end to his professional ambitions when he was struck with inspiration (Donnelly,2015). He thought that it is attainable to work out science to manage society based on his life learning of how to identify hidden patterns in the celestial heavens. Thus, he used the same science to find hidden patterns in the apparent chaos of social behavior by applying the methods of astronomy to the study of people.

In this context, Quetelet dreamed up the statue of a gladiator, supposing that sculptors make several copies of the statue. Quetelet claimed that every copy would be different due to flaws. Moreover, according to Quetelet, the average statue of 1,000 copies would be nearly identical to the original statue. In the same manner, Quetelet contended, in a striking leap of logic, that if wey average together 1,000 different soldiers, we will end up with a very close approximation of the 'One True Soldier', who exists in some Platonic realm, of which each living soldier is an imperfect representation.

Florence Nightingale adopted Quetelet's ideas in nursing while Karl Marx developed his economic theory of Communism, announcing that the 'Average Man' proved the existence of historical determinism. The physicist James Maxwell was also inspired by Quetelet's mathematics to formulate the classical theory of gas mechanics, and the physician John Snow marked the start of the field of public health by using Quetelet's ideas to fight cholera in London. Finally, Wilhelm Wundt, the father of experimental psychology, proclaimed that we could learn more psychology from statistical averages.

However, Quetelet is only half the story of how the 'Age of Average' evolved. The other half revolves on Sir Francis Galton (1822-1911) who started as one of Quetelet's most devout disciples but eventually became his most distinguished critic (Forrest, 1974). Explicitly, Galton rejected Quetelet's belief that individuals who deviated from the average represented "error." At the same time, he agreed with Quetelet's concept of types, since he believed that 'the Eminent', 'the Imbecile', and 'the Mediocre' comprised a separate type of human beings. As a result, he wanted to preserve Quetelet's idea that the average member of a group represented that group's type but rejected the idea that an individual's deviation from average represented an error. He resolved this apparent paradox by redefining 'error' as 'rank.'

Besides, Frederick Winslow Taylor (1856-1915) started in the 1890s to share a new vision for the industrial organization, suggesting that he would minimize inefficiency in the same way that the method of averages was presumed to minimize error (Kanigel, 2005). His vision, though Quetelet was the first scientist to champion standardization in government bureaucracies and scientific data collection, which was grounded on the concept of standardization. Nonetheless, Taylor argued that his inspiration for standardizing human labor came from one of his math teachers at Phillips Exeter Academy. According to Taylor, his teacher often assigned Taylor and his classmates a series of math problems, instructing them to snap their fingers and raise their hand when they completed the problems. The teacher used a stopwatch to time the students and then calculated how long it took the average boy to finish. Finally, the teacher created homework assignments by using the average time to calculate the number of problems he had to include in the assignment so that the average student should work two hours to complete the exercises.

Taylor realized his teacher's method of standardizing homework could also be used to standardize any industrial process. His earliest attempts at standardization took place at Midvale Steelworks. First, Taylor looked for ways to improve the speed of any given task in the factory. Once a task was optimized according to Taylor's satisfaction, he measured the average time it took workers to complete the task.

American factories embraced Taylor's principles of standardization and were soon posting work rules, printing books of standard operating procedures, and issuing job instruction cards, all laying out the requisite way to get things done. The worker, once celebrated as a creative craftsman, was relegated to the role of automaton.

However, standardization left the crucial question of who should create the standards that governed a business unanswered. Taylor argued that businesses should hand overall planning, control, and decision making from the workers and to a new class of 'planners' who would be responsible for overseeing the workers and determining the best way to standardize an organization's processes.

Taylor adopted the recently invented term of 'manager' to describe this new role. He laid out his ideas of standardization and management in his 1911 book 'The Principles of Scientific Management.' The book became a national and international business bestseller and almost immediately scientific management—often called "Taylorism"—swept across the world's industries.

However, all the management consultants, planning departments, and efficiency experts conducted their analyses relying on the mathematics of the average and believing that the science of Quetelet and Galton justified treating each worker like a cell on a spreadsheet. It was not very difficult to convince managers that individuality did not matter since it made their job more comfortable and secure.

Edward Thorndike (1874-1949), one of the most prolific and influential psychologists of all time, publishing more than four hundred articles and selling millions of textbooks (Joncich, 1968). William James, his mentor at Harvard, described him as a 'freak of nature." Thorndike established the mission of schools, colleges, and universities in the 'Age of Average'. He was an enthusiastic advocate of the ideas of Francis Galton arguing for the theory that if a person was talented at one thing, it was likely to be talented at most other things. He justified his belief using the biological theory of learning. He believed that some people were born with brains that learned quickly, and these fast-learning individuals would not only be successful at school, but they would also be successful in life. On the other hand, some people would struggle all lifelong as they were born with slow brains.

Thorndike answered the question about how schools should go about ranking students in his book entitled 'Individuality', where he redefined individuality according to the Galtonian definition, that is, a person's uniqueness and value stem from his deviation from the average. He agreed that we should standardize every aspect of the educational system around the average, not only because this would ensure standardized outcomes, and make it easier to measure the deviation of each student from the average.

OVERTHROWING THE AVERAGE AND THE SCIENCE OF INDIVIDUALITY

In 2003, Peter Molenaar, an H1 professor of the highest possible rank in the Dutch educational system, served as the chairman of the Department of Psychological Methods at the University of Amsterdam (2007). However, the Dutch law mandated that all H1 professors should step back from their duties at the age of sixty-two to make way for their replacements, and then retire entirely at age sixty-five. Peter Molenaar was fifty-nine in 2003, and he was not quite sure if he was ready to step down, as he was expecting to ride off into the academic sunset at the top of his game.

After a lifetime of mathematical psychology, Molenaar unexpectedly saw an unjustifiable assumption. He knew that there was a manifest error at the very heart of 'averagarianism'.

Molenaar acknowledged that there is a fatal flaw of 'averagarianism' which lies in its questionable assumption to understand individuals while ignoring their individuality. He gave the name of 'ergodic switch' to this error, after a field known as ergodic theory. According to ergodic theory, we can use a group average to make predictions about individuals if two conditions are true (Cunha, 2013):

- Every member of the group is identical.
- Every member of the group will remain the same in the future.

If a particular group of entities fulfills these two conditions, the group is 'ergodic', in which case it is fine to use the average behavior of the group to make predictions about an individual.

Furthermore, contrary to the mathematics of 'averagarianism' which is known as statistics because it is a math of static values, Molenaar argues that to understand individuals we should turn to dynamic systems (Van Geert, 2011).

All-embracing, we might argue that research moves toward analyzing individual patterns of variability. In this context, Todd Rose (2015) shares three principles, drawn from the science of the individual that can replace the reliance on the average (Todd Rose, 2016):

- The jaggedness principle.
- The context principle.
- The pathways principle.

The jaggedness principle of individuality argues that jaggedness is not just about human size; as every human characteristic is jagged. It continues to argue that we cannot apply one-dimensional thinking to understand something 'jagged'. Moreover, the jagged quality must consist of multiple dimensions, which are related weakly to one another.

The context principle attributed to Yuichi Shoda personality research who thought there is a third way to think about personality, not in terms of traits or situations, but in terms of how traits and situations interact (Shoda, 1994). Shoda's results repudiate situation theory since his data demonstrated that any given situation affects each person differently. He summarized his ideas in the book entitled 'The Person in Context: Building a Science of the Individual'. Shoda provides an alternative to essentialist thinking he calls "if-then signatures." According to Shoda's theory, If we want to understand a coworker we should mention the following descriptions:

- If he is in the office, then he is very extroverted.
- If he is in a large group of strangers, then he is mildly extroverted.
- If he is stressed, then he is very introverted.

Finally, the third principle of individuality, namely the pathways principle argues that there is not a single, normal pathway for *any* human development. The principle makes two assertions:

- There are reasonably compelling ways to reach the same outcome in all aspects of our lives.
- The optimal pathway depends on the individuality.

The first point is grounded in the powerful concept of equifinality. The concept is drawn from the mathematics of complex systems and argues that there are multiple ways to get from one point to another in a multidimensional system. The second point states that individuals diverge in the pace of progress, and the sequences they follow to reach an outcome.

REASONS FOR THE EMERGENCE OF THE SCIENCE OF INDIVIDUALITY IN HEALTHCARE

Applying linear theory in medicine had led to many of its accomplishments. So far, the methods of data analysis are linear. However, due to their complex dynamic nature, nonlinear behavior commonly occurs within human systems. As a result, nonlinear thinking is growing among healthcare professionals, although it has not been able to explain all of the complexity present in human systems. However, it is helping to explain system behaviors that linear systems cannot.

We define a complex nonlinear system as 'a system or whole consisting of a huge and variable number of parts, where the individual components display marked variability over time and are characterized by a high degree of connectivity or interdependence between variables' (Seely & Christou, 2000). However, most complex nonlinear systems manifest the 'attractors' states rather than exhibiting random behavior. That leads to 'emergence' which describes the order that arises from what on initial inspection appears to be disorder (Lewin, 1999).

James Clerk Maxwell was the first to discuss the idea of infinitely small variations leading to a future unstable system behavior (Hunt &York, 1993). Further, Henri Poincare concluded that a comparable influence, at different times, does not result in similar effects (Persson & Wagner, 1996). Edward Lorenz, a mathematician meteorologist working at the Massachusetts Institute of Technology in 1961, observed what he believed was order masquerading as randomness (Gleick,1997). That observation was the earliest reference to chaos theory. Finally, Robert May wrote about chaos concerning deterministic nonlinear behavior in 1974, but he credits James Yorke with using the term 'chaos' to describe behavior manifesting similar features (May,1974; Li & Yorke, 1975).

However, nonlinear systems theory only recently has been seriously investigated within the biological sciences. In this context, there are three types of element behavior, within a system, which have been described as (Higgins, 2002):

- periodic or orderly behavior
- random behavior
- chaotic behavior

Periodic or orderly behavior describes behavior which tends toward a particular state(s), random behavior is that in which each item of the element is described by a uniform or non-uniform probability distribution, and the chaotic behavior describes dynamic behavior that is sensitive to initial conditions and parameter changes.

A general definition of chaos is 'Chaos is defined as the quality of a deterministic mathematical system in which an extreme sensitivity to initial conditions exists'(Skinner, 1994) while elements that exhibit chaos behavior often have a multiplicity of components, existing across different scales of organization (Philippe & Mansi, 1998).

Applications of chaotic behavior in medicine occur within the basic and clinical sciences while many researchers believe that behavior governed by chaos theory underlies many human systems (Rossler & Rossler, 1994). Que et al. (2001) have demonstrated increased variability in respiratory impedance in patients with asthma while use sensitivity to initial conditions to convert a chaotic pattern of arrhythmia (unstable) to a low-order periodic pattern (stable). Besides, other researchers argue that by altering period and amplitude modulation, it is possible to move from non-chaos to chaos.

As mathematics is frequently used to model physiology, investigators have been able to apply models of chaos to living systems. However, the enthusiasm must be tempered by the knowledge that models can never replicate precisely the real world.

On the other hand, the doctor-patient relationship can be seen as a social mechanism with salubrious impact on the patient's well-being (Benedetti, 2011). The critical point is why this social interplay is necessary in order to stimulate the endogenous mechanisms that are responsible for expectation and placebo outcomes. However, the reason a social mechanism of that kind surfaced in the course of evolution appears to be reasonable. There are numerous benefits in altruism, and social partnership as suppression of psychological uneasiness by human interactions warrants a robust mechanism to recover, at least in part. In this context, following evolutionary theory, the healthcare system can be more complicated and can acquire the qualities of an actual endogenous system. According to Humphrey (2002), the ability to stimulate expectation in addition to placebo mechanisms following the doctor-patient encounter is a new quality and essential feature of the 'natural healthcare service'. Humphrey (2002) claims that patient's body together with the brain have a considerable role for healing themselves, but that capacity for self-cure is not revealed spontaneously, as the influence of the doctor can trigger it. Therefore, the pivotal point is to realize why the patient-doctor encounter is necessary to initiate the self-cure mechanisms.

The conceptualization of an endogenous healthcare system by Humphrey (2002) is extremely useful to know why the doctor-patient encounter is necessary in order to trigger expectation in addition to placebo mechanisms in the patient's brain. Doctors and health professionals represent environmental variables that act on the patient's brain by inducing expectancies of benefit and hope. Health professionals are a crucial point in this process, as they promise treatment and induce expectations and hope for the patient's future well-being. The patient's expectations also play a crucial role. If the patient wants to consult a physician, this is because of his own beliefs about the doctor's healing skills. Therefore, the 'healer' is the environmental variable that triggers endogenous mechanisms of self-cure. From both an evolutionary, neuroscientific and patient-centered care perspective, it is evident that the therapist belongs to the system and has a pivotal role in triggering all mechanisms that take place in the patient's brain.

Moreover, the population health management concept requires extensive data, which currently flows from the beneficiaries towards data centers. Such data include a multitude of health and well-being information collected manually or automatically (Moumtzoglou & Pouliakis, 2018). Algorithms are required to process such information and alert when health-related actions should be taken. On the other hand, nowadays, there are technologies which provide both the data storage and processing capacity while the mobile device (especially the mobile phone), as well as inter-connectable devices (health gadgets), may serve as data acquisitions points on the individual level.

However, there is a significant deficiency of contemporary medicine which is reflected by the use of experts to make recommendations or guidelines for a large proportion of decisions for which no or minimal data exists. These guidelines are published in major specialty journals which have a pronounced impact, as they are believed to represent the standard of care. Overall, there is too much literature which is evidenced by the statistic that only 0.5 per cent of the 38 million published papers are cited more than two hundred times, and half were never cited. Moreover, when pooled analyses of prior studies are published, many relevant papers are excluded (Topol, 2012).

That should be considered 'eminence-based medicine.' (Topol, 2012). Better studies might be part of the solution. However, as we can accrue more meaningful data and information for individuals, the hope is that we can override our dependence on such recommendations. We need evidence which is built not on populations but individuals.

Fortunately, our capacity to get just that information is rapidly arising. An era which is characterized by the right drug and dose, at the right cost and timing has begun (Topol, 2012). Medicine for the common good is not sufficient. A rebooted life science, instead of a mass-population-directed strategy, would leverage the science of individuality, getting the relevant digital readout from an individual to shape a therapy. We now, for the first time, have the devices to promote a level of prescription precision we have never seen before (Topol, 2012).

The era of individualized medicine ultimately promises to do away with terms like 'cryptogenic' and 'essential,' fully recognizing the uniqueness of the individual who needs to be seen and treated with utter respect for his or her individuality. It will not be long until digitizing a person unlocks the cause for what is wrong, creating valuable knowledge that can save a life or markedly improve the quality of life. That is a significant outgrowth of the science of individuality.

In this context, the entire classification system of medical conditions and diagnoses is about to be rewritten. Instead of our current reductionist model for which individuals are unwisely assigned to such categories as one of two types of diabetes or cancer of a particular organ, the science of individuality will promote a new molecular taxonomy that invokes the primary biologic basis, regarding genes or pathways.

Overall, there is an essential need for health services to recognize that patients experience their condition in a unique way. Recognizing and responding to the needs of patients forms a critical underpinning to the concept of personalization and the development of responsive service.

THE IMPACT OF THE SCIENCE OF INDIVIDUALITY ON HEALTHCARE QUALITY & PATIENT SAFETY

Just as reductionism has influenced the scientific investigation to adopt the classical Newtonian viewpoint, so have traditional management models tended to view organizations as machines (Mikulecky,1996). In that model, effective leadership relates to the introduction of best practices via a top-down approach and any resistance. Likewise, any variation in practice from a predetermined norm can be eliminated via the imposition of protocols and guidelines. When a real consensus exists as to what constitutes best practice, then such an approach may be perfectly valid. However, more frequently, uncertainty may exist as to how to meet a particular challenge. It is in these situations that we might adopt complexity theory.

By viewing an organization as a complex system, then a greater focus is placed upon the connections between individual components which lead to the emergence of novel, unpredictable outcomes. That situation introduces the idea and use of 'minimum specifications' (Zimmerman, Lindberg & Plsek, 1998), a management strategy where the emphasis is placed upon 'direction pointing', setting 'boundaries' and 'resources', and giving 'permission' for the system to generate its solutions.

Minimum specifications theory perfectly adapts to the idea of initial conditions and parameter changes of complexity theory. Furthermore, as variation is natural in complex systems, it overthrows the idea statistical process control and helps us sort out the paradox of desirable and undesirable variation. As a sequel, statistical process control relegates to issues of high certainty regarding the outcome.

In this context, we could easily consider the integration of linear and non-linear theories in healthcare, as we can draw the initial conditions of chaotic behavior from the clinical guidelines of the linear theory.

It is also essential to realize that we still cannot capture all the multidimensional variables that run parallel to, intersect with, diverge from and converge with the evolution of e-health (Kastania & Moumtzoglou, 2012). Small deviations are being carried through the interaction and result in magnified impact, which is amplified when the incompatible worlds of a patient, family, and visitor join the world of healthcare professionals. On the other hand, the patient safety movement needs to advocate for the free flow of information in order to fertilize organizational learning and nourish worker intelligence (Wheatley, 1999). However, information cannot be disentangled from e-health initiatives. Information technology provides alternative methods for making health information accessible to consumers while research shows an improvement of health awareness, high user satisfaction, evidence of more significant benefit for under-served people and beneficial impact on health behavior (Gaston &Mitchell, 2005; Murray et al., 2005; Santo et al., 2005; Wofford et al., 2005). Mobile e-health, defined as 'mobile communications and web technologies for healthcare (Istepanian et al. 2006), can better reach areas, people, and healthcare professionals with limited exposure to certain aspects of healthcare. As a result, it enables personalized care, which relates to the integrated practice of medicine and patient care based on one's unique life characteristics, behavior, and surroundings. However, personalized care relates to personalized medicine, which emphasizes customization of healthcare. Personalized medicine is a conceptual paradigm, with only a few clinical practices, so far. Nevertheless, personalized treatment is anticipated because of the increased consciousness of the shortcomings in the delivery of drugs, molecular understanding, and increased demand for integrating genetic information into the drug development process (Lesko, 2007). The core issue of personalized medicine is tailoring individualized therapies by using an individual's specific biological characteristics. Personalized genomics is the critical input to consumer personalized medicine, although biomarkers, personalized indicators, predictive biosimulation, which translates into using biological data as well as mathematical modeling, are of great importance.

These applications not only facilitate care but also interact with other technologies and shape how patients are treated. They emphasize active involvement of patients (Chetney, 2003; Montfort & Helm, 2006) and can be thought as a current transformer of health care (Berg & Mol, 1998; Webster, 2002). Their primary characteristic is that health care can be provided at a distance, thus replacing face-to-face contacts by technology-mediated interactions. Consequently, they affect the critical dimensions of traditional health care delivery, physical proximity and narrative proximity (Malone, 2003). They also challenge the traditional paternal model of medicine by facilitating digital proximity that provides patients with practical tools for self-care (Oudshoorn, 2009).

Overall, the patient safety movement should not deal with the longstanding and widespread tradition of person approach or system approach. The active failures and latent conditions, which hold a central position in the system approach (Reason, 2000), are no longer the only driver. Risk perception comes into play through personalized self-care.

CONCLUSION

The application of linear models to human systems and healthcare management and quality has improved our understanding of their system structure and function. However, such models often fall short of explaining experimental results or predicting future abnormalities in complex nonlinear systems which help in dissecting and analyzing individual system components. Nonlinear models may better explain how the individual components collectively act and interact to produce a dynamic system in constant flux. They also assist in filling in some of the results which are not adequately explained by linear models.

However, as not all medicine is nonlinear, linear modeling should not be abandoned, as the use of both models is complementary and leads to a complete understanding of system behavior.

Chaos theory also provides new insights in standard as well as abnormal behavior within systems. Applications of chaos, especially fractals, may detect disease in its early stages and proves valuable in managing illness while the pursue of complexity theory provides new insights regarding the genetic encryption of the environment in the context of biological evolution, cellular automata, and modulation of protein production using biological pulse signals (Lewin, 1999).

In this context, we could easily consider the integration of linear and non-linear theories in healthcare quality and management, as we can draw the initial conditions of chaotic behavior from the standardization of the linear theory. Moreover, we can distinguish between desirable and undesirable variation relegating statistical process control only to issues of high certainty regarding the outcome.

REFERENCES

Bardsley, M. (2016). *Understanding analytical capability in health care: Do we have more data than insight?* The Health Foundation.

Bayer, R., & Galea, S. (2015). Public health in the precision-medicine era. *The New England Journal of Medicine*, *373*(6), 499–501. doi:10.1056/NEJMp1506241 PMID:26244305

Benedetti, F. (2011). *The Patient's Brain: The neuroscience behind the doctor-patient relationship*. Oxford, UK: Oxford University Press.

Berg, M., & Mol, A. (Eds.). (1998). *Difference in Medicine; Unravelling Practices, Techniques, and Bodies*. Durham, NC: Duke University Press.

Chetney, R. (2003). The Cardiac Connection Program. *Home Healthcare Nurse*, *21*(10), 680–686. doi:10.1097/00004045-200310000-00007 PMID:14557707

Cunha, A. (2013). Understanding the Ergodic Hypothesis Via Analogies. *Physica E, Low-Dimensional Systems and Nanostructures*, *10*, 9–12.

Donnelly, K. P. (2015). *Adolphe Quetelet, Social Physics and the Average Men of Science, 1796–1874*. London: Pickering & Chatto. doi:10.4324/9781315653662

Evans, H. (2018). *Does the public see tax rises as the answer to NHS funding pressures?* London: The King's Fund.

Forrest, D. W. (1974). *Francis Galton: The Life and Work of a Victorian Genius*. New York: Taplinger.

Frey, C. B., & Osborne, M. A. (2017). The Future of Employment: How susceptible are jobs to computerisation? *Technological Forecasting and Social Change*, *114*, 254–280. doi:10.1016/j.techfore.2016.08.019

Gaston, C. M., & Mitchell, G. (2005). Information giving and decision-making in patients with advanced cancer: A systematic review. *Social Science & Medicine, 61*(10), 2252–2264. doi:10.1016/j.socscimed.2005.04.015 PMID:15922501

Gleick, F. (1997). *Chaos: the Amazing Science of the Unpredictable*. London: Minerva.

Greenhalgh, T., Wherton, J., Papoutsi, C., Lynch, J., Hughes, J., A'Court, C., ... Shaw, S. (2017). Beyond Adoption: A New Framework for Theorizing and Evaluating Nonadoption, Abandonment, and Challenges to the Scale-Up, Spread, and Sustainability of Health and Care Technologies. *Journal of Medical Internet Research, 19*(11), e367. doi:10.2196/jmir.8775 PMID:29092808

Higgins, J. (2002). Nonlinear Systems in Medicine. *The Yale Journal of Biology and Medicine, 75*, 247–260. PMID:14580107

Holt-Lunstad, J., Smith, T. B., Baker, M., Harris, T., & Stephenson, J. (2015). Loneliness and Social Isolation as Risk Factors for Mortality: A Meta-Analytic Review. *Perspectives on Psychological Science, 10*(2), 227–237. doi:10.1177/1745691614568352 PMID:25910392

Humphrey, N. (2002). *The mind made flesh*. Oxford, UK: Oxford University Press.

Hunt, B. R., & York, J. A. (1993). Maxwell on chaos. *Nonlinear Sci. Today, 3*, 1–4.

Istepanian, R., Laxminarayan, S., & Pattichis, C. (Eds.). (2006). *M-Health: Emerging Mobile Health Systems*. New York: Springer. doi:10.1007/b137697

Joncich, G. (1968). *The Sane Positivist: A Biography of Edward L. Thorndike*. Middletown: Wesleyan University Press.

Kanigel, R. (2005). *The One Best Way: Frederick Winslow Taylor and the Enigma of Efficiency*. Cambridge, MA: MIT Press Books.

Kastania, A., & Moumtzoglou, A. (2012). Is there a Quality linkage of E-health? *International Journal of Reliable and Quality E-Healthcare, 1*(1), i–iv.

Laugesen, K., Baggesen, L. M., Schmidt, S. L. J., Glymour, M. M., Mathias, L., Arnold, M., & .... (2018). Social isolation and all-cause mortality:a population-based cohort study in Denmark. *Scientific Reports, 8*(1), 4731. doi:10.103841598-018-22963-w PMID:29549355

Lesko, L. J. (2007). Personalized Medicine: Elusive Dream or Imminent Reality? *Clinical Pharmacology and Therapeutics, 81*(6), 807–816. doi:10.1038j.clpt.6100204 PMID:17505496

Lewin, R. (1999). *Complexity: Life at the Edge of Chaos*. Chicago: The University of Chicago Press.

Li, T., & Yorke, J. A. (1975). Period three implies chaos. *The American Mathematical Monthly*, *82*(10), 985–992. doi:10.1080/00029890.1975.11994008

Lovell, N., & Bibby, J. (2018). *What makes us healthy? An introduction to the social determinants of health*. London: The Health Foundation.

Malone, R. E. (2003). Distal nursing. *Social Science & Medicine*, *56*(11), 2317–2326. doi:10.1016/S0277-9536(02)00230-7 PMID:12719184

May, R. M. (1974). Biological populations with nonoverlapping generations: Stable points,stable cycles, and chaos. *Science*, *186*(4164), 645–647. doi:10.1126cience.186.4164.645 PMID:4412202

Mikulecky, D. C. (1996). Complexity, communication between cells, and identifying the functional components of living systems: Some observations. *Acta Biotheoretica*, *44*(3-4), 179–208. doi:10.1007/BF00046527 PMID:8953209

Mindell, D. A. (2015). *Our robots, ourselves: robotics and the myths of autonomy*. Viking.

Mitchell, C., Hobcraft, J., McLanahan, S. S., Siegel, S. R., Berg, A., Brooks-Gunn, J., ... Notterman, D. (2014). Social disadvantage, genetic sensitivity,and children's telomere length. *Proceedings of the National Academy of Sciences of the United States of America*, *111*(16), 5944–5949. doi:10.1073/pnas.1404293111 PMID:24711381

Molenaar, P. (2007). On the Implications of the Classical Ergodic Theorems: Analysis of Developmental Processes Has to Focus on Intra-Individual Variation. *Developmental Psychobiology*, *50*(1), 60–69. doi:10.1002/dev.20262 PMID:18085558

Montfort, A.P.W.P., & van der Helm, M.H.J. (2006). Telemonitoring of Patients with Chronic Heart Failure. *Disease Management & Health Outcomes*, *14*(1), 33–35.

Moumtzoglou, A., & Pouliakis, A. (2018). Populatin health Management & the Science of Individuality. *International Journal of Reliable and Quality E-Healthcare*, *7*(2), 1–25. doi:10.4018/IJRQEH.2018040101

Murray, E., Burns, J., See Tai, S., Lai, R., & Nazareth, I. (2005). Interactive Health Communication Applications for people with chronic disease. *Cochrane Database of Systematic Reviews*, *CD004274*(4). PMID:16235356

Notterman, D. A., & Mitchell, C. (2015). Epigenetics and understanding the impact of social determinants of health. *Pediatric Clinics of North America*, *62*(5), 1227–1240. doi:10.1016/j.pcl.2015.05.012 PMID:26318949

Office for National Statistics. (n.d.). *Which occupations are at highest risk of being automated?* Retrieved June 3, 2019, from www.ons.gov.uk/employmentandlabourmarket/peopleinwork/employmentandemployeetypes/articles/whichoccupationsareathighestriskofbeingautomated/2019-03-25

Oudshoorn, N. (2009). Physical and digital proximity: Emerging ways of health care in face-to-face and telemonitoring of heart-failure patients. *Sociology of Health & Illness*, *31*(3), 390–405. doi:10.1111/j.1467-9566.2008.01141.x PMID:19144084

Pantell, M., Rehkopf, D., Jutte, D., Syme, S. L., Balmes, J., & Adler, N. (2013). Social isolation: A predictor of mortality comparable to traditional clinical risk factors. *American Journal of Public Health*, *103*(11), 2056–2062. doi:10.2105/AJPH.2013.301261 PMID:24028260

Persson, P. B., & Wagner, C. D. (1996). General principles of chaotic dynamics. *Cardiovascular Research*, *31*(3), 332–341. doi:10.1016/S0008-6363(96)00006-5 PMID:8681321

Philippe, P., & Mansi, O. (1998). Author. *Theoretical Medicine and Bioethics*, *19*(6), 591–607. doi:10.1023/A:1009979306346 PMID:10051792

Que, C. L., Kenyon, C. M., Olivenstein, R., Macklem, P. T., & Maksym, G. N. (2001). Homeokinesis and short-term variability of human airway caliber. *Journal of Applied Physiology (Bethesda, Md.)*, *91*(3), 1131–1141. doi:10.1152/jappl.2001.91.3.1131 PMID:11509508

Reason, J. (2000). Human error: Models and management. *British Medical Journal*, *320*(7237), 768–770. doi:10.1136/bmj.320.7237.768 PMID:10720363

Rose, T. (2015). *The End of Average: How We Succeed in a World That Values Sameness*. New York, NY: HarperOne.

Rossler, O. E., & Rossler, R. (1994). Chaos in physiology. *Integrative Physiological and Behavioral Science*, *29*(3), 328–333. doi:10.1007/BF02691336 PMID:7811652

Santo, A., Laizner, A. M., & Shohet, L. (2005). Exploring the value of audiotapes for health literacy: A systematic review. *Patient Education and Counseling*, *58*(3), 235–243. doi:10.1016/j.pec.2004.07.001 PMID:16054796

Seely, A. J., & Christou, N. V. (2000). Multiple organ dysfunction syndrome: Exploring the paradigm of complex nonlinear systems. *Critical Care Medicine*, *28*(7), 2193–2200. doi:10.1097/00003246-200007000-00003 PMID:10921540

Shoda, Y., Mischel, W., & Wright, J. C. (1994). Intraindividual Stability in the Organization and Patterning of Behavior: Incorporating Psychological Situations into the Idiographic Analysis of Personality. *Journal of Personality and Social Psychology*, *67*(4), 674–687. doi:10.1037/0022-3514.67.4.674 PMID:7965613

Skinner, J. E. (1994). Low-dimensional chaos in biological systems. *Biotechnology*, *12*, 596–600. PMID:7764948

Topol, E. (2019). High-performance medicine: The convergence of human and artificial intelligence. *Nature Medicine*, *25*(1), 44–56. doi:10.103841591-018-0300-7 PMID:30617339

Topol, E. J. (2012). *The creative destruction of medicine: how the digital revolution will create better health care*. New York: Basic Books.

Trust, W. (2019). *The ethical, social and political challenges of using artificial intelligence in healthcare*. Retrieved June 3, 2019 from https://wellcomeac.uk/funding/ethical-social-and-political-challenges-using-artificial-intelligence-healthcare

Van Geert, P. (2011). The Contribution of Complex Dynamic Systems to Development. *Child Development Perspectives*, *5*(4), 273–278. doi:10.1111/j.1750-8606.2011.00197.x

Watts, N., Amann, M., Arnell, N., Ayeb-Karlsson, S., Belesova, K., Berry, H., ... Costello, A. (2018). The 2018 report of the Lancet Countdown on health and climate change: Shaping the health of nations for centuries to come. *The Lancet Review.*, *392*(10163), 2479–2514. doi:10.1016/S0140-6736(18)32594-7 PMID:30503045

Webster, A. J. (2002). Innovative health technologies and the social: Redefining health, medicine and the body. *Current Sociology*, *50*(3), 443–457. doi:10.1177/0011392102050003009

Wheatley, M. J. (1999). *Leadership and the new science: Discovering order in a chaotic world.* San Fransisco: Berrett-Koehler.Wofford.

Willis, M., Duckworth, P., Coulter, A., Meyer, E. T., & Osborne, M. (2019). The Future of Health Care: Protocol for Measuring the Potential of Task Automation Grounded in the National Health Service Primary Care System. *JMIR Research Protocols*, *8*(4), e11232. doi:10.2196/11232 PMID:30964437

Wolfe, B., Evans, W., & Seeman, T. E. (Eds.). (2012). The Biological Consequences of Socioeconomic Inequalities. Russell Sage Foundation.

Woolford, J., Smith, E., & Miller, D. (2005). The multimedia computer for office-based patient education: A systematic review. *Patient Education and Counseling*, *59*(2), 148–157. doi:10.1016/j.pec.2004.10.011 PMID:16257619

Zimmerman, B. J., Lindberg, C., & Plsek, P. E. (1998). *Edgeware: insights from complexity science for health care leaders*. Irving, TX: VHA Publishing.

KEY TERMS AND DEFINITIONS

Average: A number expressing the central or typical value in a set of data.

Chaos Theory: The study of apparently random or unpredictable behaviour in systems governed by deterministic laws.

Complexity Theory: A set of concepts that attempts to explain complex phenomena which traditional theories do not explain.

Healthcare Quality: The degree to which health care services for individuals and populations increase the likelihood of desired health outcomes. In 1999, the Institute of Medicine released six domains to measure and describe healthcare quality, that is, safety, effectiveness, patient-centered care, timeliness, efficiency, equitability.

Linear Models: Models which describe a continuous response variable as a function of one or more predictor variables.

Nonlinear Models: A model which is not linear in at least one parameter.

Patient Safety: The prevention of harm to patients. Emphasis is placed on the system of care delivery that prevents errors, learns from the errors, and is built on a culture of safety.

Science of Individuality: The science which acknowledges that each human needs to be seen and treated with utter respect for his or her individuality.

Statistical Process Control: A method of quality control which employs statistical methods to monitor and control a process.

Variation: A change or slight difference in condition, amount, or level, typically within specified limits.

Chapter 2
Population Health Management, Emerging Technologies, and the Science of the Individual

Anastasius S. Moumtzoglou
https://orcid.org/0000-0002-5899-1033
P. & A. Kyriakou Children's Hospital, Greece

Abraham Pouliakis
https://orcid.org/0000-0002-0074-3619
2nd Department of Pathology, National and Kapodistrian University of Athens, Greece

ABSTRACT

Population health management (PHM) has been a discipline that studies and facilitates care delivery across a group of individuals or the general population. In the context of PHM, the life science industry has had no motivation to design drugs or devices and even offer treatment of patient management that is only effective for a distinct population segment. The primary outgrowth of the science of individuality, as well as the rising 'wiki medicine', fully recognizes the uniqueness of the individual. Cloud computing, big data, m-health, and recently, internet of things can offer the resources to deal with numerous shortcomings such as data collection and processing, of the PHM approach, as they facilitate the propagation of the science of individuality.

DOI: 10.4018/978-1-7998-2390-2.ch002

INTRODUCTION

Public health connotes a relatively narrow field with activities carried out by agencies granted with official functions. 'Population health' a term with broader content, is related to a field relevant to the study of several important factors for health. As a result, it involves many terms, such as outcomes, disparities, determinants, and risk factors (Kindig, 2007).

Notwithstanding the term 'population health' combines the concepts of both health and population, every term has an essential meaning of its own. The population is related to a group of persons being organized into numerous different units of analysis. Similarly, the term health was defined negatively, i.e., the absence of disease. Nowadays, modern understanding stresses the positive aspects as well, and health is considered to be related to all life issues. Summarizing, today it is debated whether population health and public health are different or identical. Nevertheless, population health is defined as health outcomes and their distribution in a population (Kindig, 2007).

Population health management (PHM) has been defined as 'the technical field of endeavor which utilizes a variety of individual, organizational and cultural interventions to help improve the morbidity patterns (i.e., the illness and injury burden) and the health care use behavior of defined populations (Hillman, 2002). It is differentiated from disease management because it includes (Howe & Spence, 2004):

- More chronic conditions and diseases.
- Uses a single point of contact and coordination and predictive modeling across multiple clinical conditions.

Moreover, PHM is considered a broader term than disease management, as it includes (Coughlin, Pope, & Leedle(Jr), 2006):

- Intensive care management for individuals at the highest level of risk.
- Personal health management for those at lower levels of predicted health risk.

At the provider level, there are three highlighted components (Care Continuum Alliance, 2012):

- The leadership and the central care delivery role of the primary care physician.
- The importance of patient activation.
- The expansion of care coordination.

In this context, to successfully achieve all of these requirements, an organization should provide proactive, preventive and chronic care services to all managed patients. Furthermore, this should take place both during encounters of patients with the healthcare system and in between. Therefore, providers should maintain regular contact with their patients and support them in the management of their health. Additionally, providers must manage patients at high risk, to prevent the deterioration of their health and avoid the development of complications. Finally, evidence-based protocols for the diagnosis and treatment of patients, consistently and cost-effectively, are also required if a provider-based PHM approach is followed.

The Federal Agency for Healthcare Research and Quality (AHRQ) developed the concept of 'practice-based population health' (PBPH) and defined it as "an approach to care that uses information on a group of patients within a primary care practice or group of practices to improve the care and clinical outcomes of patients within that practice.' (Cusack, Knudson, Kronstadt, Singer, & Brown, 2010).

The implementation of health IT is among the essential components and requirements for planning and implementing PHM. The adoption of Electronic Health Records is just the first step toward the creation of the requisite infrastructure. However, a wide range of other IT applications to automate PHM, track results and engage the patients in their health care is required. Additionally, IT systems should repeatedly be evaluated because of rapid technological changes, new government regulations and new approaches to patient management (Moumtzoglou & Pouliakis, 2015).

AHRQ recommends health IT tools for the stratification and monitoring of populations, as follows:

- Target patients being in greatest need of health services by stratifying the patients and narrowing subpopulations.
- Make patient-related data actionable by generating alerts to the patients.
- Make data actionable by generating alerts towards health providers about patient care needs.

Conclusively, population health management is designed around the collective. However, nowadays, to truly drive high-quality care at a lower cost, these endeavors must work for the individual, align with their personal goals and intermix with their reality. In this context, the objective of the chapter is twofold. First, it will deal with the greatest misconception about population health, that is, population health is not about the population. Ultimately, it is about the individual. Secondly, it will show how to connect the dots from the science of individuality to improving health on a massive scale - a bottom-up approach that uses the technologies of cloud computing, Big Data, M-Health and Internet of Things (IoT).

THE SCIENCE OF THE INDIVIDUAL

Traditional models assume that the population insights automatically apply to all individuals(Molenaar, 2013). As a result, they analyze statistical averages, providing descriptions about global regularities which are poor substitutes for an exact science of individuality.

On the contrary, modern science assumes that individuals change dramatically over time and even moment-to-moment (Fischer & Bidell, 2006; Mischel, 1973; van Geert & van Dijk, 2002), as a function of context and irrespective of culture and age. That assumption of individual variability presents a challenge for most traditional models, regardless of the field of study, because, so far, models focus on population stability, ignoring the variability of the individual (Anastasi, 1937; Chomsky, 1957; Fodor, 1983). Consequently, the object of interest, in all fields of study which try to understand individuals, is not the statistical average but individual variability (Bergman & Vargha, 2013; Levsky & Singer, 2003; Murray, 1938). Individual variability is thought to be extensive at every level of analysis, including the cells (Dawson, 1988), the genomes(Chen et al., 2012), the mind (Siegler, 2007), and brain(Mazziotta et al., 2009).

In this context, since the mid-twentieth century, various fields of study have gone through a dramatic shift, moving from traditional static perspectives to a dynamic perspective that analyzes individual variability in growth processes and moment-to-moment activity. The essence of this new approach is dynamic systems theory, which represents a flexible set of concepts and nonlinear mathematical models uniquely suited to the analysis of complex phenomena.

Several researchers have emphasized on the individuality, and have sought to explain both stability and variability of individuals(Fischer & Bidell, 2006; Molenaar, 2013; Thelen & Smith, 2006; van Geert & van Dijk, 2002). As a result, a science-centered on individual variability has emerged as an essential perspective in many fields(Blau & Liakopoulou, 2013; Garrett et al., 2013; Nesselroade, Gerstorf, Hardy, & Ram, 2007; Stahlberg, Kubista, & Aman, 2011).

However, individual modeling demands massive amounts of data that a decade ago would have been both difficult and expensive to collect(King, 2011). Likewise, the population health management concept requires extensive data, which currently flows from the beneficiaries towards data centers. Such data include a multitude of health and well-being information collected manually or automatically. Moreover, algorithms are required to process such information and alert when health-related actions should be taken. On the other hand, nowadays, there are technologies which provide both the data storage and processing capacity while the mobile device (especially the mobile phone), as well as inter-connectable devices (health gadgets), may serve as data acquisitions points on the individual level.

However, there is a significant deficiency of contemporary medicine, which is reflected by the use of experts to make recommendations or guidelines for a large proportion of decisions for which no or minimal data exists. These guidelines are published in major specialty journals which have a pronounced impact, as they are believed to represent the standard of care. Overall, there is too much literature, which is evidenced by the statistic that only 0.5 percent of the 38 million published papers are cited more than two hundred times, and half were never cited. Moreover, when pooled analyses of prior studies are published, many relevant papers are excluded (Topol, 2012).

That should be considered 'eminence-based medicine.' (Topol, 2012).

Better studies might be part of the solution. However, as we can accrue more meaningful data and information for individuals, the hope is that we can override our dependence on such recommendations. We need evidence which is built not on populations but individuals.

Fortunately, our capacity to get just that information is rapidly arising. An era which is characterized by the right drug and dose, at the right cost and timing has begun (Topol, 2012). Medicine for the common good is not sufficient. A rebooted life science, instead of a mass-population-directed strategy, would leverage the science of individuality, getting the relevant digital readout from an individual to shape a therapy. We now, for the first time, have the devices to, promote a level of prescription precision we have never seen before (Topol, 2012).

The era of individualized medicine ultimately promises to do away with terms like 'cryptogenic' and 'essential,' fully recognizing the uniqueness of the individual who needs to be seen and treated with utter respect for his or her individuality. It will not be long until digitizing a person unlocks the cause for what is wrong, creating valuable knowledge that can save a life or markedly improve the quality of life. That is a significant outgrowth of the science of individuality.

In this context, the entire classification system of medical conditions and diagnoses is about to be rewritten. Instead of our current reductionist model for which individuals are unwisely assigned to such categories as one of two types of diabetes or cancer of a particular organ, the science of individuality will promote a new molecular taxonomy that invokes the primary biologic basis, regarding genes or pathways.

THE TECHNOLOGIES OF INDIVIDUALITY

The data for how many patients search for health websites is staggering (Topol, 2012). Although this trend represents an outlier in many respects and an extreme of patient activism, these cases also demonstrate that the current level of being informed is not adequate. Furthermore, they capture a sense of inspiration and independence, the hunt for innovation, and the primacy of the individual. In essence, they are the precursors for the next phase of medicine, in which powerful digital tools will provide data that was heretofore unavailable.

Whether it is sequencing the genome of cancer tissue to determine a specific mutation or being able to anticipate the likelihood of a fatal disease before it has ever manifested, our capabilities greatly expand based on the following technologies.

CLOUD TECHNOLOGIES

Cloud computing has emerged rapidly as an exciting new paradigm that offers a challenging model of computing and services. Leveraging cloud computing technology, bioinformatics tools, can be made available as services to anyone, anywhere, and through any device. The use of large bio-datasets, the highly demanding algorithms, and the hardware for sudden computational resources make large-scale bio-data analysis an attractive test case for cloud computing" (Hsu, Lin, Ouyang, & Guo, 2013). Cloud computing is a concept related to numerous computers that use Internet infrastructure to communicate producing shared resources such as software, hardware, and storage. Nowadays, cloud computing is not widely used for the various tasks related to medicine; however, there are numerous fields that it could be employed; thus, cloud computing is an emerging field having the potential to change the everyday practice of medicine.

Cloud systems are categorized into three different groups according to the offered service type:

- Infrastructure as a Service (**IaaS**), i.e. offering hardware, storage and physical devices through the Internet.
- Software as a Service (**SaaS**), i.e. offering software and hosted applications over the Internet.
- Platform as a Service (**PaaS**), i.e. offering the capability to deploy applications created via programming languages, libraries, services, and tools owned and supported by the provider.

For cloud computing, the user/consumer does not manage or control the underlying cloud infrastructure. However, he has control over the deployed applications as well as the offered services (i.e. storage, networking, and processing power). Clouds, according to their hosting, may be public, private, hybrid, and community, uniquely adapted to the medical field:

- **Public Clouds** are for general use. The cloud owners are responsible for information hosting; public clouds are rarely utilized in the area of medicine and case of use, data are encrypted.
- **Private Clouds** are only for in-hospital use and are dealing with confidential patient data. The owners or the hospital premises are responsible for information hosting.
- **Hybrid Clouds** are hosting non-confidential information on public Clouds and confidential information in a private domain.
- **Community Clouds** are hosting information among members of the same community. Laboratories and hospitals can create a community Cloud while sharing the same infrastructure and software.

There are three fundamental aspects of Cloud-based services (Soman, 2011):

1) Browser-based applications

Browser-based applications are different from native applications since they are executed mainly on the computer on which they are hosted while browser-based applications run through the web browser and consume mainly computational resources located remotely. A native application uses mainly the computing resources and storage of the computer which was used to launch the application (note that newer native applications are cloud-aware and can consume remote resources as well). Conversely, browser-based applications are applications that run from within Internet Browsers; however, the consumed resources are located on one or more servers. They are conceptually similar to client-server applications, which require a powerful central computer, but there are two distinct characteristics:

- Browser-based applications are invoked from inside a standard browser.
- The Client and the Server do not necessarily reside simultaneously in a Local Area Network; in contrast, they can be on remote networks accessible through the Internet Protocol.

2) Optimal utilization of server resources

It is well known that cloud services observe variable levels of the utilization of their services. This variability has two parts: a) the number of concurrent users accessing the service is different at different times, and b) the processing and storage of resources required by any particular user are never constant. Thus, technologies for scaling and resource partitioning are at the heart of cloud services; otherwise, the Cloud business model would not be feasible. Cloud service providers apply extensively load balancing, a mechanism for balanced or even distribution of load across multiple physical resources, such as servers, storage devices or communication links.

3) Data centers

A data center is a collection of resources where the user's data is processed and stored. Important design considerations for data centers are as below (Moumtzoglou, 2014; Soman, 2011):

- Data centers are typically located in places where the risk of natural disasters and human-made disasters is low, data centers have been installed even at the bottom of the sea.
- Buildings used to house data centers typically do not accommodate other offices and businesses. The area around the data center is well-lit and comfortable to monitor. It is easy to control access to the premises where the data center is housed.
- Data centers have areas with raised flooring to allow for cable management and reduction of damages in cases of flooding.
- Data centers have to own air-condition and other systems for removing generated heat.
- Data centers have different levels of physical security and access control.
- Data centers have assured a stable electric supply, uninterruptable power supply and electric power generators.
- Data centers have state of the art fire prevention and fire protection systems and are equipped with numerous detectors for heat, humidity, smoke etc.

From a networking perspective (Moumtzoglou, 2014; Soman, 2011):

- Data centers have high-bandwidth data pipes with various levels of redundancy.
- Data centers have all the elements installed that are required to run Intranet services continually.
- Data centers achieve the most advanced network security tools including intrusion detection, firewalls, antivirus systems, and systems that guard against spamming, Denial of Service Attacks, and all known malware.

Lastly, (Moumtzoglou, 2014; Soman, 2011):

- Data centers employ qualified system administrators.
- Data centers support systems and processes in place to keep smooth functioning 24x7 and throughout the year.
- Data centers have a disaster recovery plan.

HEALTHCARE AND CLOUD COMPUTING

The healthcare industry is very delicate and different from most other industries since several entities have to deal with healthcare data including regulatory bodies, care providers, hospital administration staff, payers such as insurance organizations or the patients, and patients themselves as service recipients. Key differences between the healthcare industry and other industries, in which cloud-based systems have been used, include (Soman, 2011):

- **High-risk industry**

The healthcare industry impacts individuals to a great extent, even though it is not used frequently by individuals.

- **Highly regulated**

Numerous regulations govern the provision of healthcare.

- **Multiple stakeholders**

There is a large number of interested parties in healthcare which include the patients, the physicians, the nurse practitioners, all hospitals' departments, their administrative staff members, the payers/ insurance companies, employers, pharmaceutical companies, technology vendors and creators, device manufacturers, government bodies, and many others.

- **Slow Pace of Adoption**

The healthcare industry has traditionally been slow to adopt IT, especially the smaller clinics and individual physician practices

- **Small and Large Providers**

Small providers typically do not have the resources to evaluate or experiment with advanced IT systems. On the other hand, there are several large multi-specialty hospitals whose IT requirements are distinctly different from those of office practitioners.

- **Long-Term Relationships**

Changing IT systems often, especially in large oganisations, is not secure, and there is, therefore, an assumption that any adopted product would be advantageous if planned to be used for several years. Such a hypothesis does not follow the need for both the IT systems and individuals to adapt.

Given all of these differences, it is not clear that Cloud-based systems would work as well in the healthcare industry as they have in other industry verticals unless Cloud-based healthcare solutions address these specific attributes of the industry.

From a clinical perspective, an EMR (electronic medical record) leads to improvement in the quality of care provided to patients. Cloud-based EMRs, therefore, seems to be the critical component of any Cloud-based healthcare offering. Electronic Medical Records are created and maintained by care providers when a patient avails service from the vendor.

The following critical pieces of medical information are a part of virtually all EMR systems (Soman, 2011):

- Patient Identification information.
- Information about Patient Allergies and Habits.
- Immunization Record.
- Medical History.

There are significant advantages to using EMR when compared to the traditional paper-based files and charts (Soman, 2011):

- Storage.
- Usage in Emergency.
- Duplication and Transportation costs.
- Uniformity.
- Risks.
- Audit/Reporting.

- Integration.
- Efficiency.
- Ability to apply automated algorithms to suggest treatment and avoid malpractice.

Cloud-based EMR systems have all the features and capabilities of in-house EMR systems. There are many cloud-based systems with an easy-to-use user interface along with the ability to customize the fields in the records. Cloud-based EMR systems make it even easier to access or transfer medical information to any point, for example, to the point of care in an emergency (Witzke & Specht, 2017). Cloud-based EMR systems also make it simpler to provide access to the records of the patient via patient portals.

A Cloud-based medical practice management application enables a healthcare provider to manage and streamline business management tasks and workflows. A 'workflow' is a series of steps followed to achieve a specific purpose. Provision of healthcare involves the implementation of various workflows within the practice, mirroring the movement of the patient within the system. Medical Practice Management relates to the operation of various workflows within the practice while Medical Practice Management Systems are the key to ensuring that all transactions within the practice run smoothly and efficiently.

Cloud-based Practice Management software supports features such as (Soman, 2011):

- Appointment scheduling of patients.
- Eligibility and authorization.
- Physician scheduling, scheduling surgery or other procedures for patients.
- Tracking patient referrals.
- Patient account management.
- Managing patients as they move from admission to discharge, including information on hospital rounds.
- Managing patient recall.
- Claims submission and processing, automated follow-ups, collections, and remittance advice.
- Managing the schedules of employees of the clinic.
- Managing the inventory of medical supplies and office materials.
- Inter and Intra clinic/location communication.
- HIPAA compliance.
- Patient portal.

In a Cloud-based Practice Management solution, the software is accessed through a browser over the Internet, which is why continuous Internet availability is crucial. Cloud-based Practice Management solutions can be customized, although admittedly to a limited extent when compared to on-site solutions. However, Cloud-based solutions can effectively compete with on-site solutions regarding functionality and features.

A patient portal is essentially a website on which patients can log in and access most portions of their medical records. In a patient portal, the information is presented in a manner which makes it easy for the patient to understand the nature of his conditions and his treatment. Most Patient Portals also provide some level of interactivity with the healthcare provider.

Patient Portals represent one of the critical advantages of Cloud-based systems over in-house systems. Patient Portal interfaces with sensitive, private information of individuals should be securely available and web-accessible at all times. It is, therefore, best if the responsibility of managing the patient portal is assigned to an entity that has the expertise, the infrastructure, the resources, and experience to develop and achieve high availability, high-security information systems. Most clinics or physician practices do not have this capability, nor is it practically feasible to invest in infrastructure and human resources to undertake such capability. It is, therefore, best to opt for a cloud-based Patient Portal.

Many Practice Management systems and EMR systems include ePrescription capability as a part of their overall functionality. An ePrescription system is a computerized system in which the prescription is either entered by the physician/ nurse practitioner or generated by the information available to the system. The prescription can be automatically communicated to pharmacies associated with the healthcare provider. Further, ePrescription systems also have inbuilt rules/databases about drug-drug allergies and appropriateness of each drug in the context of various health conditions.

An ePrescription system brings several benefits (Soman, 2011):

- It eliminates the possibility of a prescription being incorrectly interpreted due to poor handwriting, thereby reducing medical errors.
- It reduces the occurrence of drug-drug allergies and the possibility of the inappropriate drug being administered in the view of the patients' comprehensive medical history.
- It makes ordering refills easier since prior prescriptions can be easily accessed electronically.
- ePrescriptions are also found to increase compliance by patients merely because they are more convenient.

A Cloud-based ePrescription system is likely to be much more highly available and secure and thus be able to communicate prescriptions to pharmacies with higher reliability than an in-house system. Secondly, a Cloud-based system is more likely to cooperate with more and more pharmacy chains over time, enhancing the number of pharmacies the ePrescriptions can be sent to.

Even if a clinic does not use Cloud-based systems for practice management, it is a brilliant idea to consider Cloud-based systems for data backup and secondary storage.

The way most Cloud-based backup systems work is as follows (Soman, 2011).

There is software installed on one or more of the computers within the facility (called the backup client) connected to the primary storage. The backup client tracks the changes to the data stored on the primary storage at regular intervals and communicates the changes to the Cloud-based storage space of the service provider.

The backup client is responsible for encrypting all information before it is transmitted to cloud storage. Secondly, bandwidth requirements are significantly reduced because the client only transmits the changes that have occurred in the data since the last backup run, rather than transmitting all the details again.

A notable particular case of a data backup system, due to the large sizes of medical images, is the Picture Archival and Communication System ('PACS'). In the process of administering health care, various images, graphs, pictures, and scans are generated. That includes images from X-Rays, ultrasound machines, MRI and CT scans, endoscopy, mammograms, computed radiography, etc. Even scanned images of paper documents are often required to be stored when legacy paper-based data is digitized via scanning. To ensure uniformity, a standard format used to store and communicate pictorial information has been defined—the Digital Imaging and Communications in Medicine ('DICOM').

Cloud-based laboratory solutions are available for various functions such as microbiology, histology and cytology processes, Synoptic/Antibiogram reporting, Image/Document capture, Inventory Management, Voice recording, Blood bank. They have all the functionality of on-site solutions.

Cloud-based Radiology systems are similar to PACS systems. These systems support basic Radiology workflows where physicians can register examination requests for existing or new patients, and select appropriate billing rules. It is also possible to interface laboratory devices directly to Cloud-based systems. That means that the readings from instruments or captured images are directly uploaded to the cloud.

Overall, cloud-based healthcare IT systems are easier to get started; distinctly cost-effective when compared to on-site solutions; more convenient, especially for smaller clinics and private physician practices, while allowing doctors to collaborate on any medical data efficiently, and work on the system from anywhere, including from home.

Cloud Computing is a novelty that rapidly showed tremendous opportunities for application in medicine and health care improvement (Archondakis, Pouliakis, Margari, & Karakitsos, 2014; Eugster, Schmid, Binder, & Schmidberger, 2013; Glaser, 2011; Kuo, 2011; Lupse, Vida, & Stoicu-Tivadar, 2012; Mirza & El-Masri, 2013; Moumtzoglou & Kastania, 2014; Patel, 2012; Pouliakis, A., Archondakis, Karakitsou, & Karakitsos, 2014; Pouliakis, A., Spathis, et al., 2014; Rosenthal et al., 2010; Waxer, Ninan, Ma, & Dominguez, 2013; Webb, 2012). It is forecasted that there will be an increase in cloud computing market for medical images which is mainly due to the growing volume of medical images and the increasing costs of the ownership for owning Picture Archiving and Communication Systems (PACS).

BIG DATA

Big Data is a terminology which is used to describe a collection of datasets being so broad and complicated that it becomes challenging to process them using the standard and on-hand database management tools or the available traditional data processing software applications. Although there is no single formal definition of Big Data, most definitions seem to associate to four Vs, which include volume, velocity, variety, and veracity. Volume relates to the unusually large data which are produced, collected and exchanged; velocity refers to an often requirement for real-time analysis; variety indicates the different forms of data being difficult to integrate and veracity emphasizes the issues which are related to trust and uncertainty. However, not all data that occupy a large volume are considered big. Thus, when defining Big Data, the size is not the primary characteristic; the most appropriate characteristic is the number of independent data sources (separate databases), each one having the potential to interact and be interconnected with one or more data sources.

According to the newest market studies (Market Research Future, 2017; Markets and Markets, 2017), the revenue of Big Data by 2020 and 2021 is estimated in the range of 25-35 billion USD. Thus, the Big Data market is continuously increasing. It is a very competitive market, and many stakeholders have presented innovative products and services dealing with Big Data. The Big Data ecosystem has several discrete areas: a) storage and management including data servers, software, networking, monitoring, administration and data management b) tools and technologies specialized for Big Data analytics that generate insight from collected data c) healthcare intelligence for the organization and d) embedding the Big Data framework into the organization's business intelligence infrastructure (Koumpouros, 2015).

There are several Big Data solutions, either open source or commercial ones. Open platforms have advantages as they come at no cost for software acquisition and permit the use of various tools for data analytics. However, they require significant effort to install and setup by specialists. The Apache Hadoop framework is the pioneering and mostly used open platform. Other open-source systems include NoSQL databases: MongoDB and Cassandra, among others. The Hadoop framework with proper scaling can support the analysis of petabytes of data. In this arena, another platform, Red Hat Enterprise Linux, in companion with the OpenStack hybrid cloud, supports Big Data applications. In the commercial product arena, InfoSphere is one of the products offered by IBM, another platform based on the Hadoop system. It includes data warehouse and stream computing software to perform real-time analysis on vast volumes of streamed data. Cisco offers the Cisco Common Big Data Platform, which is based on Cisco's Unified Computing Architecture and concept. Due to the company's networking history, it integrates computing, networking and storage capabilities. Other Big Data platform and services vendors include Cloudera, Hortonworks, Platfora, DataStax, 10Gen, and Amazon, being supporters of Hadoop and NoSQL. As well as Hadapt, Platfora, Splunk, Datameer, and Karmasphere.

One of the primary Big Data and cloud service providers is Amazon. The leading service is the Elastic MapReduce (EMR), a Hadoop based platform that scales to thousands of nodes per cluster. There is support for easy to use mission-critical, real-time applications, a petabyte-scale warehouse service. Finally, it includes business intelligence tools and can operate on datasets of a few hundred gigabytes to petabytes.

Healthcare is probably one of the leading areas in the Big Data arena because significant amounts of personal and sensitive, health-related data are continuously collected from patients since the beginning of their life. In the medical field, those data are collected by different actors, in different locations, for various purposes and is used/viewed differently by each information consumer (Koumpouros, 2015). For the medical specialists, to reach the best possible diagnosis, and subsequently, the appropriate therapeutic approach, accurate and complete information is required; without Big Data, this is not feasible.

Evidence-based medicine (EBM), is another factor that stresses the need for Big Data in healthcare, as it relies on large scale data sets, usually distributed (Beckmann & Lew, 2016; Sniderman, LaChapelle, Rachon, & Furberg, 2013). EBM is used by the physicians as well as by health care management and insurance organizations, paving the way for the acceptance of Big Data.

As far as population health management is concerned, there is already an application of Big Data (Wells, Ozminkowski, Hawkins, Bhattarai, & Armstrong, 2016). Specifically, the application is mainly based on the U.S. Medicare insurance program. Within this application, data from diverging lines of evidence are used:

- Demographic and contact details along with insurance coverage.
- Insurance claims, submitted by doctors, hospitals, and other providers to Medicare; those data include standardized codes for medical diagnoses and procedures, place of treatment, amounts billed, as well as whether service was provided:
  1) in the emergency room
  2) inpatient service
  3) ambulatory service iv)
  4) laboratory
  5) long-term care unit
  6) ancillary service
- Prescribed pharmaceuticals that include the drug name and class, a drug code identifier (applied at the national level), drug dosage, dates, and the number of days for drug usage. It is worth noting that this is a separate database linkable to the medical claims and administrative data from Medicare.
- A questionnaire is measuring experiences with health plans of Medicare, which includes the health status, satisfaction, and experiences from healthcare services.
- U.S. Census data which are related to the zip code and are used to identify differences by in the geographic regions.
- Data from Dartmouth Atlas which describes the supply of healthcare services in a geographically geographical context.
- The AmeriLINK Data Sourcing system, which indicates the social and economic status of members.

The processed Medicare data were around 4 million records, and the results of health analytics proved to be very interesting. The aim was to 'get the right person to the right care at the right time.' Individuals that filled the questionnaire had two times more probability of using a Medicare service while increased time in care coordination was linked with fewer hospital readmissions. Thus, those individuals were more likely to visit a physician's office than return to the hospital and increase healthcare costs. Improved depression management enabled the reduction of depression symptoms in about 60% of engaged individuals in the program. Finally, Big Data analytics-enabled suggestions for participation in a wellness program.

However, there are still numerous issues in the Big Data arena, especially in healthcare. By 2020, experts predict that data will be produced at a rate of about 40 trillion gigabytes per day. Current information technology is not capable of storing and processing such large volumes. Also, there is a shortage of skilled personnel to collect, manage and process these data. Furthermore, there is resistance from health providers and administrators, as they do not understand the benefits of Big

Data and especially for population health management. For data collected from the medical facilities, systems' time and technical diversity seem to be a barrier for data collection.

Moreover, medical systems are continually changing, as they adapt to new technological and scientific advances, as well as to emerging organizational and regulatory requirements and newly developed standards. As a sequel, even in a single hospital, there are several information systems, and often a bridge is required to ensure interoperability. Despite the evolution in medical standards, it seems that several efforts are still needed. Within the healthcare facilities, the replacement of existing systems depends on the willingness and financial capacity of healthcare providers. Additional barriers will emerge due to the application of M-Health; whereas data collection will be more intense, individuals are already able to collect them from their own devices.

There are somewhat limited published resources for Big Data and population health management (Moumtzoglou & Pouliakis, 2015, 2018; Wells et al., 2016). Moreover, the evaluation of the applications is scarce. Recently a review (Wells et al., 2016) concluded that the use of Big Data in the management and evaluation of population health programs led to several improvements. The program management, reporting, and evaluation processes generate additional data that are useful. However, the analysis is not always easy. When analyzed, the outcome can help to continuous refinement of the program implementation and quality. Moreover, the authors of this study (Wells et al., 2016) suggested, as improvements, the incorporation and enhanced integration of social service programs. These are expected to generate their data streams for further analyses and further improvement of health and wellbeing.

M-HEALTH

M-Health describes the use of a broad range of telecommunication and multimedia technologies within the wireless care delivery design and can be broadly defined as the provision of healthcare services via non-wired communication devices (Dimitriou et al., 2017; Metelmann & Metelmann, 2017; Rana, 2017). M-Health establishes healthcare communities in which every stakeholder can participate (O'Connor, Heavin, & O'Donoghue, 2015). However, it disrupts the traditional service model where healthcare information, security, and access is centrally managed, maintained and limited, transforming the health sector and destroying components that are slow to adapt.

M-Health interventions range from simple to complex applications and systems that remotely coordinate and actively manage patient care (Moumtzoglou, 2016; Pouliakis, A, Archondakis, Margari, & Karakitsos, 2016; Pouliakis, A., Karakitsou,

& Margari, 2019; Pouliakis, A., Margari, Archondakis, Karakitsou, & Karakitsos, 2016; Tamposis, Pouliakis, Fezoulidis, & Karakitsos, 2016). In this context, M-health is an elegant solution to the problem of accessing the right information where and when it is needed within highly fluid, distributed organizations. Moreover, it removes geography and time as barriers to care by establishing connectivity with remote locations and remote workers, creates new points of contact with patients, and changes the frequency and intensity of health care delivery. It also establishes effective new treatment modalities like telehealth, remote patient monitoring, self-care, and home health while it blurs the boundaries between professional medical advice and self-care. Overall, M-Health blends three bodies of knowledge: high technology, life sciences, and human factors.

M-Health could also be thought of as the practice of medicine and public health supported by mobile devices. The use of mobile computing and communication devices, such as mobile phones, tablet computers and personal digital assistants (PDAs), by health professionals, is nowadays rapidly growing. Wireless networks are the answer for the interconnection of ubiquitous devices. However, wireless communications increase security challenges, privacy concerns, and trust issues for the wireless network, the mobile devices, the connected medical devices and e-health applications (Grami & Schell, 2004). Wireless, mobile nodes is a new challenge in the distributed systems which carry out functions like packet forwarding, routing, and network management (Chlamtac, Conti, & Liu, 2003). Various protocols and algorithms are available for mobile ad-hoc networks (Chlamtac et al., 2003) while the quality of service models for mobile ad-hoc networks and network security are significant challenges to be surveyed (Chlamtac et al., 2003). As a result, different quality of service constraints for various services illustrates the need for an automatic wireless technology option (Janevski, 2009; Kitanov, Monteiro, & Janevski, 2016). An additional characteristic of the M-Health application is the rapid deployment time. This is a reality not only for the applications but also for the terminal devices. Notably, since there is no need for wire installations, the mobile device is almost ready to be used just when it is out of the box.

Moreover, applications via the use of centralized repositories are installed within a few minutes. A major issue could be the unavailability of centralized resources such as the base stations. However, even in this case and especially in emergencies, mobile base stations can be transferred to specific locations to increase coverage.

Currently, the generations of mobile phone networks (3G/UMTS, 4G and the predecessor of 5G, i.e., 4.5G) are packet-based architectures (Kastania & Moumtzoglou, 2012). Mobile telephony since 3G technology enabled the seamless delivery of web content to mobile consumers (Wilson, 2006). Users' management involves subscriptions and profiles for different terminals (cell phone, PDA, laptops, desktops) (Hong & Leon-Garcia, 2005) while the choice of a cell/mobile device is heavily influenced by the provided mobile services and device capabilities.

Existing cellular and Wi-Fi networks that have, nowadays, merged with the Internet, represent the 4th Generation (4G) and the predecessor of 5G (i.e., 4.5G) wireless, mobile Internet networks (Gani, Li, Yang, & Zakaria, 2008). 4G generation of wireless enhanced and replaced the 3G systems. 4G is a mobile network, IP-based, providing a connection via always the best available network using seamless roaming and free radio spectrum technologies. In 4G mobile systems, different access technologies are combined, in the best possible way, for various radio environments and service requirements. 4G technologies have already implemented much more extensive data rates supporting full mobility while enabling wireless connection and access to multimedia services with high-quality voice and high-definition video. 4G wireless telecommunication supports smart multi-media providing higher bit rate and broader bandwidth, 3D image technology, streamed HD TV with remote control, video multimedia and advanced multimedia messaging service. The mobile multimedia provision requires a modern mobile communication system to make ubiquitous communication using mobile characteristics. High-quality voice, video, and data services can be delivered to a metropolitan using Wi-Fi (IEEE 802.11a/b/g/n/ac) as a transition towards 5G. Mobile WiMAX, while expected to fulfill the goals of 4G technology offering full broadband for all services, is not, nowadays, the technology of choice. In this context, global roaming and open interconnection interfaces are essential functions of 4G communications systems.

According to many researchers, mobile applications ensure seamless mobile services for end-users, anywhere, and on any device. However, the shifts towards more advanced networking systems depend on the development of wireless radio access technologies and networking technologies.

Services adding to 4G include 5G, which is expected to be a more intelligent technology for the whole interconnection world without limits. 5G technology is currently implemented and is the standard of mobile telecom providers; it is synonym with the LTE Advanced (Long Term Evolution) and MIMO (multiple input / multiple outputs) technologies that enable the multiplication of capacity and frequency use along with optimization in the urban and indoor environments to handle multipath effects.

5G is planned to provide additional services and have more advantages, related to energy consumption, network coverage, spectrum handling, bandwidth use, and allows users to participate in a fully distributed or cellular-controlled fashion. All IP-based services for heterogeneous wireless access technologies, assisted by mobile IP, are to be provided by 5G mobile communication networks. 5G aims at a higher capacity and simultaneously, a higher density of mobile users.

Moreover, it supports device-to-device, and machine to machine reliable communications (i.e., mobile ad-hoc networks / MANETs). Thus, 5G aims at lower latency than the 4G equipment and lower battery consumption and is an enabling technology for the Internet of things. Nowadays, there is no standard for the deployment of 5G. However, the expected characteristics include:

- Tens of megabits per second, simultaneously for dozens of thousands of users.
- More than 100 megabits per second for metropolitan networks.
- 1 Gb per second, simultaneously available to all users on the same building floor.
- Capacity for hundreds of thousands of simultaneous connections for the implementation of the Internet of Things.
- Spectral efficiency / i.e., more Mbps for the same frequency slot.
- Improved coverage.
- Significantly reduced latency.

MEDICAL APPLICATIONS FOR THE NEXT GENERATION OF MOBILE DEVICES AND NETWORKS

Mobile web services represent the integration of web services between mobile devices without any centralized entities (Srirama, Jarke, Zhu, & Prinz, 2008). Factors influencing mobile hosts are network characteristics, searching capability of the services and computational resources (Srirama, 2006) while collaborative sharing of peer resources is possible for Mobile Hosts in P2P (Srirama, 2006). Mobile Host in JXME JXME allows collaboration, image sharing, and location-based services (Srirama, 2006). Each Mobile Host can provide some services in the wireless network acting, through the cell phone, as both web service client and provider (Srirama, Jarke, & Prinz, 2007). The quality of service (QoS) for the Mobile Host is critical regarding security and scalability.

A mobile phone is a communications device offering wide-area networking capabilities (Roussos, Marsh, & Maglavera, 2005). Cell phones can serve as control devices for ubiquitous systems and information service endpoints with a focus on protecting the user's information (Roussos et al., 2005). Many mobile phones interact with other nearby devices due to the availability of wireless networking capabilities (Itani, Kayssi, & Chehab, 2016; Roussos et al., 2005). Visual tag clicking on camera phone allows user interaction with a mobile service (Toye et al., 2007) while mobile content can be downloaded, in commercially available products scanning visual tags (Toye et al., 2007). Moreover, data rates increase web browsing and offer reduced access times. However, there are constraints associated with small mobile displays and keypads (Toye et al., 2007), while more significant data rates increase energy consumption and complexity of the device.

Overall, the smart Internet phone lets the mobile phone select the best connections (Janevski, 2009). Furthermore, all smartphones (cell phones that include PDA functionality) are equipped with the functionality to access high-speed data through a variety of networks including those supported by mobile phone networks (3G and 4G+), local networks (WiFi) and personal area networks (Bluetooth and NFC). Applications for the next generation of cell phones will provide localized, real-time services and localized information services. However, confirmation is needed for the services provided by smartphones in a wireless network (Srirama et al., 2007).

Handheld computing has already numerous applications such as:

- Ambulatory medicine (Banitsas, K., Perakis, Koutsouris, Konis, & Tachakra, 2005; Banitsas, K. A., Perakis, Tachakra, & Koutsouris, 2006; Kiselev, Gridnev, Shvartz, Posnenkova, & Dovgalevsky, 2012; Pavlopoulos, Kyriacou, Berler, Dembeyiotis, & Koutsouris, 1998; Rosales Saurer, Mueller-Gorchs, & Kunze, 2009; Zerth, Besser, & Reichert, 2012).
- Diabetes management (Quinn et al., 2011; Ribu et al., 2013; Skrovseth, Arsand, Godtliebsen, & Hartvigsen, 2012; Spat et al., 2013).
- Asthma management (Finkelstein, Hripcsak, & Cabrera, 1998; Gupta, Chang, Anyigbo, & Sabharwal, 2011).
- Control of obesity (Patrick et al., 2009).
- Smoking control (Ghorai, Akter, Khatun, & Ray, 2014; Ybarra, Holtrop, Prescott, & Strong, 2014).
- Seizure management (Pandher & Bhullar, 2014).
- Stress management (Clarke et al., 2014)
- Helping new mother to treat newborns (Feroz, Perveen, & Aftab, 2017; Shorey, Yang, & Dennis, 2018) and
- Treatment of depression (Burns et al., 2011).

In the field of M-Health most applications are fitness related (43%) followed by health resource (15.0%) and diet/caloric intake (14.3%,), while user engagement has the form of self-monitoring and training (74.8%) (Sama, Eapen, Weinfurt, Shah, & Schulman, 2014). On the other hand, despite the applications which target patients, currently, there are somewhat limited applications targeting physicians and doctor-patient interactions (Martin, 2012). The pioneering field seems to be radiology consultation for X-rays and mostly Computer Tomography (Choudhri et al., 2012; Choudhri et al., 2013; Johnson et al., 2012; Toomey et al., 2010) and ECG transmission (Vaisanen, Makijarvi, & Silfvast, 2003).

However, the mobile device has emerged recently as a technology gadget collecting biomedical data, either in the form of the mobile phone or as a specialized appliance, usually in the shape of a wrist attached device. This plethora of devices has created a new movement called quantified self (QS) (Fawcett, 2015). QC involves ordinary and usually healthy people that record and process aspects of their lives with the help of (usually) self-collected data. This QS movement has attracted the interest of commercial companies offering products and services (hardware and software). The M-Health applications being of interest to physicians, patients, and the science of individuality include the following.

Mobile MIM (MIM Software, 2017) is a software application for viewing MRI, PET and CT data using mobile devices compatible with the Apples' iPhone series operating system (iPad®, iPhone®, and iPod touch®). MRI, PET, and CT images are transmitted using the software, and it is possible to measure the image intensity and distances.

MobiUS™ is an image-based series of products (Mobisante Inc., 2017) supporting ultrasound (US) imaging. That is smartphone and tablet-based and is cheaper than traditional US systems, being equipped with specialized monitors. Moreover, this system supports sharing of images among patients and clinicians.

Gyromaniac (Subversus Interactive, 2011) uses the iPhone gyroscope electronic components to help physicians practice spatial orientation: for example, to assist gastroenterologists during training how to perform a colonoscopy (Iltifat, 2010).

There are, as well, software platforms for connected wearables, and non-obtrusive ECG data (cardiac) monitoring. Such solutions can be of help for cardiologists to monitor and manage patients with angina, infarction of the myocardium, cardiac interventions such as stents, pacemakers, and bypass, as well as cardiac failures and ambulatory medicine. Such devices have been in service for gynecologists for fetus monitoring (Medical design, 2013; Su & Chu, 2014). That avoids frequent visits to the outpatient department for follow up, the unnecessary waiting time and anxiety for patients. That system also aids proactive management of complications, identifying them with intelligent analysis as and when they occur and addressing them based on evidence.

A recently announced device (Wavelet Health, 2017) incorporates a photoplethysmograph (PPG) sensor; a pulse oximeter illuminating the skin and measuring changes in light absorption; such a device is capable to continuously monitor perfusion of blood to the dermis as well as subcutaneous tissue; therefore, it can detect heart rate as well as blood oxygen levels.

Recent announcements (University of Illinois College of Engineering, 2017) are related to a lab on a chip device that when coupled with a smartphone, can perform lab-grade medical diagnostics. Such tests usually require extensive, specialized and expensive instruments. However, the developed inexpensive microchip incorporates technology prevailing in the three top categories of medical diagnostics. The microchip promises to perform thousands of already available tests. It is based on the mobile phone camera that is used as a spectrometer. Specifically, the biological sample should be in a fluid form; this is illuminated by the cell phone's white LED flash. Subsequently, the light from the fluidic sample is collected by an optical fiber and after being captured by the phone's internal camera can be evaluated by the use of the software. Such technology enables the application of advanced biological tests in remote areas, often in the developing world, and personalized tests at the individual patient level.

In the field of otolaryngology, some applications can determine reference sound levels with a minimum variation; therefore, it is feasible to conduct a hearing screening on devices calibrated with a predefined reference noise level (Masalski, Kipiński, Grysiński, & Kręcicki, 2016).

Also, the advanced communication capabilities allow voice and video conferencing features for patient/doctor and doctor/doctor interactions as well as seamless transmission of captured images and video.

Portable electroencephalograph (EEG) is another area that mobile devices may become a commodity. Emotiv Insight Brainware® (see Figure 1) is a channel EEG device that can capture brain signals and transmit them via Bluetooth interface to the mobile phone (EMOTIV, 2017). Such commercial and portable EEG devices have already been used to measure auditory potential on children and adults (Barham et al., 2017). They are used to convert brain signal to computer commands, and some identify the mental status and record it for archiving purposes.

Figure 1. A commercial portable EEG device capable of communicating via Bluetooth with the mobile phone

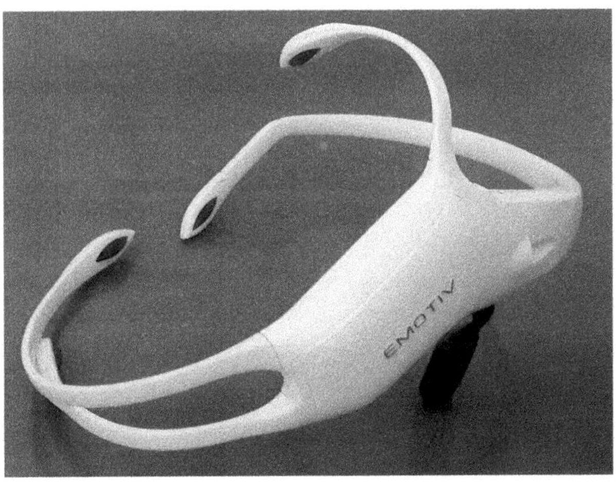

Furthermore, modern high-end mobile phones are coupled with sensors that can measure life signals and communicate with commercial devices that measure health signals such as blood glucose. For instance, some cell phones have integrated heart rate sensors with high accuracy and step counters. They also have applications (Figure 2) that measure and store data to the cloud, such as exercise and sports activity, heart rate, stress, sleeping duration, consumption of food and liquids, weights and glucose when coupled with appropriate medical devices or when the user wishes to supply such information.

Other applications include provisioning of care continuation from antenatal and childbirth to the postnatal period in order to reduce maternal and neonatal morbidity and mortality. The postpartum period is very critical; however, it is the most neglected phase for mothers and the newborns. This period begins immediately after childbirth and usually extends for about six weeks for the mother's body to return to its initial state. The postpartum period poses substantial risks for both mothers and newborn infants; this is the period that most maternal and infant mortalities and morbidities occur. The World Health Organization estimates that more than 300,000 women died as a result of pregnancy and childbirth-related complications, and more than 2.5 million newborns died after birth in 2015 (World Health Organization, 2015). Therefore, application of postnatal care apps constitutes a promising approach.

Conclusively, the recent advances of the mobile telephony have contributed to the conversion of the mobile telephones into smartphones; due to the sophisticated operating systems and the plethora of easy to use accompanying applications. Notably, during the previous last years, hardware components enriching cell phones became available, including more processing power (8 or more processors), high-definition

Figure 2. A display of mobile phone applications for the measurement of health and well-being data

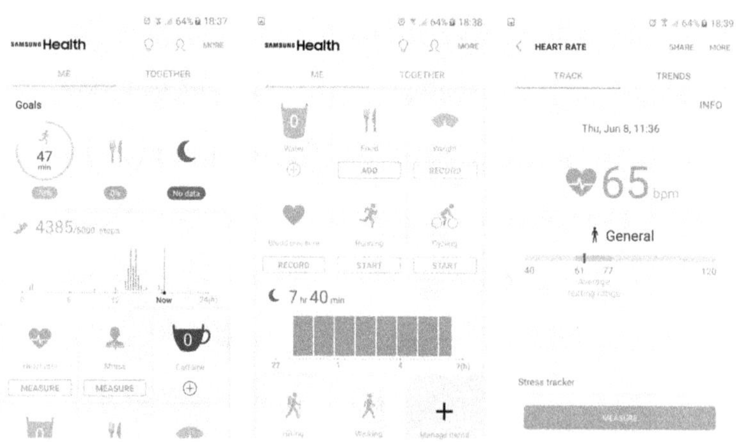

cameras (more than 20Mpixel) and large display resolutions. Moreover, the 4.5G and WiFi connectivity have created an always open, rather inexpensive, communication channel with the Internet. Today, there is no more the trend to shrink the telephone; in contrast, mobile phones are becoming larger and complete tablets regarding size and weight; they are easy to use and have capabilities similar to computers available five years ago. It seems that mobile devices have now the maturity of computers that were used in the health sector five years ago.

INTERNET OF THINGS

The **Internet of things (IoT)** is the extension of Internet connectivity into physical devices and everyday objects. Nowadays, Internet connectivity has become embedded with electronics (see Figure 3), and when combined with other forms of hardware such as sensors and actuators, these electronic devices get the capability to communicate and moreover interact over the Internet. Thus, they can be monitored and controlled remotely and on a global scale. Such progress is moreover combined usually at a little cost. Thus, IoT has opened a plethora of new possibilities in medicine which can be understood by merely considering that a medical device when connected to the Internet, it can collect additional data and allow instant diagnosis and problem resolution or provide additional insight into symptoms and patient trends. IoT seems to be a catalytic technology for personalized medicine since the electronic health devices are attached to specific persons (healthy or not healthy) and generally give patients more control over their treatment and lives.

The applications of IoT in healthcare are countless; some are presented in the sequel:

During a randomized clinical trial, 357 patients were treated for head and neck cancer; within this trial, a Bluetooth-enabled device was used for weight and blood pressure monitoring. The device was further coupled with an app which was tracking symptoms and sending data to patients' physicians (Peterson et al., 2013). Patients that used this monitoring system (known as CYCORE) experienced less severe symptoms relevant to cancer and treatment when compared to a control group.

There are other applications which have become "commodities". Diabetes is a very fertile ground for such developments, affects about 10% of the adults, and moreover requires continuous monitoring and treatment. Some devices perform Continuous Glucose Monitoring (CGM) and help people with diabetes to monitor their blood glucose by taking readings at regular intervals. Such systems have already been approved by the US FDA since, and today there are numerous CGMs available in the market. These smart CGMs send data from glucose measurements to apps. Thus, the device wearer can quickly check information, detect trends and receive

Figure 3. An electronic board capable of communicating via WiFi with nearby smartphones or directly to the Internet. An antenna is visible at the left side, a USD port at the right side, and at the top, the bottom is a series of pins allowing connection of inputs and outputs. The device is equipped with a microcontroller capable of being programmed to perform specific tasks — device with about 8 cm.

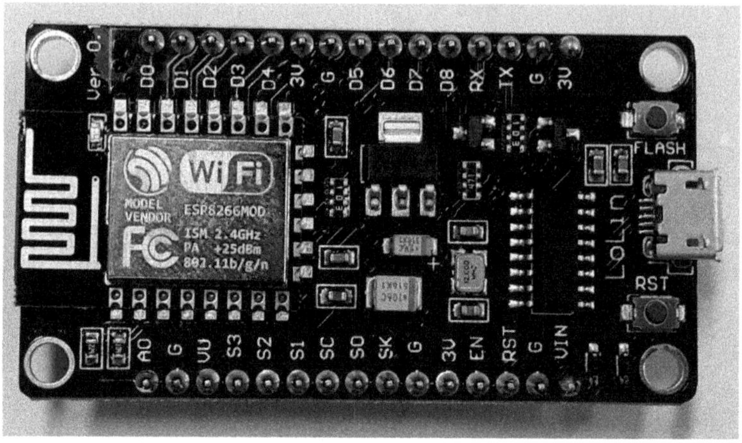

medication on appropriate dosage. The connectivity allows remote monitoring by caregivers, including parents of diabetic children are relatives of elderly patients. In the same arena smart insulin pens are now capable to automatically record the amount, time, amount and type of insulin that should be injected in a dose, and moreover, recommend the appropriate insulin type for injection at the right time and the right dosage. As expected, such smartpen devices interact with the app that not only stores long-term data to help diabetes patients calculate their insulin details but can allow patients to record and propose meals. This combination of three smart devices, the smartphone, the CGM and the smartpen along with the Internet connectivity, seem to revolutionize diabetes management and improve individuals' lives and reduce complications.

According to WHO (World Health Organisation, 2003), about 50% of the medicines are not taken as prescribed by the patients. That is an essential issue for treatment efficiency and can have a severe impact on the patient's health. Today there are pills that when dissolved in the stomach produce a week but adequate signal being picked up by a wearable sensor. An app in a smartphone is then capable of receiving this information and either store it or relay it to confirm not only that the drug was used and additionally to confirm the time that was received. This approach has been used in trials for treating uncontrolled hypertension, type II diabetes, and antipsychotic medication.

Moreover, such traceable pills have been already approved by the US FDA. This approach could help to track and improve the regularity of medication intake, allow the patients to have a more informed dialogue with their physician and alert patients if the medication was not received in time. The high percentage of medication misuse (or not use) makes the application of such a system attractive especially in those patients, that discontinue sharing information with their physicians and more critical for patients that opt out of a treatment program altogether.

The primary issue in IoT applications in healthcare, unfortunately, is related to security. Manufacturers often do not consider the risks of these devices connected to the Internet. There is always a possibility that the exploitation of the vulnerability in a medical device could cause injury or even death to the user(Chacko & Hayajneh, 2018). These vulnerabilities have been identified by the US FDA (FDA, 2019a, 2019b). Consequently, guidelines have been issued and medical device manufacturers should alleviate such cyber vulnerabilities. Despite the tremendous opportunities and benefits, security seems to be the most intriguing issue of IoT in healthcare.

Issues, Controversies, Problems

First, we must recognize that by centering population health efforts on the patients, we are overlooking those who are not patients. Even for those who are exceptionally engaged patients, their interaction with the healthcare system is a mere fraction of health and well-being influences. Consequently, if we design population health efforts solely around patients, we fail to address the enormously significant social determinants of health, which include environmental, economic, and cultural factors.

Instead, we need a proactive, holistic, longitudinal, without walls, profoundly personal approach to population health management. That means the approach should include not only the care of sick but also well being of healthy individuals, as the goal should be lifelong health and quality of life support. That also includes proactively reaching out to hard-to-reach populations. Moreover, the approach should:

- Address the range of psychological, biological and social factors that influence health and wellness.
- Leverage the patient as a source of continuity by engaging him or her as an integral member of the care team.
- Recognize that supporting an individual's lifelong health and well-being cannot be relegated to any one particular setting.
- Take into account the personal goals, strengths, and challenges as primary drivers of care management, planning and decision-making.

While 'Big Data' has its place for identifying patterns and gaps in care and predictive analysis, and IoT is the platform that can provide a plethora of such data, the most relevant data regarding the science of individuality are self-reported data. In this context, the population health management strategies will fail to engage patients, reduce costs, and improve outcomes if they are implemented without the underpinning of person-centered care. Ultimately, the health of a population has nothing to do with data and technology but with the individuals that make up the population. Poor acceptance of technology would be inhibitory towards that goal.

To this direction, and due to the sensitivity of the stored and transferred information, data security for all of the associated technologies is of essential importance (Spyra, Buchanan, Cruickshank, & Ekonomou, 2014). In this context, the US FDA has issued guidelines, and in the legal systems, the European Union approved (in April 2016) the General Data Protection Regulation (GDPR); the most significant change in the European legal framework the last twenty (20) years. The GDPR has a direct application in all member states since May 25, 2018, and its enforcement is assured by hefty fines on non-compliant organizations. However, the implementation of the GDPR, in no small scale, might be a big issue, as information flowing across the EU borders and data storage in non-EU countries could be essential, taking into account that non-EU countries are not obliged to apply the GDPR. As a result, services offered by organizations residing outside the EU could be vital for e-health applications targeting individuals.

FUTURE RESEARCH DIRECTIONS

The future of population health management is tied to the rise of cognitive computing. Cognitive computing is the simulation of human thought processes in a computerized model and uses parallel processing and artificial intelligence to convert unstructured into structured data, search the medical literature, and find connections among multiple types of evidence, in short, it creates knowledge.

The goal of cognitive computing is to build automated IT systems that are capable of solving problems without requiring human assistance and exploit a vast amount of data originating from diverse resources. The cognitive computing systems:

- Use natural language processing and machine learning algorithms.
- Mine the data for information.
- Refine the way they search for patterns
- Resolve security risks

to become capable of anticipating new problems and modeling solutions.

Heretofore, cognitive computing is used in the following artificial intelligence (AI) applications:

- Expert systems.
- Natural language programming.
- Neural networks.
- Robotics.
- Virtual and augmented reality.

CONCLUSION

Population health management (PHM) has been, so far, a discipline which studies and facilitates care delivery across a group of individuals or the general population. In the context of population health management, the life science industry has no motivation to design drugs or devices that are only effective for a distinct segment of the population. At the same time, the regulatory agencies are entirely risk-averse and are suppressing remarkable innovative and even frugal opportunities to change medicine.

However, the significant outgrowth of the science of individuality, as well as the rising 'wiki medicine', that is, the individualized medicine which respects individuality, fully recognize the uniqueness of the individual. In this regard, it will not be long until digitizing a person unlocks the root cause for what is wrong, creating valuable knowledge that can save or markedly improve the quality of life.

Cloud computing, Big Data, M-Health and IoT technologies offer the resources to succeed in dealing with the shortcomings of the population health management approach. Specifically, while population health management focuses on what happens on the bed or a doctor's office, the technologies above facilitate the collection, propagation and storage of the science of individuality by taking the challenges of wellness, prevention, and lower cost. Finally, cognitive computing is considered the future of population health management as the processing of this vast amount of information is impossible by humans.

REFERENCES

Anastasi, A. (1937). *Differential psychology: Individual and group differences in behavior*. New York, NY: Macmillan.

Archondakis, S., Pouliakis, A., Margari, N., & Karakitsos, P. (2014). The Implementation of Cloud-Based Telemedical Applications for External Quality Control Purposes in the Field of Cytopathology. *International Journal of Reliable and Quality E-Healthcare*, *3*(3), 22–36. doi:10.4018/ijrqeh.2014070102

Banitsas, K., Perakis, K., Koutsouris, D., Konis, G., & Tachakra, S. (2005). Ambulance 3G. *Conference Proceedings; ... Annual International Conference of the IEEE Engineering in Medicine and Biology Society. IEEE Engineering in Medicine and Biology Society. Conference*, *1*, 371–374. doi:10.1109/IEMBS.2005.1616422 PMID:17282191

Banitsas, K. A., Perakis, K., Tachakra, S., & Koutsouris, D. (2006). Use of 3G mobile phone links for teleconsultation between a moving ambulance and a hospital base station. *Journal of Telemedicine and Telecare*, *12*(1), 23–26. doi:10.1258/135763306775321335 PMID:16438775

Barham, M. P., Clark, G. M., Hayden, M. J., Enticott, P. G., Conduit, R., & Lum, J. A. G. (2017). Acquiring research-grade ERPs on a shoestring budget: A comparison of a modified Emotiv and commercial SynAmps EEG system. *Psychophysiology*, *54*(9), 1393–1404. doi:10.1111/psyp.12888 PMID:28497557

Beckmann, J. S., & Lew, D. (2016). Reconciling evidence-based medicine and precision medicine in the era of big data: Challenges and opportunities. *Genome Medicine*, *8*(1), 134. doi:10.118613073-016-0388-7 PMID:27993174

Bergman, L. R., & Vargha, A. (2013). Matching method to problem: A developmental science perspective. *European Journal of Developmental Psychology*, *10*(1), 9–28. doi:10.1080/17405629.2012.732920

Blau, C. A., & Liakopoulou, E. (2013). Can we deconstruct cancer, one patient at a time? *Trends in Genetics*, *29*(1), 6–10. doi:10.1016/j.tig.2012.09.004 PMID:23102584

Care Continuum Alliance. (2012). *Advancing the Population Health Improvement Model*. Retrieved from http://www.fiercehealthit.com/story/hennepin-health-project-looks-build-countywide-ehr-program-national-implica/2012-01-10

Chacko, A., & Hayajneh, T. (2018). Security and Privacy Issues with IoT in Healthcare. *EAI Endorsed Transactions on Pervasive Health and Technology, 4*(14).

Chen, R., Mias, G. I., Li-Pook-Than, J., Jiang, L., Lam, H. Y., Chen, R., ... Snyder, M. (2012). Personal omics profiling reveals dynamic molecular and medical phenotypes. *Cell*, *148*(6), 1293–1307. doi:10.1016/j.cell.2012.02.009 PMID:22424236

Chlamtac, I., Conti, M., & Liu, J. J. N. (2003). Mobile ad hoc networking: Imperatives and challenges. *Ad Hoc Networks*, *1*(1), 13–64. doi:10.1016/S1570-8705(03)00013-1

Chomsky, N. (1957). *Syntactic structures*. The Hague, The Netherlands: Mouton.

Choudhri, A. F., Carr, T. M. III, Ho, C. P., Stone, J. R., Gay, S. B., & Lambert, D. L. (2012). Handheld device review of abdominal CT for the evaluation of acute appendicitis. *Journal of Digital Imaging*, *25*(4), 492–496. doi:10.100710278-011-9431-9 PMID:22146833

Choudhri, A. F., Norton, P. T., Carr, T. M. III, Stone, J. R., Hagspiel, K. D., & Dake, M. D. (2013). Diagnosis and treatment planning of acute aortic emergencies using a handheld DICOM viewer. *Emergency Radiology*, *20*(4), 267–272. doi:10.100710140-013-1118-8 PMID:23525945

Clarke, J., Proudfoot, J., Birch, M. R., Whitton, A. E., Parker, G., Manicavasagar, V., ... Hadzi-Pavlovic, D. (2014). Effects of mental health self-efficacy on outcomes of a mobile phone and web intervention for mild-to-moderate depression, anxiety and stress: Secondary analysis of a randomised controlled trial. *BMC Psychiatry*, *14*(1), 272. doi:10.118612888-014-0272-1 PMID:25252853

Coughlin, J. F., Pope, J. E., & Leedle, B. R. Jr. (2006). Old Age, New Technology, and Future Innovations in Disease Management and Home Health Care. *Home Health Care Management & Practice*, *18*(3), 196–207. doi:10.1177/1084822305281955

Cusack, C. M., Knudson, A. D., Kronstadt, J. L., Singer, R. F., & Brown, A. L. (2010). *Practice-Based Population Health: Information Technology to Support Transformation to Proactive Primary Care* (pp. 44). Retrieved from https://pcmh.ahrq.gov/sites/default/files/attachments/Information%20Technology%20to%20Support%20Transformation%20to%20Proactive%20Primary%20Care.pdf

Dawson, P. S. S. (1988). The 'average cell'— A handicap in bioscience and biotechnology. *Trends in Biotechnology*, *6*(5), 87–90. doi:10.1016/0167-7799(88)90063-7

Dimitriou, M., Giazitzi, K., Stavridi, E., Palisidis, G., Karathanos, V., & Boskou, G. (2017). Evaluation of an Electronic Application for Nutritional Information in Food Service Outlets: A Pilot mHealth Application. *International Journal of Reliable and Quality E-Healthcare*, *6*(1), 46–58. doi:10.4018/IJRQEH.2017010104

EMOTIV. (2017). *Emotiv insight Brainware®*. Retrieved 2 Sept., 2017, from https://www.emotiv.com/insight/

Eugster, M. J., Schmid, M., Binder, H., & Schmidberger, M. (2013). Grid and cloud computing methods in biomedical research. *Methods of Information in Medicine*, *52*(1), 62–64. doi:10.1055-0038-1627052 PMID:23318694

Fawcett, T. (2015). Mining the Quantified Self: Personal Knowledge Discovery as a Challenge for Data Science. *Big Data*, *3*(4), 249–266. doi:10.1089/big.2015.0049 PMID:27441406

FDA. (2019a). *Cybersecurity*. Retrieved 20 August, 2019, from https://www.fda.gov/medical-devices/digital-health/cybersecurity

FDA. (2019b). *The FDA'S role in medical device cybersecurity: Dispelling Myths and Understanding Facts*. Retrieved 20 August, 2019, from https://www.fda.gov/media/103696/download

Feroz, A., Perveen, S., & Aftab, W. (2017). Role of mHealth applications for improving antenatal and postnatal care in low and middle income countries: A systematic review. *BMC Health Services Research*, *17*(1), 704. doi:10.118612913-017-2664-7 PMID:29115992

Finkelstein, J., Hripcsak, G., & Cabrera, M. (1998). Telematic system for monitoring of asthma severity in patients' homes. *Studies in Health Technology and Informatics*, *52*(Pt 1), 272–276. PMID:10384460

Fischer, K. W., & Bidell, T. R. (2006). Dynamic development of action and thought. In W. Damon & R. M. Lerner (Eds.), Theoretical models of human development. Handbook of child psychology (6th ed.; Vol. 1, pp. 313–399). New York, NY: John Wiley & Sons.

Fodor, J. (1983). *The modularity of mind: An essay on faculty psychology*. Cambridge, MA: MIT Press. doi:10.7551/mitpress/4737.001.0001

Gani, A., Li, X., Yang, L., & Zakaria, O. (2008). Radio frequency combination for TCP/IP suite protocol improvement in 4G mobile internet networks. *International Journal of Communication*, *2*(1), 27–36.

Garrett, D. D., Samanez-Larkin, G. R., MacDonald, S. W., Lindenberger, U., McIntosh, A. R., & Grady, C. L. (2013). Moment-to-moment brain signal variability: A next frontier in human brain mapping? *Neuroscience and Biobehavioral Reviews*, *37*(4), 610–624. doi:10.1016/j.neubiorev.2013.02.015 PMID:23458776

Ghorai, K., Akter, S., Khatun, F., & Ray, P. (2014). mHealth for Smoking Cessation Programs: A Systematic Review. *Journal of Personalized Medicine*, *4*(3), 412–423. doi:10.3390/jpm4030412 PMID:25563359

Glaser, J. (2011). Cloud computing can simplify HIT infrastructure management. *Healthcare Financial Management, 65*(8), 52–55. PMID:21866720

Grami, A., & Schell, B. H. (2004). *Future trends in mobile commerce: Service offerings, technological advances and security challenges.* Paper presented at the the Second Annual Conference on Privacy, Security and Trust.

Gupta, S., Chang, P., Anyigbo, N., & Sabharwal, A. (2011). mobileSpiro: accurate mobile spirometry for self-management of asthma. *Proceedings of the First ACM Workshop on Mobile Systems, Applications, and Services for Healthcare.* 10.1145/2064942.2064944

Hillman, M. (2002). *Testimony before the Subcommittee on Health of the House Committee on Ways and Means, Hearing on Promoting Disease Management in Medicare.* Retrieved 10 June, 2015, from http://waysandmeans.house.gov/Legacy/health/107cong/4-16-02/4-16hill.htm

Howe, R., & Spence, C. (2004). *Population Health Management: Healthways. In PopWorks* (Vol. 2, pp. 291–297). HCT Project. Retrieved from http://mthink.com/article/population-health-management-healthways-popworks/

Hsu, C. H., Lin, C. Y., Ouyang, M., & Guo, Y. K. (2013). Biocloud: Cloud computing for biological, genomics, and drug design. *BioMed Research International, 909470.* doi:10.1155/2013/909470

Iltifat, H. (2010). Gyromaniac app for iPhone could help gastroenterologists when learning how to perform a colonoscopy. *iMedicalApps.* Retrieved 20 Aug., 2017, from https://www.imedicalapps.com/2010/06/gastroenterologists-iphone-4-medical-spatial-orientation/#

Itani, W., Kayssi, A., & Chehab, A. (2016). Wireless Body Sensor Networks: Security, Privacy, and Energy Efficiency in the Era of Cloud Computing. *International Journal of Reliable and Quality E-Healthcare, 5*(2), 1–30. doi:10.4018/IJRQEH.2016040101

Janevski, T. (2009). *5G Mobile Phone Concept.* Paper presented at the 2009 6th IEEE Consumer Communications and Networking Conference.

Johnson, P. T., Zimmerman, S. L., Heath, D., Eng, J., Horton, K. M., Scott, W. W., & Fishman, E. K. (2012). The iPad as a mobile device for CT display and interpretation: Diagnostic accuracy for identification of pulmonary embolism. *Emergency Radiology, 19*(4), 323–327. doi:10.100710140-012-1037-0 PMID:22450843

Kastania, A. N., & Moumtzoglou, A. (2012). Quality Implications of the Medical Applications for 4G Mobile Phones. *International Journal of Reliable and Quality E-Healthcare, 1*(1), 58–67. doi:10.4018/ijrqeh.2012010106

Kindig, D. A. (2007). Understanding population health terminology. *The Milbank Quarterly, 85*(1), 139–161. doi:10.1111/j.1468-0009.2007.00479.x PMID:17319809

King, G. (2011). Ensuring the data-rich future of the social sciences. *Science, 331*(6018), 719–721. doi:10.1126cience.1197872 PMID:21311013

Kiselev, A. R., Gridnev, V. I., Shvartz, V. A., Posnenkova, O. M., & Dovgalevsky, P. Y. (2012). Active ambulatory care management supported by short message services and mobile phone technology in patients with arterial hypertension. *Journal of the American Society of Hypertension, 6*(5), 346–355. doi:10.1016/j.jash.2012.08.001 PMID:22995803

Kitanov, S., Monteiro, E., & Janevski, T. (2016). *5G and the Fog — Survey of related technologies and research directions.* Paper presented at the 2016 18th Mediterranean Electrotechnical Conference (MELECON).

Koumpouros, Y. (2015). Big Data in Healthcare. In A. Information Resources Management (Ed.), Healthcare Administration: Concepts, Methodologies, Tools, and Applications (pp. 23-46). Hershey, PA: IGI Global. doi:10.4018/978-1-4666-6339-8.ch002

Kuo, A. M. (2011). Opportunities and challenges of cloud computing to improve health care services. *Journal of Medical Internet Research, 13*(3), e67. doi:10.2196/jmir.1867 PMID:21937354

Levsky, J. M., & Singer, R. H. (2003). Gene expression and the myth of the average cell. *Trends in Cell Biology, 13*(1), 4–6. doi:10.1016/S0962-8924(02)00002-8 PMID:12480334

Lupse, O. S., Vida, M., & Stoicu-Tivadar, L. (2012). Cloud computing technology applied in healthcare for developing large scale flexible solutions. *Studies in Health Technology and Informatics, 174*, 94–99. PMID:22491119

Market Research Future. (2017). *Global Big Data in Healthcare Market Promises a Striking Revenue of USD 35 Billion By 2021.* Retrieved 27 Aug., 2017, from http://www.prnewswire.com/news-releases/global-big-data-in-healthcare-market-promises-a-striking-revenue-of-usd-35-billion-by-2021-300472980.html

Markets and Markets. (2017). *Healthcare Analytics Market worth 24.55 Billion USD by 2021*. Retrieved 25 Aug., 2017, from http://www.marketsandmarkets.com/PressReleases/healthcare-data-analytics.asp

Martin, T. (2012). Assessing mHealth: Opportunities and barriers to patient engagement. *Journal of Health Care for the Poor and Underserved, 23*(3), 935–941. doi:10.1353/hpu.2012.0087 PMID:24212144

Masalski, M., Kipiński, L., Grysiński, T., & Kręcicki, T. (2016). Hearing Tests on Mobile Devices: Evaluation of the Reference Sound Level by Means of Biological Calibration. *Journal of Medical Internet Research, 18*(5), e130. doi:10.2196/jmir.4987 PMID:27241793

Mazziotta, J. C., Woods, R., Iacoboni, M., Sicotte, N., Yaden, K., Tran, M., ... Toga, A. W. (2009). The myth of the normal, average human brain--the ICBM experience: (1) subject screening and eligibility. *NeuroImage, 44*(3), 914–922. doi:10.1016/j.neuroimage.2008.07.062 PMID:18775497

Medical Design. (2013). *Platform makes possible remote fetal monitoring and cardiac care*. Retrieved 10 Aug., 2017, from http://medicaldesign.com/business/platform-makes-possible-remote-fetal-monitoring-and-cardiac-care

Metelmann, C., & Metelmann, B. (2017). Can a Mobile Video Communication Improve Patient Safety in Prehospital Emergency Medicine? *International Journal of Reliable and Quality E-Healthcare, 6*(4), 27–36. doi:10.4018/IJRQEH.2017100104

Mirza, H., & El-Masri, S. (2013). National Electronic Medical Records integration on Cloud Computing System. *Studies in Health Technology and Informatics, 192*, 1219. PMID:23920993

Mischel, W. (1973). Toward a cognitive social learning reconceptualization of personality. *Psychological Review, 80*(4), 252–283. doi:10.1037/h0035002 PMID:4721473

Mobisante Inc. (2017). *MobiSante Inc. web site*. Retrieved 19 Aug., 2017, from http://www.mobisante.com

Molenaar, P. C. M. (2013). On the necessity to use person-specific data analysis approaches in psychology. *European Journal of Developmental Psychology, 10*(1), 29–39. doi:10.1080/17405629.2012.747435

Moumtzoglou, A. (2014). Demystifying Quality of Healthcare in the Cloud. In M. Anastasius & N. K. Anastasia (Eds.), *Cloud Computing Applications for Quality Health Care Delivery* (pp. 284–301). Hershey, PA: IGI Global. doi:10.4018/978-1-4666-6118-9.ch015

Moumtzoglou, A. (Ed.). (2016). *M-Health Innovations for Patient-Centered Care.* Hershey, PA: IGI Global. doi:10.4018/978-1-4666-9861-1

Moumtzoglou, A., & Kastania, A. (Eds.). (2014). *Cloud computing applications for quality health care delivery.* Hershey, PA: IGI Global. doi:10.4018/978-1-4666-6118-9

Moumtzoglou, A., & Pouliakis, A. (2015). Mapping Population Health Management Roadmap into Cervical Cancer Screening Programs. *International Journal of Reliable and Quality E-Healthcare, 4*(3), 1–18. doi:10.4018/IJRQEH.2015070101

Moumtzoglou, A., & Pouliakis, A. (2018). Population Health Management and the Science of Individuality. *International Journal of Reliable and Quality E-Healthcare, 7*(2), 1–26. doi:10.4018/IJRQEH.2018040101

Murray, H. A. (1938). *Explorations in personality:Aclinical and experimental study of fifty men of college age Press.* New York, NY: Oxford University.

Nesselroade, J. R., Gerstorf, D., Hardy, S. A., & Ram, N. (2007). Focus Article: Idiographic Filters for Psychological Constructs. *Measurement: Interdisciplinary Research and Perspectives, 5*(4), 217–235. doi:10.1080/15366360701741807

O'Connor, Y., Heavin, C., & O'Donoghue, J. (2015). Review of Key Stakeholders for an mHealth Pilot Study in Malawi Motivations and Expectations. *International Journal of Reliable and Quality E-Healthcare, 4*(2), 51–66. doi:10.4018/IJRQEH.2015040105

Pandher, P. S., & Bhullar, K. K. (2014). Smartphone applications for seizure management. *Health Informatics Journal.* doi:10.1177/1460458214540906 PMID:25038202

Patel, R. P. (2012). Cloud computing and virtualization technology in radiology. *Clinical Radiology, 67*(11), 1095–1100. doi:10.1016/j.crad.2012.03.010 PMID:22607956

Patrick, K., Raab, F., Adams, M. A., Dillon, L., Zabinski, M., Rock, C. L., ... Norman, G. J. (2009). A text message-based intervention for weight loss: Randomized controlled trial. *Journal of Medical Internet Research, 11*(1), e1. doi:10.2196/jmir.1100 PMID:19141433

Pavlopoulos, S., Kyriacou, E., Berler, A., Dembeyiotis, S., & Koutsouris, D. (1998). A novel emergency telemedicine system based on wireless communication technology--AMBULANCE. *IEEE Transactions on Information Technology in Biomedicine*, *2*(4), 261–267. doi:10.1109/4233.737581 PMID:10719536

Peterson, S. K., Shinn, E. H., Basen-Engquist, K., Demark-Wahnefried, W., Prokhorov, A. V., Baru, C., ... Patrick, K. (2013). Identifying early dehydration risk with home-based sensors during radiation treatment: A feasibility study on patients with head and neck cancer. *Journal of the National Cancer Institute. Monographs*, *2013*(47), 162–168. doi:10.1093/jncimonographs/lgt016 PMID:24395986

Pouliakis, A., Archondakis, S., Karakitsou, E., & Karakitsos, P. (2014). Cloud Computing for Cytopathologists. In A. Moumtzoglou & A. Kastania (Eds.), *Cloud computing applications for quality health care delivery* (pp. 250–271). Hershey, PA: IGI Global. doi:10.4018/978-1-4666-6118-9.ch013

Pouliakis, A., Archondakis, S., Margari, N., & Karakitsos, P. (2016). From telecytology to mobile cytopathology: Past, present and future. In A. Moumtzoglou (Ed.), *M-Health Innovations for Patient-Centered Care*. Hershey, PA: IGI Global. doi:10.4018/978-1-4666-9861-1.ch012

Pouliakis, A., Karakitsou, E., & Margari, N. (2019). Cytopathology and the Smartphone: An Update. In M. Anastasius (Ed.), *Mobile Health Applications for Quality Healthcare Delivery* (pp. 136–164). Hershey, PA: IGI Global. doi:10.4018/978-1-5225-8021-8.ch007

Pouliakis, A., Margari, N., Archondakis, S., Karakitsou, E., & Karakitsos, P. (2016). Emerging Technologies Serving Cytopathology. Big Data, the Cloud and Mobile Computing. In I. E. Naqa (Ed.), *Handbook of Research on Emerging Developments and Practices in Oncology* (pp. 114–152). Hershey, PA: IGI Global.

Pouliakis, A., Spathis, A., Kottaridi, C., Mourtzikou, A., Stamouli, M., Archondakis, S., ... Karakitsos, P. (2014). Cloud Computing for BioLabs. In A. Moumtzoglou & A. Kastania (Eds.), *Cloud computing applications for quality health care delivery* (pp. 228–249). Hershey, PA: IGI Global. doi:10.4018/978-1-4666-6118-9.ch012

Quinn, C. C., Shardell, M. D., Terrin, M. L., Barr, E. A., Ballew, S. H., & Gruber-Baldini, A. L. (2011). Cluster-randomized trial of a mobile phone personalized behavioral intervention for blood glucose control. *Diabetes Care*, *34*(9), 1934–1942. doi:10.2337/dc11-0366 PMID:21788632

Rana, A. (2017). The Immense Potential of M-Care in India: Catering Better to Patients Needs in the Context of a Fragmented Healthcare System. *International Journal of Reliable and Quality E-Healthcare*, *6*(4), 1–3. doi:10.4018/IJRQEH.2017100101

Ribu, L., Holmen, H., Torbjornsen, A., Wahl, A. K., Grottland, A., Smastuen, M. C., ... Arsand, E. (2013). Low-intensity self-management intervention for persons with type 2 diabetes using a mobile phone-based diabetes diary, with and without health counseling and motivational interviewing: Protocol for a randomized controlled trial. *JMIR Research Protocols*, *2*(2), e34. doi:10.2196/resprot.2768 PMID:23978690

Rosales Saurer, B., Mueller-Gorchs, M., & Kunze, C. (2009). Scenario-based design of an ICT platform for mobile information services in ambulatory care nursing. *Studies in Health Technology and Informatics*, *146*, 64–68. PMID:19592810

Rosenthal, A., Mork, P., Li, M. H., Stanford, J., Koester, D., & Reynolds, P. (2010). Cloud computing: A new business paradigm for biomedical information sharing. *Journal of Biomedical Informatics*, *43*(2), 342–353. doi:10.1016/j.jbi.2009.08.014 PMID:19715773

Roussos, G., Marsh, A. J., & Maglavera, S. (2005). Enabling pervasive computing with smart phones. *IEEE Pervasive Computing*, *4*(2), 20–27. doi:10.1109/MPRV.2005.30

Sama, P. R., Eapen, Z. J., Weinfurt, K. P., Shah, B. R., & Schulman, K. A. (2014). An evaluation of mobile health application tools. *JMIR mHealth and uHealth*, *2*(2), e19. doi:10.2196/mhealth.3088 PMID:25099179

Shorey, S., Yang, Y. Y., & Dennis, C. L. (2018). A Mobile Health App-Based Postnatal Educational Program (Home-but not Alone): Descriptive Qualitative Study. *Journal of Medical Internet Research*, *20*(4), e119. doi:10.2196/jmir.9188 PMID:29674314

Siegler, R. S. (2007). Cognitive variability. *Developmental Science*, *10*(1), 104–109. doi:10.1111/j.1467-7687.2007.00571.x PMID:17181707

Skrovseth, S. O., Arsand, E., Godtliebsen, F., & Hartvigsen, G. (2012). Mobile phone-based pattern recognition and data analysis for patients with type 1 diabetes. *Diabetes Technology & Therapeutics*, *14*(12), 1098–1104. doi:10.1089/dia.2012.0160 PMID:23035775

Sniderman, A. D., LaChapelle, K. J., Rachon, N. A., & Furberg, C. D. (2013). The necessity for clinical reasoning in the era of evidence-based medicine. *Mayo Clinic Proceedings*, *88*(10), 1108–1114. doi:10.1016/j.mayocp.2013.07.012 PMID:24079680

Software, M. I. M. (2017). *MIM Software web site*. Retrieved 20 Aug., 2017, from https://www.mimsoftware.com

Soman, A. K. (2011). Cloud-based solutions for healthcare IT. Enfield, NH: Science Publishers. doi:10.1201/b10737

Spat, S., Holl, B., Petritsch, G., Schaupp, L., Beck, P., & Pieber, T. R. (2013). Automatic system testing of a decision support system for insulin dosing using Google Android. *Studies in Health Technology and Informatics*, *186*, 187–191. PMID:23542995

Spyra, G., Buchanan, W. J., Cruickshank, P., & Ekonomou, E. (2014). Cloud-Based Identity and Identity Meta-Data: Secure and Control of Data in Globalization Era. *International Journal of Reliable and Quality E-Healthcare*, *3*(1), 49–66. doi:10.4018/ijrqeh.2014010105

Srirama, S. (2006). *Publishing and discovery of mobile web services in peer to peer networks.* Paper presented at the First International Workshop on Mobile Services and Personalized Environments.

Srirama, S., Jarke, M., & Prinz, W. (2007). *Mobile web service discovery in peer to peer networks.* Paper presented at the 5th International Workshop on Ubiquitous Mobile Information and Collaboration Systems.

Srirama, S., Jarke, M., Zhu, H., & Prinz, W. (2008). *Scalable Mobile Web Service Discovery in Peer to Peer Networks.* Paper presented at the Third International Conference on Internet and Web Applications and Services. 10.1109/ICIW.2008.52

Stahlberg, A., Kubista, M., & Aman, P. (2011). Single-cell gene-expression profiling and its potential diagnostic applications. *Expert Review of Molecular Diagnostics*, *11*(7), 735–740. doi:10.1586/erm.11.60 PMID:21902535

Su, C. J., & Chu, T. W. (2014). A mobile multi-agent information system for ubiquitous fetal monitoring. *International Journal of Environmental Research and Public Health*, *11*(1), 600–625. doi:10.3390/ijerph110100600 PMID:24452256

Subversus Interactive. (2011). *Gyromaniac*. Retrieved 16 Aug., 2017, from http://subvers.us

Tamposis, I., Pouliakis, A., Fezoulidis, I., & Karakitsos, P. (2016). Mobile Platforms Supporting Health Professionals: Need, Technical Requirements and Applications. In A. Moumtzoglou (Ed.), *M-Health Innovations for Patient-Centered Care*. Hershey, PA: IGI Global. doi:10.4018/978-1-4666-9861-1.ch005

Thelen, E., & Smith, L. B. (2006). Dynamic systems theories. In W. Damon & R. M. Lerner (Eds.), Theoretical models of human development. Handbook of child psychology (6th ed.; Vol. 1, pp. 258–312). New York, NY: John Wiley & Sons.

Toomey, R. J., Ryan, J. T., McEntee, M. F., Evanoff, M. G., Chakraborty, D. P., McNulty, J. P., ... Brennan, P. C. (2010). Diagnostic efficacy of handheld devices for emergency radiologic consultation. *AJR. American Journal of Roentgenology, 194*(2), 469–474. doi:10.2214/AJR.09.3418 PMID:20093611

Topol, E. J. (2012). *The creative destruction of medicine: how the digital revolution will create better health care.* New York: Basic Books.

Toye, E., Sharp, R., Madhavapeddy, A., Scott, D., Upton, E., & Blackwell, A. (2007). Interacting with mobile services: An evaluation of camera-phones and visual tags. *Personal and Ubiquitous Computing, 11*(2), 97–106. doi:10.100700779-006-0064-9

University of Illinois College of Engineering. (2017). *New handheld spectral analyzer uses power of smartphone to detect disease.* Retrieved 10 Aug., 2017, from https://www.eurekalert.org/pub_releases/2017-08/uoic-nhs081017.php

Vaisanen, O., Makijarvi, M., & Silfvast, T. (2003). Prehospital ECG transmission: Comparison of advanced mobile phone and facsimile devices in an urban Emergency Medical Service System. *Resuscitation, 57*(2), 179–185. doi:10.1016/S0300-9572(03)00028-5 PMID:12745186

van Geert, P., & van Dijk, M. (2002). Focus on variability: New tools to study intra-individual variability in developmental data. *Infant Behavior and Development, 25*(4), 340–374. doi:10.1016/S0163-6383(02)00140-6

Wavelet Health. (2017). *Wavelet Health web site.* Retrieved 14 Aug., 2017, from https://wavelethealth.com

Waxer, N., Ninan, D., Ma, A., & Dominguez, N. (2013). How cloud computing and social media are changing the face of health care. *The Physician Executive Journal, 39*(2), 58-60, 62.

Webb, G. (2012). Making the cloud work for healthcare: Cloud computing offers incredible opportunities to improve healthcare, reduce costs and accelerate ability to adopt new IT services. *Health Management Technology, 33*(2), 8–9. PMID:22397112

Wells, T. S., Ozminkowski, R. J., Hawkins, K., Bhattarai, G. R., & Armstrong, D. G. (2016). Leveraging big data in population health management. *Big Data Analytics, 1*(1), 1. doi:10.118641044-016-0001-5

Wilson, J. (2006). 3G to Web 2.0? Can Mobile Telephony Become an Architecture of Participation? *Convergence, 12*(2), 229–242. doi:10.1177/1354856506066122

Witzke, K., & Specht, O. (2017). M-Health Telemedicine and Telepresence in Oral and Maxillofacial Surgery: An Innovative Prehospital Healthcare Concept in Structurally Weak Areas. *International Journal of Reliable and Quality E-Healthcare*, *6*(4), 37–48. doi:10.4018/IJRQEH.2017100105

World Health Organisation. (2003). *Adherence to long-term therapies. Evidence for action.* Retrieved 23 July, 2019, from https://www.who.int/chp/knowledge/publications/adherence_report/en/

World Health Organization. (2015). *Postnatal Care for Mothers and Newborns Highlights from the World Health Organization 2013 Guidelines.* Retrieved July 25, 2019, from https://www.who.int/maternal_child_adolescent/publications/WHO-MCA-PNC-2014-Briefer_A4.pdf

Ybarra, M. L., Holtrop, J. S., Prescott, T. L., & Strong, D. (2014). Process evaluation of a mHealth program: Lessons learned from Stop My Smoking USA, a text messaging-based smoking cessation program for young adults. *Patient Education and Counseling*, *97*(2), 239–243. doi:10.1016/j.pec.2014.07.009 PMID:25103183

Zerth, J., Besser, J., & Reichert, A. (2012). Effectiveness and efficiency for ambulatory care assisted by mobile technological devices. *Biomedizinische Technik. Biomedical Engineering*, *57*(Suppl 1.). doi:10.1515/bmt-2012-4062 PMID:23096280

KEY TERMS AND DEFINITIONS

Big Data: The term used for the collection of data sets so large and complex that it becomes difficult to process using on-hand database management tools or traditional data processing applications.

Cloud Computing: A large number of computers connected through a network, capable of running an application on many computers and of configuring virtual servers which do not have physical presence and can be moved around and scaled up or down without being noticed by end-users.

Internet of Things (IoT): The interconnection and the created network via the Internet of devices embedded in everyday objects. This interconnection adds bidirectional communication capability to these devices enabling them to send and receive data.

Mobile Health (mHealth): The practice of medicine and public health supported by mobile devices.

Population Health: A term with broader content, which is related to a field relevant to the study of several important factors for health. As a result, it involves many terms, such as outcomes, disparities, determinants, and risk factors

Population Health Management: The aggregation of patient information (data) across multiple resources related to health information, the analysis of the data into a single patient record, and the outcome of the actions of health care providers which can improve clinical and economic outcomes.

Public Health: A term which connotes a relatively narrow field with activities carried out by agencies granted with official functions.

Chapter 3
Digital Transformation Challenges for the Implementation of Quality Electronic Medical Records

Dimitrios G. Katehakis
https://orcid.org/0000-0002-3763-191X
Foundation for Research and Technology – Hellas, Greece

Angelina Kouroubali
https://orcid.org/0000-0002-3023-8242
Foundation for Research and Technology – Hellas, Greece

ABSTRACT

The purpose of this work is to analyze the digital transformation challenges related to the implementation of quality electronic medical record systems in Greece, within the wider frame of the European digital single market. The authors explore characteristics of quality, interoperable and secure electronic medical records, and provide an overview of the challenges and factors affecting their adoption, implementation, and operation. Key challenges relate to linking electronic medical records with the workflow, building trust and acceptance by making the best use of champions and key stakeholders, and financing the digital transformation transition and sustainability. The foreseen benefits include better support of medical decisions across all stages of the patient pathway, patients empowered to carry with them clinically significant information, fostering research, and unlocking the full potential of vendors to implement innovative tools to support continuity of care.

DOI: 10.4018/978-1-7998-2390-2.ch003

INTRODUCTION

Healthcare systems worldwide face significant challenges that relate to increasing costs, increasing demand for the provision of quality services in an aging society and improvement of outcomes (Herrmann et al., 2018). It has been shown that despite the fact that medicine becomes increasingly high-tech, the standards of care often remain low compared to cost (Porter et al., 2006). Digital transformation in healthcare can modify operations, reduce costs and improve the quality of patient services and care.

Data is a key enabler to achieve digital transformation and drive health systems towards seamless information flows. Currently, health data is not available in the same formats nor managed in the same way across European Union (EU) member states or even within national health systems. Citizens, public authorities, medical professionals and researchers do not usually have access to all the data that would help them manage their health, deliver better diagnosis, treatment or personalized care. When health data exist in digital form, they often depend on technologies that are not interoperable, thus hindering wider use.

Lack of key information results in limited health systems optimization and difficulty to implement digital health and care solutions to support cross-border use of health services in the EU. In addition, the uptake of digital solutions for health and care remains slow and varies greatly across EU member states. The Digital Single Market in this area cannot achieve the envisioned results for citizens and health professionals. Market fragmentation and lack of interoperability across health systems hinder an integrated approach to disease prevention, care and cure. Appropriate regulatory frameworks and high quality data are necessary to realize and safeguard the rights of individuals and society. Secure access to a comprehensive electronic health record (EHR) anywhere in the EU will enable citizens to share their health data for medical treatment, preventive services, and research, irrespective of where the data is located and in line with data protection legislation (Katehakis et al., 2017b).

The national health system (NHS) is responsible for the provision of healthcare services in Greece. The execution of the operational program for implementing the information society strategy for Greece (2000-2010) resulted in the introduction of modern information technology (IT) systems for the vast majority of hospitals in the country (Katehakis et al., 2011). Foreseen benefits included an upgraded quality of services to citizens through business process re-engineering and reduction of medical errors, secure exchange of medical information, and efficient access to the EHR.

Following the introduction of integrated IT systems at the hospitals, a multitude of eHealth services has been introduced, in line with EU priorities, to control costs and improve services in a secure manner. These include: ePrescription; electronic dispensation (eDispensation) and electronic referral (eReferral) for primary care (https://www.e-prescription.gr/); electronic confirmation (eConfirmation) for insurance status verification (https://www.atlas.gov.gr/ATLAS/Pages/Home.aspx); eReimbursement (http://www.eopyy.gov.gr); electronic appointment (eAppointment) for booking doctors' appointments for primary care (https://www.e-syntagografisi.gr/p-rv/p); and a business intelligence system (Bi-Health, http://portal.bi.moh.gov.gr/) that automates online retrieval of operational data for the Hellenic Ministry of Health (MoH).

The country participates actively in the cross-border services development projects for ePrescription/ eDispensation and patient summary and a national contact point for eHealth (NCPeH) is already in place for the country. However, there are still many challenges to face to allow for a broad uptake of digital solutions for better patient care (European Court of Auditors, 2019).

Despite the fact that significant progress has been made to effectively link hospitals, regional health systems, and primary care, still no uniform access to EHR is available nationwide (Katehakis, 2018).

The objective of this work is to present and discuss on digital transformation challenges relevant to the implementation of quality electronic medical record (EMR) systems. EMR characteristics are outlined and relevant initiatives are examined. Both the national as well as the European perspectives are presented together with key factors contributing to EMR adoption. The intention of the chapter is not to discuss the challenges of the Greek healthcare system but rather challenges related to EMR implementation within the context of the Greek NHS. The authors propose specific directions for the implementation of quality EMRs in the country, in line with international developments, and discuss on prospective issues. They also make recommendations for future work.

BACKGROUND

Definitions

EMRs are digital versions of paper charts maintained in clinical settings (physician offices, clinics, and hospitals). The notes and information that goes in the EMRs are mostly used for diagnosis and treatment. EMRs enable providers to track data over time, identify patients for preventive visits and screenings, monitor patients, and improve healthcare quality (Habib 2010; Kierkegaard, 2011; HiMSS, 2011).

EHRs are inclusive of a broader view of a patient's care that goes beyond standard clinical data collected in clinical settings. EHRs contain the information collected from all the clinicians involved in a patient's care and can be accessed by all authorized clinicians to provide care to that patient. EHRs also share information with other healthcare providers and systems, such as specialists and laboratories. EHRs follow patients – to the specialist, the hospital, the nursing home, or even across the country. It is not difficult for any health professional to see the direct benefits of using EHR and having both administrative and clinical data that are accessible, comparable, communicable, and confidential (Iakovidis, 1998). Streamlining patient information flow and its accessibility to other healthcare providers through national, regional and/ or patient controlled services has the potential to improve care quality and patient safety over time.

Unlike the EMR and the EHR, the personal health record (PHR) refers to a representation of health records related to the care of the patient that is managed by the patient (Tang et al., 2006). With the growth of mobile computing, the number of records regarding personal health is increasing exponentially. That leads to the need for an integrated method of storing health-related data that healthcare providers and patients can use (Roehrs et al., 2017). As health systems undergo paradigm changes, EHRS and PHRs have to advance as well to meet the related interoperability challenges (Blobel, 2018). Connecting to the EMR requires establishing interfaces to link islands of information based on certain workflows, and semantically homogenizing the produced information.

The following paragraphs clarify EMR characteristics, and further explain the concepts of EHR and PHR. Authors present relevant initiatives in connection to the European Digital Single Market. They also present factors mentioned in the literature as contributing to EMR and EHR adoption.

Characteristics

The EMR consists of electronic copies of medical records produced in a physician's office, a clinic or a hospital. It can include patient, hospital, and healthcare professional details, encounter details, clinical information, diagnoses, medication, operations, treatments, etc. The most important quality EMR systems characteristic is related to access to information in a secure and legitimate manner.

The purpose of EMRs are to create legible and organized recordings and to access clinical information about individual patients and can serve as a data source for an EHR. The EHR is an essential tool for improving both the safety and quality of healthcare. However, physicians must actively use these systems to accrue the benefits (Ajami & Bagheri-Tadi, 2013). The gains from EHR systems depend on meaningful sharing and rely on access to information regardless of place and time, and from re-using information for multiple purposes (Dobrev et al., 2010; Prey et al., 2016). That results in less time searching for information and more quality time with patients. Improved organizational efficiency and secondary uses of data are typically amongst the most commonly expected benefits (Black 2011). The EHR usually reflects the partial view of a healthcare provider without the ability for patients to control or interact with their data.

The EMR can be used to compose the EHR and is patient centric. Physicians use EMRs and EHRs to improve the quality of care and contain costs. Whereas EMR is usually considered an internal organizational system, the EHR is defined as an inter-organizational system. The EHR is primarily episodic and could be longitudinal. It incorporates administrative, financial, and clinical data. The concept of EHR extends beyond the boundaries of a healthcare provider and includes the concept of timelessness. Main advantage of EHR is the availability of cross-provider medical information.

The use of EHR requires the presence of a certain user and system attributes, and numerous organizational and environmental facilitators. That is why the EMR in a public hospital cannot be easily shared today among several hospitals. In many cases, this information exchange cannot be made electronically even within the boundaries of a single hospital.

Healthcare providers play a critical role in the adoption and utilization of health IT, including EMRs in hospitals (Cresswell et al., 2015). However, many healthcare professionals, from nurses to ambulatory care physicians, are still reluctant to utilize the available technologies, leading to limited system use and, eventually, system failure (Bowens et al., 2010; Linder et al., 2006).

Recently, a digital platform for patient-centered medical care known as PHR was introduced, as an enabler for self-management of medical records. PHRs are online systems used by patients, supporting a person-centered functionality, and could be cradle-to-grave. They support the shift from institution-centered care to citizen-centered care, paying emphasis on continuity of care from prevention to management of chronic conditions (Katehakis et al. 2017a). PHR information is expected to be sent, received, or exchanged from multiple systems, including: EHR systems, insurer systems, payer systems, public health systems, clinical trials systems, and/ or collaborative care systems (HL7 International, 2014). The PHR, on the contrary to EMRs and EHRs is not a legal record. PHR enables integration of main information components in the EMR and EHR systems.

EHR is the favored nomenclature for a sophisticated, generic term covering several concepts (Katehakis & Tsiknakis, 2006). It consists of components implemented according to measurable and realistic benefits, including PHR information, and includes wellness information and nontraditional links to external knowledge, like guidelines, protocols, and genetic information, contrasting EPR. It extends beyond the boundaries set by a single healthcare organization (in contrast to EMR), and is primarily created and managed by healthcare professionals (in contrast to PHR).

EMRs, EHRs, and PHRs can reside on different platforms under various technologies and standards. Although EMRs contain local information and provide fast and accurate delivery, the major advantage of EHR in medical practice is the availability of cross-provider medical information. Medical information integration leads to a dramatic change in personalized care but also poses serious challenges and threats to security and privacy (Heart et al., 2017).

Several countries are already moving towards the development of national infrastructures to support legitimate access to EHR information for all involved stakeholders by means of standardized protocols. Some prominent examples include the following:

- Kind Messages for Electronic Healthcare Record in Belgium (KMEHR, https://www.ehealth.fgov.be/);
- Elektronisches Petientendossier in Switzerland (EPD, https://www.e-health-suisse.ch/);
- Kanta digital services in Finland (https://www.kanta.fi/);
- elektronische Gesundheitsakte in Austria (ELGA, https://www.gesundheit.gv.at/);
- L' interopérabilité des systèmes d' information de santé in France (Interop'Santé, http://www.interopsante.org/);
- eHealth Exchange in the United States (https://sequoiaproject.org/ehealth-exchange/);
- My Health Record in Australia (https://www.digitalhealth.gov.au/); and
- eHealth Digital Service Infrastructure by the European Commission Connecting Europe Facility (CEF eHDSI, https://ec.europa.eu/cefdigital/wiki/display/EHOPERATIONS/eHealth+DSI+Operations+Home)

Foreseen benefits of EHR systems can be considered as clinical, organizational, and societal. Quality of care, reduced errors and continuity of care are some of the clinical outcomes. Improvements in financial and operational performance are seen as organizational outcomes. While, societal outcomes include research and public health (Menachemi & Collum, 2011).

The great value of EHRs lies in the fact that they allow the distributed collection of clinical data as part of the overall workflow. The information is collected once and stored so that it is then available for multiple uses to serve different medical and administrative needs. For example, the staff can collect pricing data, the physician to see trends in the effectiveness of the treatments, the nurse to report an undesirable side effect, and the investigator to analyze the efficacy of drugs in patients with co-morbidity. In contrast, the use of individual non interoperable ICT systems limits healthcare professionals to manage patient data locally and separately with an incomplete picture of patient condition.

National implementations of EHRs offer the ability to exchange health information electronically throughout healthcare structures in the public health sectors. EHR benefits can be summarized below:

- Quality and accurate information at the point of care
- Access to patient information from different sources to support continuity of care
- Role based security sharing of information with patients and clinicians
- Enhanced decision support for diagnosis reducing medical errors and providing safer care
- Communication and interaction improvement between patients and providers
- Safer and reliable prescriptions
- Promotion of completeness, accuracy, and legibility of patient information documentation
- Cost reduction through reduced duplication, paperwork and improvement of quality and safety

In order to achieve these benefits, the systems that feed information to the EHR should be responsive to the complexity of the environment, tailored to the needs of the users, as well as communicating with each other in the context of the automation of operational processes.

Implementation in Greece

During the period 2000-2006, in the frame of the 3rd Community structural assistance programme, Greece started developing IT solutions for the majority of the –at that time- seventeen Health Regions. More than 60% of the NHS hospitals of Greece were covered by the programme and had purchased integrated information systems that included all basic key EMR components, to support the regional health authorities they belonged to. A detailed analysis of the implementations and the key challenges are described in the papers by (Katehakis et al., 2011; Katehakis et al., 2018).

In November 2010, Law 3892/2010 put in place the national ePrescription system and the obligation to submit prescription and dispense medications electronically. The law describes duties of doctors and pharmacists, as well as access rights including for patient access to own information. The transition from the handwritten to the ePrescription system has many benefits. It contributes to the eradication of the geographical dispersion of the points of creation and filling of prescriptions. Also, it contributes to the development of a stable electronic system which offers quality and safety in healthcare, a clear picture of the patient's medical history, ensuring the protection of personal data and the ability of recording, in the system, of the population that is in need of pharmaceutical care. One of the major achievements of ePrescription has been to consolidate (linking and interoperation) all national social security funds through a fully integrated electronic prescription platform. In addition, it has contributed to the effective control and rationalisation of the expenditure and the subsequent reduction of costs in the areas of medical and pharmaceutical care by coordinating a large number of bodies and stakeholder with different interests.

The system has presented several benefits also for stakeholders within the prescription continuum. Patients are assisted through the immediate receipt of prescriptions and medication, and the reduced hassle related to insurance coverage of prescriptions. Pharmacists avoid errors resulting from misinterpretation of handwritten prescriptions while at the same time simplifying the compensation process related to medication. Doctors enjoy on-line access to the patient's history, the ability to better apply the pharmacopoeia, electronic notification of drug interactions, and the ability to control prescription cost. Health authorities face less red tape as a result of reduced time with regard to bureaucratic procedures, a reduction in the cost of drugs, while supporting prescription of generic drugs, and direct information on the prescribing histories of doctors and the state of health of citizens.

Greek eHealth policy (2014-2020) set as priorities the restructuring of primary healthcare, pooling of financial resources, introducing new managerial and administrative methods, adopting cost effectiveness and monitoring mechanisms, and developing policies for better resource allocation. The Ministry of Health (MoH) has the overall responsibility for electronic health (eHealth) in Greece. The development of an electronic patient record is a major objective and a priority of the National Health System (Milieu Ltd and Time.lex, 2013; EU Directorate-General for Health and Food Safety, 2014).

In February 2019, Law 4600/2019 established the national EMR for primary care for Greek citizens (AHFY). AHFY contains the health history of each recipient of health services within the NHS, as well as data, assessments and information of any kind related to the condition and clinical development of that person during the healthcare process. The content of the AHFY is uniform, mandatory, and maintained at a national level for life.

As of June 2019, Croatia, Czechia, Estonia, Finland, Luxembourg, Malta, and Croatia have received approval to launch the productive operation of specific cross-border services under eHDSI (https://ec.europa.eu/cefdigital/wiki/display/EHOPERATIONS/eHDSI+Deployment+Plans), as they comply with any remedies that remain pending concerns the readiness of their contact points (NCPeH). Upon completion of Wave 1, the road opens for countries in Wave 2, including Greece.

The HiMSS EMR Adoption Model

There are many barriers to data analytics adoption in a hospital environment. Barriers such as isolation of data stores, end users' resistance, low data quality, lack of focus on integration, are recurrent in this area (Carvallo et al., 2016). Using a maturity model, can help the health managers to evaluate its HIS in order to determine in which maturity level it resides and how it can continuously improve to a higher maturity. One of the most prominent models is the HiMSS Maturity Model for EMR used to identify EMR stages of maturity from the limited departmental systems to paperless EMR environment (HiMSS Analytics, 2019). The HiMSS EMR Adoption Model (EMRAM) consists of eight stages, described in Table 1. It determines the level of EMR implementation in a healthcare organization (i.e. a hospital) in a scale from 0 to 7. Level 7 corresponds to a fully paperless hospital (i.e. all patient records kept in electronic form). That enables the managers of such establishments to see what level they are on and what steps they would have to take to improve their score.

Table 1. The EMR Adoption Model cumulative capabilities

Stage	Description	Cumulative Capabilities
7	Complete EMR, data analytics to improve care	The hospital no longer uses paper charts to deliver and manage patient care and has a mixture of discrete data, document images, and medical images within its EMR environment. Data warehousing used to analyze patterns of clinical data to improve the quality of care and patient safety and care delivery efficiency. Clinical information can be readily shared via standardized electronic transactions with all entities that are authorized to treat the patient. The hospital demonstrates summary data continuity for all hospital services (e.g. inpatient, outpatient, emergency department, and with any owned or managed ambulatory clinics). Blood products and human milk are included in the closed-loop medication administration process. Continuity of care realized throughout the hospital.
6	Physician documentation (templates), full clinical decision support systems (CDSS), closed loop medication administration	Full physician documentation with structured templates and discrete data implemented for progress notes, consult notes, discharge summaries or problem list, and diagnosis list maintenance. Level three of clinical decision support guides all clinician activities related to protocols and outcomes in the form of variance and compliance alerts. The closed loop medication administration with the bar coded unit dose medications environment is fully implemented. The electronic medication administration record application (EMAR) and bar coding or other auto identification technology are implemented and integrated with computerized practitioner order entry (CPOE) and pharmacy to maximize point of care patient safety processes for medication administration. The "five rights" of medication administration are verified at the bedside with the scanning of the bar code on the unit does medication and the patient identification (ID).
5	Full radiology PACS	A full complement of radiology PACS provides medical images to physicians via an intranet and displaces all film-based images. Intrusion detection extended to intrusion prevention.

continues on following page

Table 1. Continued

Stage	Description	Cumulative Capabilities
4	CPOE; clinical decision support (clinical protocols)	CPOE for use by any clinician licensed to create orders added to the nursing and clinical data repository (CDR) environment along with the second level of clinical decision support capabilities related to evidence-based medicine protocols. Where publicly available, clinicians have access to national or regional databases and registries to support decision-making. Precautions for EMR downtime and network intrusion detection implemented.
3	Clinical documentation, CDSS for error checking	Nursing/ clinical documentation (e.g. vital signs, flow sheets, nursing notes). EMAR implemented and integrated with the CDR for at least one inpatient service in the hospital. First level of CDSS implemented to conduct error checking with order entry (i.e., drug/ drug, drug/ food, drug/ lab conflict checking normally found in the pharmacy information system). Medical image access from PACS is available for physicians for access outside the radiology department.
2	CDR, controlled medical vocabulary, basic CDS, health information exchange (HIE) capable	A clinical data repository (CDR) enables full interoperability between the aforementioned units, supported by a controlled vocabulary and a clinical decision support (CDS) rule engine for rudimentary conflict checking. Basic security services such as access control and usage management, encryption, mobile security, etc. implemented. The hospital may be HIE capable at this stage and can share information it has in the CDR with other patient care stakeholders.
1	Ancillaries: lab, rad, pharmacy all installed	All three major ancillary clinical systems installed (i.e., pharmacy, laboratory, and radiology).
0	All three ancillaries not installed	The organization does not have neither a general LIS, nor an RIS, nor a pharmacy information system.

HiMSS vision, besides facilitating the development of IT solutions in order to systematically improve quality, safety, and efficiency, includes the creation of mutually interconnected and harmoniously co-functioning EMRs of patients, which would connect distinct entities on the market and service providers (Katehakis, 2018).

Factors Contributing to EMR and EHR Adoption

It is commonly agreed, that information contained in the EHR is critical to support clinical care and the longitudinal EHR is of high value. Still, the vision of seamless flow of data amongst digital systems and patient access to this information any time and from anywhere is particularly challenging. Current business trends show that the patient is expected, over the next years, through patient-generated data (via e.g. wearables or other tools and gadgets) and health records owned and managed by him/ herself to be further empowered (HiMMS Analytics, 2018).

The development of a mature national EMR is a prerequisite for the transition to patient empowerment projects. Successful digital transformation is a team play requiring collective effort, and expanded skill sets. In the digital transformation of the healthcare sector, EU member states are advancing at different speeds, and countries that are succeeding in digitalizing their healthcare systems feature an effective strategy, strong political leadership and a coordinating institution with a clear national mandate (Thiel et al., 2019). Promoting acceptance for professionals and patients through strategies such as co-creation measures is essential to success.

The European Digital Single Market

The European Digital Single Market strategy is built on three main objectives: (i) to provide better access to digital goods and services across Europe; (ii) to create the necessary conditions for digital networks and innovative services; and (iii) to maximize the growth potential of the digital economy. In line with this strategy, the European Commission has created policy guidelines towards digital transformation of health and care to empower citizens and build a healthier society. These guidelines give direction to EU activities in this field for the coming years. (European Commission, 2018) identifies three priorities: (i) citizens' secure access to their health data; (ii) personalized medicine through shared infrastructure; and (iii) citizen empowerment with digital tools for user feedback and person-centered care (see Table 2).

The interoperability of EHR systems of member states can be supported, beyond ePrescriptions and patient summaries, with the development and adoption of the European EHR exchange format (EHRxF), which is based on open standards, taking into consideration the potential use of data for research and other purposes (European Commission, 2019). The framework includes: (i) a set of principles that should govern access to and exchange of EHRs across borders in the EU; (ii) a set of common technical specifications for the cross-border exchange of data in certain health information domains, which should constitute the baseline for an EHRxF; and (iii) a process to take forward the further elaboration of a EHRxF. The European EHRxF has the potential to facilitate the cross-border interoperability of EHR systems. Incentives for its wider adoption and other measures to tackle lack of interoperability will help promote the strategic priorities of the digital single market in this area.

Table 2. Areas enabling the digital transformation of care

EU Priority	Details
Secure access to health data	to enable citizens to securely access their health data nationally and across borders in the EU
Personalized medicine	to allow researchers and other professionals to pool resources across the EU, such as data, expertise, computing processing and storage capacities towards personalized medicine
Citizen empowerment	to empower citizens to take care of their health, engage in prevention activities and enable feedback and interaction with healthcare providers with digital tools

The New European Interoperability Framework (EIF)

The new EIF promotes the secure free flow of data within the EU for public services across member states. It provides principles and guidelines that facilitate the establishment of advanced interoperability structures. Interoperability across healthcare services will enhance benefits such as time and cost savings, transparency, data availability and quality, as well as satisfaction, compliance and improved decision-making. Digital cooperation can in turn promote the development of cost effective, quality and competitive solutions. The framework maps the necessary processes towards the development of a European public services ecosystem. All involved stakeholders, including owners, designers and users of systems and services develop a culture towards collaboration and seamless information flow within national and across national borders to support a digital single market in Europe (Kouroubali & Katehakis, 2019).

Based upon the Tallin Declaration (Ministers in charge of eGovernment policy and coordination from 32 countries of the EU and EFTA, 2017), the new EIF requires systems to follow certain principles throughout their lifecycle, from conception, to design, to implementation:

- Digital-by-default, providing services and data preferably via digital channels;
- Cross-border-by-default, accessible for all citizens in the EU;
- Open-by-default, enabling reuse, participation, access and transparency;
- Privacy-by-design and security-by-design to secure infrastructure and building blocks compliant with the legal requirements and obligations regarding data protection and privacy; and
- Interoperability-by-design as a standard approach for the design and operation of European public services.

As stated within the official document of the new EIF (European Commission, 2017): *The lack of interoperability is a major obstacle to progress on the digital single market. Using the EIF to steer European interoperability initiatives contributes to a coherent European interoperable environment, and facilitates the delivery of services that work together, within and across organisations or domains.*

Relevant interoperability principles and a clear implementation roadmap act as facilitators for the development and implementation of EMRs, to enable healthcare providers to share health data outside their organization.

To realize the benefits of integrated information systems in healthcare, appropriate interoperability governance needs to be in place. Interoperability governance establishes the mechanisms of the application of interoperability rules across the care continuum. Strategic and policy decision making needs to incorporate interoperability governance to align strategic objectives with implementation of interoperability initiatives (European Commission, 2017). To establish the appropriate governance framework a thorough knowledge of organizational structures, roles, responsibilities and decision-making processes is required. Interoperability governance establishes enablers to ensure alignment with the overall interoperability objectives at policy level. Interoperability governance proposes and guides the change management practices that need to be implemented, and establishes the foundations for the sustainability of interoperability initiatives at present and future times (Kouroubali & Katehakis, 2019).

DIGITAL TRANSFORMATION CHALLENGES

The three main challenges in Greece for implementing quality EMRs relate to linking information systems with the clinical and operational workflow, the engagement of champions and key stakeholders and securing the financial means for the digital transformation and sustainability. The following sections focus on these factors for effective exploitation of EMRs in the hospitals of the NHS in Greece and in other similar health systems globally (Figure 1).

Link With The Workflow

Usually, hospital infrastructures are closed networks restricted for administrative and clinical support. In order to support integrated workflows, it is vital that health IT systems adopt nationally accepted data standards that facilitate semantic interoperability. Besides the need for having established a national infrastructure, all relevant legal and regulatory enablers need also to be in place as well.

Data entered once, used anywhere is the key concept. That requires fully interfaced ICT solutions in a stable and standardized manner. Fundamental principles to follow include the exploitation of available open standards and best practices, the adoption of an interoperability framework tailored to national needs, and implementation based on planning. This will allow for the development of quality EMRs, the development, maintenance and evolution of a scalable, secure, and affordable infrastructure to support incremental evolution building upon existing investments, while adding new capabilities as new needs arise.

Trust and security is a critical area in which healthcare presents demanding and challenging needs. IT security in healthcare systems, services, and applications is positioned as a major concern due to the high privacy and confidentiality requirements of sensitive healthcare data (ENISA, 2015; ENISA, 2016). Private data needs to be accessed by professionals having a qualified role, with the consent of the patient and under strict audit controls. Medical data must only be disclosed or shared after the patient is identified and authenticated with sufficient accuracy.

Today the means for establishing patient identification in Greece is based on AMKA, which is the social security number issued in the country. Common national identification approach should be followed in line with European Regulation (EU) No 910/2014, commonly known as eIDAS (Melin et al., 2016; Nguyen, 2018). In the future, a combination of national identity providers may provide the means towards proper end user authentication for EMRs. In order to enable workflow automation for the effective sharing of clinically significant information EMR data will have to be shared with well-defined processes, EMRs must contain reliable content, and use agreed semantics, i.e. common terminology. That is expected to effectively facilitate, amongst other, organized referrals, e.g. from primary healthcare to hospital physicians.

Today health data are stored in silos (i.e. hospital EMRs, national infrastructures, etc.). In order to address heterogeneity and fragmentation effectively it is crucial for a common framework to be in place. Efforts are currently made towards that direction for the creation of the National eHealth Interoperability Framework (Katehakis & Kouroubali, 2019) to support standardized interfaces which is expected to focus not only at a cross-border, national, or regional level but also within certain healthcare organizations (i.e. hospitals) and also to provide for reaching citizens at home, based on certain use cases. Potential sources for use cases:

Antilope project (https://www.antilope-project.eu/resources/),
eHealth Exchange use cases (https://sequoiaproject.org/wp-content/uploads/2017/01/eHealth-Exchange-Use-Case-Webinar-2017Jan13-Finalv2.pdf),
HIMSS interoperability use cases (https://www.himss.org/library/interoperability-standards/adoption-implementation/use-cases), and
IHE use case repository (https://usecase-repository.ihe-europe.net/).

This is a strategic approach that needs to be further supported at all levels starting from technical, to semantic, organizational, as well as legal. This effort should be aligned with available best practices, current experience, and available standards and guidelines (eHealth Network, 2015; European Commission, 2017; European Commission, 2019). However, key to shaping digital transformation is taking realistic steps driven by expected benefits for patients and the healthcare delivery alike.

Make the Best Use of Champions

Innovative technologies alone cannot lead to revolutionary changes. What is needed is cultural transformation and a new healthcare providers' cooperation model that does away with existing information silos. EHRs should not be looked as a side-process or administrative tool, but rather as an inseparable part of the healthcare process. Although it is the physician and the payer that frequently control the type and quality of care patient receives (Petru, 2016), implementing the smart hospital vision requires considering continuous adaptation, clinical outcome, efficiency in the supply chain and care processes and enhancement of own capabilities in regard to patient services (Kharbanda et al., 2017). Qualified human resources are a key ingredient for success. Education, training and continuous professional development for all, including for those citizens and patients which are capable and motivated to become engaged in their own care, should be strongly promoted (Stroetmann et al., 2011).

An important factor influencing user adoption is user confidence. Professionals should be encouraged with a clear motivation system and an explicit presentation of realistically envisioned benefits. Effective communication can facilitate engagement and acceptance for professionals and patients through strategies such as co-design measures. Individual initiatives should not be rejected, but, if they meet certain quality criteria, should be exploited to become part of the solution.

Trust and acceptance of data sharing solutions need to overcome cultural barriers, such as the traditional maintenance of patient data in the healthcare professionals' own files. Overall, a culture of sharing, trust and collaboration with other healthcare professionals and patients still needs further building. Resistance to the changes inflicted by digitization is common in many countries (Thiel et al., 2019). Physicians, in particular, often act as veto players.

A clear framework that fosters acceptance and drives developments towards better patient treatment, generates benefits for the patients themselves and for those engaging in secondary use. Therefore, continuous training and education in the logic of the continuous improvement of available standards and processes is considered to be essential. Clear strategic objectives need to include emphasizing and adopting best practices, providing support to users, improving the quality of available solutions and establishing co-creation processes with all stakeholders involved.

Finance, Transition, and Sustainability

Quality and secure EMR deployment do not come without cost, and therefore both initial costs, as well as the extra expenses to support operation and maintenance of such systems, should be considered. Without the right stimulation, hospitals will not improve their EMR-related competence. As already been suggested by (Fragidis & Chatzoglou, 2011), Greece needs to invest significant financial resources and work towards standards creation in order to gain the benefits of EHR for its citizens in the near future. Funding should be provided and assured, while responsibilities for sustainability should be clearly defined.

As mentioned in (Thiel et al., 2019) most funding schemes for digital healthcare solutions and services are made for an analogue age. Caregivers are paid based on the patients the see and the care they provide, without considering the value of preventing harm, reducing costs, and making better utilization of doctor's time through the provision of remote care and the use of mobile tools and apps.

As far as Greece is concerned, investments for initial acquisition and setup have already been made, as described in previous sections. EMR adoption level is still low, and no uniform way of evaluating and establishing comparable service level agreements with vendors providing technical support are in place. Without a considerable, coordinated effort, which will likely include realigning financial incentives, EMR adoption in hospitals will lag behind. In order for the EMR adoption to be successful, this will have to be combined with the quality of care incentives. Nevertheless, these investments are unlikely to pay back unless end-users, healthcare providers and patients alike, endorse them. Countries that are succeeding in digitalizing their healthcare systems feature an effective strategy, strong political leadership and a coordinating institution with a clear national mandate. As already noted by (Berg, 2001), the success of any technological healthcare innovation will be eventually decided on the work floor.

SOLUTIONS AND RECOMMENDATIONS

It is becoming increasingly clear that exchange of data can contribute to raising quality of care. Yet large parts of the actually existing digital infrastructure in the healthcare system is not, or is only to a limited extend, suitable for data exchange outside of a specific organization. This affects in particular, according to (eHealth Network, 2019), medical software used by doctors working in general practice, healthcare professionals in the outpatient sector and also many hospital information systems.

The NHS needs to seek co-operation with the private sector and software vendors specializing in the healthcare domain, in order to actively support development and investment opportunities perspectives. The main concern of such cooperation is to prepare the market for forthcoming operational changes, and the achievement of a more rational cost to the NHS. EU member states need to be open and flexible in the design of joint solutions and to be able to ensure the implementation of the decided solutions nationally.

Figure 1. Key EMR adoption challenges

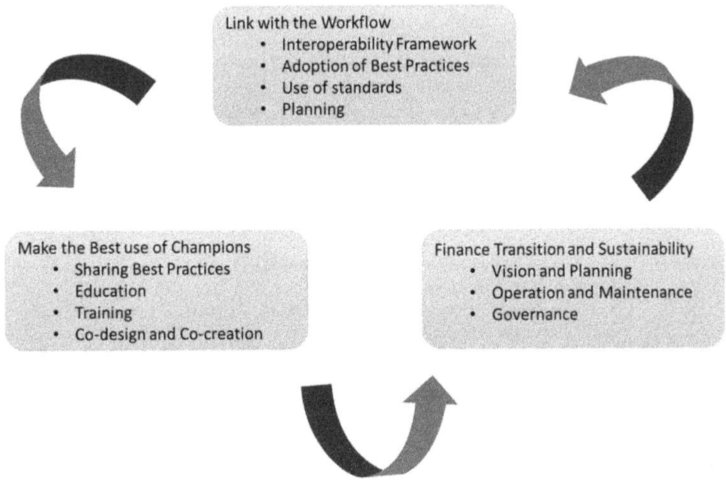

Several factors need to be taken into consideration for the successful and large scale implementations in National Health Systems (Esterle & Kouroubali, 2010). These factors are presented and explained in table 3.

Subsequent efforts should be paid towards the provision of an integrated EHR, paying emphasis on issues relevant to the protection of sensitive information and the cultivation of trust among all relevant stakeholders. The compliance of solutions with standardized requirements could be possibly certified to give vendors and providers, but also payers involved, confidence in the adoption and maturity of those solutions (Blobel, 2018).

Patients are the ones who are expected to benefit most from the use of EHRs. For this to happen EMRs must be in a position to interoperate with each other and encompass intelligence. All systems need to be build using modern clinical guidelines that identify, summarize and evaluate the highest quality evidence. Current data about prevention, diagnosis, prognosis, and therapy including dosage of medications, risk/benefit and cost-effectiveness need to be incorporated in EHRs. Decision options and relevant outcomes result from decision or computation algorithms that integrate treatment alternatives with clinical judgement and experience of practitioners.

A recent communication of the results of an open consultation (European Commission, 2018) shows that European citizens want to have access to their health data (requires interoperability and quality health data), share their health data safely, and be in a position to comment on the quality of the treatment. Social networking tools already enable patients to find each other, support each other, learn from each

Table 3. Factors influencing large scale implementations

Factor	Explanation
Leadership Governance & Vision	• Large scale implementations of EHR systems need to be part of a clearly defined vision and strategy agreed within the healthcare sector. • The vision should encompass the future of the relevant national, regional and local health economies and allow for healthcare organisational needs changing over the lifetime of the EHR implementation. • There should be a clear definition and acceptance of ambition level for the use of EHR (short and long term) to avoid different and confused ideas among stakeholders. • The vision of the future state must be held by a sponsor/leader with enough power, influence and awareness. • The leader is responsible for building a coalition of supporters and for promoting the necessary actions to overcome anticipated as well as unexpected obstacles. • Leaders must be aware of stakeholder needs, flexible to react and respond to real events, stakeholder experience feedback and adequately autonomous to be able to resist political pressures. • National EHR implementations should have strong government support towards the effort and the relevant bodies involved such as decision makers and policy makers. • Governance should be established to define clear roles for decision making, processes of agreement, monitoring, follow up, sanctions, legitimacy, roles, and means.
Clear Definition of business case, objectives, benefits & outcomes	• All EHR projects should be the subject of a clearly defined business case based on benefits and outcomes assessment across the health organisation to which all stakeholders subscribe. A clear definition of a business case allows for a sustainable change process where benefits outweigh the costs. • Outcomes, impact and quality should be considered at various levels such as clinical, financial, public health system and others. • As the implementation proceeds, there should be a formal assessment to evaluate whether the expected benefits are obtained or to understand why they are not reached. • There should also be a clear and consensual definition of the goals to be reached and the tools to be developed focusing on the added value for healthcare and citizens. • Quality assurance of the applications and the related services and project reporting need to be based on the business outcomes – not on the mechanics of delivery.
Realistic Implementation plan Change Management Health System Reform	• Projects should be realistically estimated in terms of complexity, resources, timescale, and pressure placed on staff. • Expectations for the EHR implementation need to be set appropriately and all stakeholders informed. • Implementations should be stepwise and big-bang approaches should be avoided. Projects should be broken up in manageable sub projects of not longer than 12-18 months, and budget, milestones, resources and deliverables should be established for this time. • Implementation plans should be flexible to allow for adjustments, unforeseen circumstances, time for dialog with stakeholders and a step by step process. • Change should be properly managed and as limited as possible. • EHR implementation should not be used as the main and/or unique instrument for Healthcare reform but as an enabler of reform. Introducing EHR systems in parallel with other important procedural changes for the health system can result in significant delays and/or failure. • Attention and commitment to the required process and workflow changes should be made in parallel with EHR implementation in order to ensure full realization of potential benefits. • Adoption of a senior executive-led change management programme and involvement of researchers and analysts, are vital for gaining full benefit from an EHR investment.
Evaluation & Assessment of similar initiatives	• Knowledge should be gained in EHR implementation initiatives through extensive evaluation and assessment of similar initiatives. • Documentation of success and failure of National, Regional or International initiatives should be used in future EHR design and implementation. • Use of strategic tools and continuous evaluation of an EHR implementation initiative allows for feedback that leads to changes and adaptation to accommodate emergent needs.

continues on following page

Table 3. Continued

Factor	Explanation
Stakeholder involvement	• Stakeholder engagement is vital throughout the EHR selection, decision and implementation process. Stakeholder involvement ensures system ownership and motivation towards supporting and using the EHR. • All relevant stakeholders should be involved in all parts of the implementation process to enhance communication and understanding between IT staff, healthcare professionals, policy/decision makers and management. During the process, stakeholders provide feedback communicating their needs and concerns which result in application and service improvements. • Citizens should also be involved in the process to ensure acceptance from the consumers' point of view. • Involvement raises awareness, establishes user acceptance, commitment of the senior staff, promotes public relations and trust among clinicians, citizens, informaticians and politicians. • Power struggles are carefully managed to establish a creative balance among stakeholders. • Partnerships are established allowing a continuous identification of needs and concerns. Stable partnerships between key professional stakeholders such as private public partnerships, focused on transparent governance of action plans and a defined strategy, facilitate implementation processes. • Professionals should be encouraged with a clear motivation system and an explicit presentation of realistic envisioned benefits. Professional drivers should be taken into account when defining the required incentives.
Vendor selection	• Vendor selection must be the subject of a thorough due diligence process to ensure that both the EHR software and vendor organisation are fit for purpose. • Selection should be the subject of detailed user evaluation to ensure local processes, workflows and functional needs are taken into account. • Vendors should have local and international knowledge of the market and relevant experience with the health industry and the national health system.
Infrastructure & Information-structure	• EHR systems should be delivered on an established coherent well-defined infrastructure and information-structure build on existing international health standards. • Security and privacy should be major components of the established architecture. Components include, identification services, based on a unique patient identification or equivalent, authentication services based on reliable and for free accessible authentication sources, routing services and others.
Education & Training	• Education and training for professionals and all involved users should be established at an early stage to maximise use of the system and ensure quality of data input and content of patient records. • Training should be regarded as even more important than software functionality as it allows familiarity with the EHR and facilitates change. • Education and training should be introduced in medical curricula and in vocational training. Only when health professionals understand the importance of EHRs in improving healthcare will they be able to incorporate them into their daily practice and become active advocates of EHR systems. • Training should also be established for citizens, in order to reduce the technological gap.
Resources	• Implementation, use and maintenance of applications and services should be backed up through the guaranteed flow of steady or structural resources for medium and long term time spans. • Funding should be provided and assured, while responsibilities for sustainability clearly defined. • The internal cost of a healthcare organisation's resources must be allowed for and the magnitude not underestimated if the EHR implementation is to be successful
Legislation	• EHR systems implementation should be in accordance with established laws and legislations. In the case that clear-cut laws and legislations are not in place regarding EHR systems, they should be established especially regarding data sharing and shared responsibility. • Methods for practical implementation of laws and legislations should also be considered. • A clearly defined privacy policy should be decided in advance and implemented. The discussion should involve all relevant stakeholders including citizens.

other and help each other to take decisions. All this happens outside of the healthcare system (Pitsch, 2016). From the perspective of patients, it is evident that solutions for sharing medical information electronically are needed.

Need for the development of base registries, such as those for medicinal products, as well as a terminology authority, responsible and accountable for the maintenance of relevant content. It is very important that all key stakeholders have their vision embedded in the strategy. Key actions that need to be taken on the way towards quality EHRs are the following:

- Establish a national interoperability framework and let EMRs interoperate with each other and with EHRs. Widespread adoption by physicians will require the EHR system to make their professional lives easier, not more complex, and will need to provide a clear benefit to their clinical activities. To do this implementation should be meaningful and based on appropriate technical characteristics and common implementation standards to facilitate the improvement of data quality;
- Raise awareness. Expose best practices. Inform everyone that EMR systems are available. Meet expectations. Provide guidelines and resources for quality and secure enablement. Use incentives for motivating EMR adoption and use. Build a coherent dissemination and communication strategy;
- Professionally establish robust central services in the form of core, national infrastructure services by financing standardization and quality assurance. Establish a way to monitor and control progress. A balance between long and short-term objectives should be maintained. The magnitude of the investment needed should not be underestimated if the EHR implementation is to be successful.
- Invest on human resources and the development of healthcare practitioners' digital skills and literacy. Provide appropriate education and training to facilitate the best use of digital solutions to deliver better outcomes. It would also be important to define the roles and responsibilities of the professionals participating in telemedicine pathways, identifying the person(s) leading the process.

Global practice has shown that the proliferation of public eHealth services is reinforced when the public maintains the role of a central regulator rather than when it attempts to operate them competitively to the private sector with the risk of degrading the value of the services provided in the minds of the users. Services of this type are public goods, and as such, they should have the smallest dependency on contractors and the maximum development momentum at the end user level.

FUTURE RESEARCH DIRECTIONS

Healthcare is a very complex, knowledge-driven industry that continuously creates massive amounts of clinical and financial data. Careful and attentive use of analytics in the domain can transform data into knowledge that can improve patient outcomes and operational efficiency.

The focus of current research directions in healthcare aim to support the transformation of healthcare systems in their efforts towards fair access to innovative, sustainable and high quality healthcare for everyone. Unlocking the full potential of new tools, technologies and digital solution for the provision of significant gains in healthcare outcomes is of paramount importance. Progress should inform regulatory standards and requirements, increase health industry's productivity and sustainability through innovation for the delivery of personalized services.

Digital solutions can support healthcare delivery across all stages of the patient pathway (Health First Europe, 2019). Areas of research include life coaching via digital tools, early diagnosis tools, EMRs and workflows to keep track of treatments, day-to-day symptoms and important documents, monitoring tools for citizens with chronic conditions, remote rehabilitation and post-operative car. More work needs to be done in order to realize the vision of citizen empowerment for person-centered care.

It has been demonstrated repeatedly that the use of guidelines by healthcare providers such as hospitals is an effective way of achieving objectives, such as improving effectiveness and quality of care, standardizing medical care, decreasing variations in clinical practice, and achieving the best balance between cost and effectiveness (Kredo et al., 2016). Clinical practice guidelines are usually produced at national or international levels by medical associations or governmental bodies through evolving processes. Local healthcare providers may produce their own set of guidelines or adapt them from existing top-level guidelines, while healthcare payers such as insurers practicing utilization management also publish guidelines (Moses & Feld, 2008). The application of the diagnostic and therapeutic protocols that the MoH has developed (http://www.moh.gov.gr/articles/health/domes-kai-draseis-gia-thn-ygeia/kwdikopoihseis/therapeytika-prwtokolla-syntagografhshs) together with their incorporation in the therapeutic cycle through digital tools, pose imminent challenges. Significant further research into tools for the promotion and strengthening of relevant best practices is expected.

Another target is to set up national disease registries and their interface with IT systems of the NHS for their better development and monitoring.

CONCLUSION

Connecting places where healthcare is provided and sharing of medical data is expected to close the gap that traditionally limits the provision of high-quality health services. EMR is the cornerstone for providing content to evolving eHealth services. Advancing digital transformation best focuses first on individual, well-prioritized, meaningful services rather than on large-scale, all-encompassing programs.

If we want to improve the health of the population, we need quality and secure EMRs. A major challenge for interoperability is not only to transfer patient information from one care setting to a different one but also translating it and at the same time conserving the clinical meaning of the information. Semantic interoperability, when achieved, is expected to improve quality, safety, efficiency and efficacy of healthcare delivery.

The effort has to be paid towards giving meaning to the EMR systems already available at the Greek NHS. That will require gradual implementation based on planning as well as the evolution of the already existing infrastructure. The focus should be paid on operation and interconnection of individual EMRs as well as standardizing quality, in line with international practices. To this extent, effort will be required towards testing, and possibly certification of end user applications. At the same time, the development of comprehensive policies for privacy, consent management, and access to EMRs and the EHR will be required, together with the corresponding legislation and participation incentives.

By building on existing human effort and experience and already available infrastructure, the significant funding that will be required can be controlled better. By having the entire EHR available, it will be far more possible to tailor medical care to each individual's clinical needs and empower healthcare professionals and citizens to take informed decisions. Furthermore, health IT will enable improved clinical outcomes, by linking EMRs with clinical protocols and guidelines, while improving human benefiting global research and science.

ACKNOWLEDGMENT

This research was supported by the Center for eHealth Applications and Services of the Institute of Computer Science, Foundation for Research and Technology – Hellas.

REFERENCES

Ajami, S., & Bagheri-Tadi, T. (2013). Barriers for adopting electronic health records (EHRs) by physicians. *Acta Informatica Medica, 21*(2), 129. doi:10.5455/aim.2013.21.129-134 PMID:24058254

Berg, M. (2001). Implementing information systems in health care organizations: Myths and challenges. *International Journal of Medical Informatics, 64*(2-3), 143–156. doi:10.1016/S1386-5056(01)00200-3 PMID:11734382

Black, A. D., Car, J., Pagliari, C., Anandan, C., Cresswell, K., Bokun, T., ... Sheikh, A. (2011). The impact of eHealth on the quality and safety of health care: A systematic overview. *PLoS Medicine, 8*(1), e1000387. doi:10.1371/journal.pmed.1000387 PMID:21267058

Blobel, B. (2018). Interoperable EHR Systems–Challenges, Standards and Solutions. *European Journal for Biomedical Informatics, 14*(2), 10–19. doi:10.24105/ejbi.2018.14.2.3

Bowens, F. M., Frye, P. A., & Jones, W. A. (2010). Health information technology: integration of clinical workflow into meaningful use of electronic health records. *Perspectives in Health Information Management/AHIMA, American Health Information Management Association, 7.*

ENISA. (2015). *Security and Resilience in eHealth Infrastructures and Services.* Retrieved from https://www.enisa.europa.eu/publications/security-and-resilience-in-ehealth-infrastructures-and-services

ENISA. (2016). *Cyber security and resilience for Smart Hospitals.* Retrieved from https://www.enisa.europa.eu/publications/cyber-security-and-resilience-for-smart-hospitals

Esterle, L., & Kouroubali, A. (2010), Political and organizational factors influencing large scale implementation of electronic health records: Recommendations for a realistic plan. *Report of the European Project EHR-Implement.* Retrieved from http://www.eurorec.org/files/filesPublic/EHR-I%20%20Recommendations.pdf

EU Directorate-General for Health and Food Safety. (2014). *Overview of the national laws on electronic health records in the EU Member States and their interaction with the provision of cross-border eHealth services.* Retrieved from http://ec.europa.eu/health/ehealth/docs/laws_report_recommendations_en.pdf

European Commission. (2017). *New European Interoperability Framework, Promoting seamless services and data flows for European public administrations*. Belgium: European Union.

European Commission (2018). *Communication from the Commission to the European Parliament, the Council, the European Economic and Social Committee and the Committee of the Regions on enabling the digital transformation of health and care in the Digital Single Market; empowering citizens and building a healthier society*, COM(2018) 233 final {SWD(2018) 126 final}.

European Commission (2019). *Commission Recommendation of 6.2.2019 on a European Electronic Health Record exchange format* (Text with EEA relevance), C(2019) 800 final.

European Court of Auditors. (2019). *EU actions for cross-border healthcare: significant ambitions but improved management required (pursuant to Article 287(4), second subparagraph, TFEU)*. Special Report No 7. Retrieved from https://www.eca.europa.eu/Lists/ECADocuments/SR19_07/SR_HEALTH_CARE_EN.pdf

Fragidis, L. L., & Chatzoglou, P. D. (2011, September). The use of electronic health record in greece: current status. In *2011 IEEE 11th International Conference on Computer and Information Technology* (pp. 475-480). IEEE. 10.1109/CIT.2011.42

HL7 International. (2014). *Personal Health Record System Functional Model, Release 1*. Retrieved from http://www.hl7.org/implement/standards/product_brief.cfm?product_id=88

Habib, J. L. (2010). EHRs, meaningful use, and a model EMR. *Drug Benefit Trends, 22*(4), 99–101.

Heart, T., Ben-Assuli, O., & Shabtai, I. (2017). A review of PHR, EMR and EHR integration: A more personalized healthcare and public health policy. *Health Policy and Technology, 6*(1), 20–25. doi:10.1016/j.hlpt.2016.08.002

Herrmann, M., Boehme, P., Mondritzki, T., Ehlers, J. P., Kavadias, S., & Truebel, H. (2018). Digital transformation and disruption of the health care sector: Internet-based observational study. *Journal of Medical Internet Research, 20*(3), e104. doi:10.2196/jmir.9498 PMID:29588274

HiMSS. (2011). *Electronic Health Records*. Retrieved from http://www.himss.org/library/ehr

HiMSS Analytics. (2019). *EMRAM: A strategic roadmap for effective EMR adoption and maturity*. Retrieved from: http://www.himssanalytics.org/emram

Iakovidis, I. (1998). Towards personal health record: Current situation, obstacles and trends in implementation of electronic healthcare record in Europe. *International Journal of Medical Informatics*, *52*(1-3), 105–115. doi:10.1016/S1386-5056(98)00129-4 PMID:9848407

Katehakis, D. G. (2018). Electronic Medical Record Implementation Challenges for the National Health System in Greece. *International Journal of Reliable and Quality E-Healthcare*, *7*(1), 16–30. doi:10.4018/IJRQEH.2018010102

Katehakis, D. G., Halkiotis, S., & Kouroubali, A. (2011). Materialization of Regional Health Information Networks in Greece: Electronic Health Record Barriers & Enablers. *Journal of Healthcare Engineering*, *2*(3), 389–403. doi:10.1260/2040-2295.2.3.389

Katehakis, D. G., Kondylakis, H., Koumakis, L., Kouroubali, A., & Marias, K. (2017a). Integrated care solutions for the citizen: Personal health record functional models to support interoperability. *EJBI*, *13*(1), 41–56. doi:10.24105/ejbi.2017.13.1.8

Katehakis, D. G., & Kouroubali, A. (2019). A Framework for the Consistent Management of eHealth Interoperability in Greece. *Proceedings of the 21st International Conference on Enterprise Information Systems (ICEIS 2019)*, 2, 689-695. 10.5220/0007796906890695

Katehakis, D. G., Pangalos, G., & Prentza, A. (2017b). Security Improvements for Better and Safer Cross-Border ePrescription and Patient Summary Services. *International Journal of Reliable and Quality E-Healthcare*, *6*(1), 18–28. doi:10.4018/IJRQEH.2017010102

Katehakis, D. G., & Tsiknakis, M. (2006). *Electronic health record*. Wiley Encyclopedia of Biomedical Engineering.

Kharbanda, V. C. J., Bohlin, N., Sehlstedt, U., & Treutiger, J. (2017). *Building the Smart Hospital Agenda*. Retrieved from https://www.adlittle.com/sites/default/files/viewpoints/ADL_Smart%20Hospital.pdf

Kierkegaard, P. (2011). Electronic health record: Wiring Europe's healthcare. *Computer Law & Security Review*, *27*(5), 503–515. doi:10.1016/j.clsr.2011.07.013

Kouroubali, A., & Katehakis, D. G. (2019). The new European interoperability framework as a facilitator of digital transformation for citizen empowerment. *Journal of Biomedical Informatics*, *94*, 103166. doi:10.1016/j.jbi.2019.103166 PMID:30978512

Kredo, T., Bernhardsson, S., Machingaidze, S., Young, T., Louw, Q., Ochodo, E., & Grimmer, K. (2016). Guide to clinical practice guidelines: The current state of play. *International Journal for Quality in Health Care*, *28*(1), 122–128. doi:10.1093/intqhc/mzv115 PMID:26796486

Linder, J. A., Schnipper, J. L., Tsurikova, R., Melnikas, A. J., Volk, L. A., & Middleton, B. (2006). Barriers to electronic health record use during patient visits. *AMIA ... Annual Symposium Proceedings - AMIA Symposium. AMIA Symposium*, *2006*, 499. PMID:17238391

Melin, U., Axelsson, K., & Söderström, F. (2016). Managing the development of e-ID in a public e-service context – challenges and path dependencies from a life-cycle perspective. *Transforming Government: People. Process and Policy*, *10*(1), 77–98.

Menachemi, N., & Collum, T. H. (2011). Benefits and drawbacks of electronic health record systems. *Risk Management and Healthcare Policy*, *4*, 47. doi:10.2147/RMHP.S12985 PMID:22312227

Milieu Ltd and Time.lex. (2013). *Overview of the national laws on electronic health records in the EU Member States, National Report for Greece*. Retrieved from http://ec.europa.eu/health//sites/health/files/ehealth/docs/laws_greece_en.pdf

Ministers in charge of eGovernment policy and coordination from 32 countries of the EU and EFTA. (2017). *Tallinn Declaration on eGovernment at the ministerial meeting during Estonian Presidency of the Council of the EU on 6 October 2017.* Retrieved from https://ec.europa.eu/newsroom/document.cfm?doc_id=47559

Moses, R. E., & Feld, A. D. (2008). Legal risks of clinical practice guidelines. *The American Journal of Gastroenterology*, *103*(1), 7–11. doi:10.1111/j.1572-0241.2007.01399.x PMID:18184116

Nguyen, K. (2018). Certification of eIDAS trust services and new global transparency trends. *Datenschutz und Datensicherheit-DuD*, *42*(7), 424–428. doi:10.100711623-018-0972-7

Petru, R. (2016). How to use EHRs to improve the quality of care? Interview included in "eHealth Trends & Talks". *Polish Healthcare Journal*, 69-72. Retrieved from https://www.osoz.pl/static_files/osoz/eHealth_2016.pdf

Pitsch, M. (2016). Dormant digitization. Interview included in "eHealth Trends & Talks". *Polish Healthcare Journal*, 62-64. Retrieved from https://www.osoz.pl/static_files/osoz/eHealth_2016.pdf

Porter, M., & Teisberg, E. (2006). *Redefining Health Care: Creating Value-Based Competition on Results. Watertown.* Harvard Business School Press.

Prey, J. E., Polubriaginof, F., Kuperman, G. J., Tiase, V., Collins, S. A., & Vawdrey, D. K. (2016). International perspectives on sharing clinical data with patients. *International Journal of Medical Informatics, 86*, 135–141. doi:10.1016/j.ijmedinf.2015.11.007 PMID:26631956

Roehrs, A., Da Costa, C. A., da Rosa Righi, R., & De Oliveira, K. S. F. (2017). Personal health records: A systematic literature review. *Journal of Medical Internet Research, 19*(1), e13. doi:10.2196/jmir.5876 PMID:28062391

Stroetmann, K. A., Artmann, J., & Stroetmann, V. (2011). Developing national eHealth infrastructures--results and lessons from Europe. *AMIA ... Annual Symposium proceedings. AMIA Symposium*, 1347–1354.

Tang, P. C., Ash, J. S., Bates, D. W., Overhage, J. M., & Sands, D. Z. (2006). Personal health records: Definitions, benefits, and strategies for overcoming barriers to adoption. *Journal of the American Medical Informatics Association, 13*(2), 121–126. doi:10.1197/jamia.M2025 PMID:16357345

Thiel, R., Deimel, L., Schmidtmann, D., Piesche, K., Hüsing, T., Rennoch, J., . . . Stroetmann, K. (2019). In *#SmartHealthSystems International comparison of digital strategies.* Retrieved from https://www.bertelsmann-stiftung.de/en/publications/publication/did/smarthealthsystems-1/

ADDITIONAL READING

Accenture. (2016). *Consumer Survey on Patient Engagement.* Retrieved from https://www.accenture.com/t20160629T045303__w__/us-en/_acnmedia/PDF-6/Accenture-Patients-Want-A-Heavy-Dose-of-Digital-Research.pdf

Adler-Milstein, J., DesRoches, C. M., Kralovec, P., Foster, G., Worzala, C., Charles, D., ... Jha, A. K. (2015). Electronic health record adoption in US hospitals: Progress continues, but challenges persist. *Health Affairs, 34*(12), 2174–2180. doi:10.1377/hlthaff.2015.0992 PMID:26561387

eHealth Network (2019). *EHealth Network Guidelines to the EU Member States and the European Commission on an interoperable eco-system for digital health and investment programmes for a new/updated generation of digital infrastructure in Europe.* Retrieved from https://ec.europa.eu/health/sites/health/files/ehealth/docs/ev_20190611_co922_en.pdf

European Union (2016). *Regulation (EU) 2016/679 of the European Parliament and of the Council of 27 April 2016 on the protection of natural persons with regard to the processing of personal data and on the free movement of such data, and repealing Directive 95/46/EC (General Data Protection Regulation) (Text with EEA relevance).*

HiMSS Analytics. (2018). *Annual European eHealth Survey 2018. Health-IT predictions for Europe.* Retrieved from https://www.himss.eu/himss-analytics-annual-european-ehealth-survey-2018

Johnson, J. K., & Sollecito, W. A. (2018). *McLaughlin & Kaluzny's Continuous Quality Improvement in Health Care.* Jones & Bartlett Learning.

Katehakis, D. G., & Kouroubali, A. (2019): A Framework for the Consistent Management of eHealth Interoperability in Greece. *Proceedings of the 21st International Conference on Enterprise Information Systems (ICEIS 2019)*, Heraklion, Crete, Greece, 3-5 May, 2019, Volume 2, pp. 689-695. ISBN 978-989-758-372-8. 10.5220/0007796906890695

Kouroubali, A. (2004). *Implementation of health care information systems: Key factors and the dynamics of change* (Doctoral dissertation, University of Cambridge

Kouroubali, A., Koumakis, L., Kondylakis, H., & Katehakis, D. G. (2019). An Integrated Approach Towards Developing Quality Mobile Health Apps for Cancer. In *Mobile Health Applications for Quality Healthcare Delivery* (pp. 46–71). IGI Global. doi:10.4018/978-1-5225-8021-8.ch003

Nechyporenko, T., & McKibbon, A. (2015). Review of different training approaches to facilitate successful adoption of EMR systems by physicians in hospital settings. Retrieved from https://macsphere.mcmaster.ca/bitstream/11375/20846/1/merc_wp_54.pdf

KEY TERMS AND DEFINITIONS

Digital Transformation: The process of using digital technologies to create new—or modify existing—business processes, culture, and customer experiences to meet changing business and market requirements.

Electronic Health (eHealth): The use of information and communication technologies for health.

Electronic Health Record (EHR): The Electronic Health Record (EHR) is a longitudinal electronic record of patient health information generated by one or more encounters in any care delivery setting. Included in this information are patient demographics, progress notes, problems, medications, vital signs, past medical history, immunizations, laboratory data and radiology reports. The EHR automates and streamlines the clinician's workflow. The EHR has the ability to generate a complete record of a clinical patient encounter - as well as supporting other care-related activities directly or indirectly via interface - including evidence-based decision support, quality management, and outcomes reporting.

Electronic Medical Record (EMR): An electronic record of health-related information on an individual that can be created, gathered, managed, and consulted by authorized clinicians and staff within one healthcare organization.

Health: Health is a state of complete physical, mental and social well-being and not merely the absence of disease or infirmity.

Interoperability: The ability of organizations to interact towards mutually beneficial goals, involving the sharing of information and knowledge between these organizations, through the business processes they support, by means of the exchange of data between their ICT systems.

Mobile Health (mHealth): The use of mobile and wireless devices to improve health outcomes, healthcare services and health research.

Personal Health Record (PHR): An electronic, lifelong resource of health information needed by individuals to make health decisions. Individuals own and manage the information in the PHR, which comes from healthcare providers and the individual. The PHR is maintained in a secure and private environment, with the individual determining rights of access. The PHR does not replace the legal record of any provider.

Chapter 4
Machine Learning in Healthcare:
Introduction and Real-World Application Considerations

Stavros Pitoglou
https://orcid.org/0000-0002-5309-4683
Computer Solutions SA, Greece & National Technical University of Athens, Greece

ABSTRACT

Machine learning, closely related to artificial intelligence and standing at the intersection of computer science and mathematical statistical theory, comes in handy when the truth is hiding in a place that the human brain has no access to. Given any prediction or assessment problem, the more complicated this issue is, based on the difficulty of the human mind to understand the inherent causalities/patterns and apply conventional methods towards an acceptable solution, machine learning can find a fertile field of application. This chapter's purpose is to give a general non-technical definition of machine learning, provide a review of its latest implementations in the healthcare domain and add to the ongoing discussion on this subject. It suggests the active involvement of entities beyond the already active academic community in the quest for solutions that "exploit" existing datasets and can be applied in the daily practice, embedded inside the software processes that are already in use.

DOI: 10.4018/978-1-7998-2390-2.ch004

INTRODUCTION

Machine Learning and It's Origins

One of the most quoted definitions of Machine Learning is:

The subfield of computer science that "gives computers the ability to learn without being explicitly programmed. (Samuel, 1959)

That is a compact, but also a complete description of the major paradigm shift Machine Learning brings to the world of solving problems, answering questions, and taking decisions with the use of Information Technologies. It implies that we can delegate to a computer the task to make sense out of a dataset "on its own," without needing humans defining the exact course of calculations and actions, thus without us having understood the true nature of the problem at hand and the path to its solution. That way, the machine uses the data as "learning material" in order to assess and classify new or unseen data under the same context, or predict future values, eventually developing the ability to make decisions or/and define courses of action "on its own." That human-like ability is described in a definition which was given a few decades later:

A computer program is said to learn from experience E with respect to some class of tasks T and performance measure P if its performance at tasks in T, as measured by P, improves with experience E. (Mitchell, 1997)

Taking a certain risk of oversimplification, the basic concept can be described as follows: One can take a dataset that he believes (or at least hopes) that contains the necessary information, a truth that cannot be easily discovered but is deemed essential in order to complete a specific task. He acknowledges, at the same time, the fact that, as the volume of data, the number of parameters that take part in the outcome and the complexity of their correlation increase, it becomes increasingly difficult (and at some point impossible) for the human mind to process, come up with a visible and intuitive hypothesis about the hidden patterns and model the acting causalities in order to provide means of accurate assessment and/or prediction. Then, the computer is let to create its universe out of this data, a perception of the reality in the form of multidimensional "hyperspheres", creating vectors out of every data point, and, by the application of complex mathematic principles, calculate its way to an algorithm, that "understands" the acting causalities and "captures" the underlying patterns, thus becoming capable of being applied as "knowledge" and "experience" towards solving (or helping to solve) related problems.

Why Now?

Machine Learning is not such a new idea. Already by the late 1950s, we can find a solid conceptual and theoretical background. In 1959 Dr. Arthur Samuel publishes his research about "teaching" a machine to play the game of checkers, giving at the same time a definition that is still used today (Samuel, 1959). A year before that, in 1958, faces the light of publicity, the mathematical description of the "Perceptron," the direct ancestor of contemporary Artificial Neural Networks (ANN's)(Rosenblatt, 1958).

Given this information, a completely valid question someone could ask is: "Why now?" If the background is more than 60 years old, then why is it that only in the last few years we experience this explosion (exponential growth) of interest in Machine Learning, evident by the unprecedented increase in the relative literature, the domination of the technology-related headlines, the undeclared but obvious race between all the big IT companies(Markoff & Lohr, 2016) and phenomena of "Rock Star" data scientists(Vincent, 2017).

The answer probably lies in the very basic principles of the Machine Learning concept, in terms of its "core ingredients." It is easily understood that due to their nature, Machine Learning techniques rely heavily (many times exclusively) on two information era "commodities": data and computational power. Data is the raw material, the "body of knowledge." It is often reported that having a significant volume of quality data can provide impressive results even with the use of moderate or un-optimized algorithms. On the other hand, computational power is the essential means of performing complex mathematical calculations on significant amounts of data, thus enabling the application of the underlying theoretical principles.

As far as computational power is concerned, the consistent exponential growth of the last decades has made extensive capabilities available even in the general consumer level. Processing components per spatial unit (semiconductors in integrated circuits) nearly double every single year since the 1960s. This trend, which is often named "Moore's Law" after the engineer that made this prediction(Moore, 1965) in 1965, was not only proven fairly accurate for its original 10 years' time span, but it continues until today to describe the industry advances in terms of available computational power (Mack, 2011; Waldrop, 2016).

As it seems, we are experiencing in the last few years, the result of this (additive if not multiplicative) combination of exponentially growing factors (volume of data and computational power). This effect has reached a critical level (a "boiling point" if you like) which explains the hype and presents a call for action towards the IT community /industry.

Of course, one should be aware of the fact that Machine Learning, being essentially the evolution of statistical pattern-seeking and decision making made possible by the advancements in processing power and data storage availability, is a two-edged knife. Surely enough, it facilitates attacking certain problems allowing for limited prior knowledge and substantially less effort from the data scientist, in terms of tedious data handling(feature selection, data cleaning, etc.). In the same time, somehow paradoxically, the same qualities that ensure fast, seemingly effortless and most of the time intransparent or incomprehensible pattern recognition, could result in algorithmic bias due to undetected data anomalies.

HEALTHCARE AS FIELD OF APPLICATION

Turning the spotlight on the healthcare domain, we will observe that both the need and the prerequisites are present. Healthcare as a problem space can be defined in two broad, distinct levels:

1. **Personal level**, as the process of taking necessary actions towards preserving, restoring, and/or improving the health status of an individual. This level is characterized by the immense complexity of the human body and the many interactions with the environment that could affect its operation.
2. **Social level**, as the process of providing coordinated relative services in large people groups. On this level, there is the diversion of the modern societies, as well as the complexity inherent to the process of coordinating resources, designing policies, and effectively applying them.

In this light, even without in-depth knowledge of the details, it is evident that healthcare is a relatively complex domain. As such, it presents a uniquely suitable field for the application of Machine Learning solutions.

Regarding the volume of data, many historical thresholds have been surpassed due to the widespread adoption and extensive use of software systems in healthcare providing institutions. In addition to that, there are vast amounts of data that come from diagnostic and monitoring devices, whose connectivity with software systems via well-defined and agreed-upon protocols has become a standard nowadays, as well as from personal health and activity tracking devices (wearables, etc.).

The effect of potentially successful implementations, in terms of improving the overall quality of the provided healthcare service, is evident.

On the patient's level, physicians will be able to have an invaluable ally, able to complement their skills where and when they most need it, distinguishing those tasks that they can already do well and those where they have had only limited access

(Deo, 2015). They will be able to collaborate with intelligent expert systems and extend their brain capacity to the point of making sense of vast amounts of data, e.g., inputs from sensors that operate constantly. They will be able to extend their vision to a sharpness level of spotting and evaluating even the most subtle detail of a diagnostic image, detecting and classifying anomalies that previously went unnoticed. More importantly, they will be able to provide personalized care, based not only on what is known to be effective for the average patient but also taking into consideration the individual's parameters, comparing and parallelizing with information from a continually growing body of data that contains similar cases, treatments, and outcomes. The potential is endless.

On the much broader social level, public health policymakers will be able to team up with systems that can combine heterogeneous datasets in unified information flow and find patterns that will help them forecast in a timely and precise manner, enabling them to decide the most efficient way to allocate the available resources. They will be able to predict epidemic outbursts using "smart" systems like the Real-time Outbreak and Disease Surveillance (Espino et al., 2004). The list is endless here also.

RESEARCH BACKGROUND

The purpose of this chapter is not to provide an exhaustive or a systematic research literature review. However, there is particular importance in referencing specific research examples, in order to facilitate the further study and provide the research background as a foundation for the following arguments.

Kourou et al. (Kourou, Exarchos, Exarchos, Karamouzis, & Fotiadis, 2015) present a review of recent ML approaches employed in the modeling of cancer progression. Their survey of applications covers the prediction of cancer susceptibility, recurrence, and survival. In another recent study, Kavakiotis et al. (Kavakiotis et al., 2017) provide a systematic review of the latest applications of ML in the field of Diabetes Mellitus research, concerning prediction/diagnosis, complications, genetic background, and related public health issues. These studies present the research effort (and progress) made in broad healthcare fields (diabetes and cancer), depicting the scientific community's endeavor to contribute towards the "tackling" of humanity's major health issues with the use of ML approach and techniques.

Special focus is considered appropriate in specific fields related to the study of the human brain, as a continually evolving scientific challenge, with new observations, theories and testable hypotheses presenting themselves every single week for the past years. The immense complexity (and in some aspects "chaotic" nature) of the underlying structures, the vast amount of relevant variables ("relevant" in the sense that could in principle affect the observed outcomes and qualify as predictors) and the overwhelming volume and granularity of the data to be taken into consideration (mainly due to the modern imaging and tissue-electrochemical activity cartography techniques), form a domain, in which ML methods could thrive and lead to new understanding, as well as novel predictive, diagnostic and therapeutic approaches.

Neurology/Neurosurgery

A dominant medical specialty in the domain of brain function study is neurology/neurosurgery. In recent years, new diagnostic techniques – mainly neuro-imaging modalities-, have provided the opportunity to study various aspects of the human brain with unprecedented accuracy. Magnetic Resonance Imaging (MRI) techniques (structural-sMRI, functional-fMRI or diffusion-dMRI), as well as more traditional methods (electroencephalography-EEG, magnetoencephalography-MEG), provide large datasets containing new insights into the structure, function, and connectivity of the human brain. Along with these data comes the hope of new prognostic/diagnostic methods based on them, and this has led to a growing trend in conducted studies and the relevant scientific literature (Arbabshirani, Plis, Sui, & Calhoun, 2017).

Rughani et al. (Rughani et al., 2010) trained an artificial neural network (ANN) to predict in-hospital survival following traumatic brain injury (TBI). Their study showed that ANN consistently and significantly outperformed trained experienced professionals as well as classical regression models (given the same limited clinical information).

Liu et al. (Liu et al., 2011) developed an ensemble of artificial neural networks (EANN) model to predict brain death in severe head injury patients. By establishing two models (with 11 and 14 input variables respectively) they achieved high levels of classification accuracy (~92%). Methods like this could result in significant improvement in the speed and precision of brain death diagnosis, which -in turn- is vital to the solid organ transplantation process. Speed and reliability could provide the necessary time to act before the cardiovascular collapse and somatic death that inevitably follows shortly after.

Aribisala et al. (Aribisala et al., 2010) used a support-vector-machine (SVN) (Cortes & Vapnik, 1995) modeling method to discriminate mild TBI patients from a control group of healthy individuals. As input to their model, they used advanced techniques to extract quantitative data from MRI images (T_1, T_2 mapping, and diffusion tensor MRI). Achieving sensitivity and specificity (Altman & Bland, 1994) of 88% and 75% respectively, they introduced a promising prognostic imaging method that reveals brain abnormalities where conventional neuroimaging methods fail to do so.

Choi et al. (Choi, Muizelaar, & Barnes, 1991) developed a Decision Tree (DT) (Breiman, Friedman, Olshen, & Stone, 1984) model with 23 prognostic indicators to predict the 12-months outcomes of patients with severe head injuries. Several research groups worked on this approach (the results of severe head injury using Decision Tree Analysis). Low et al. (Low et al., 2009) developed a model based on microdialysis (MD) data and brain tissue oxygenation (BptO2), achieving predictive accuracy ~90% (with an F-ratio of ~0.94).

Precision Psychiatry

It is commonly accepted that the devastating collateral damage and soaring costs of psychiatric disease prompt a global challenge for our societies (Gustavsson et al., 2011). The study of psycho-pathological disorders is another very appropriate and promising field of ML methods' application as:

- it involves "unlocking" brain function "mysteries," in a relevant (although not directly analogous) sense as mentioned above,
- patient-level predictive analytics might help psychiatry to move from a firm reliance on symptom phenomenology to catch up with biology-centered decision-making in other medical specialties (Kapur, Phillips, & Insel, 2012)

Professors Bzdok and Meyer-Lindeberg have elaborated on the potential use of ML techniques in precision psychiatry (Bzdok & Meyer-Lindenberg, 2017).

Galatzer-Levy et al. (Galatzer-Levy, Ma, Statnikov, Yehuda, & Shalev, 2017) used the support vector machine (SVM) technique (Statnikov, Alexander, Aliferis, Hardin, & Guyon, 2011) to model interactions between biological and environmental factors that underlay post-traumatic psychopathology. The study identified the substantial role of the neuroendocrine response (e.g., cortisol levels) as a biomarker panel for predictive modeling of post-traumatic stress responses. It also described sub-populations for which the observed effects are more relevant. This study is an excellent example of using ML driven pattern recognition to reveal a correlation between biomarkers and psychopathology, which can be utilized not only to create successful predictive models but also to suggest paths of (chemical) clinical intervention in order to deal with psychological implications.

Salvador et al. (Salvador et al., 2017), exploring MRI-based diagnostic prediction in psychosis, investigate the discriminative power of commonly used ML algorithms among three groups (patients with schizophrenia, patients with bipolar disorder and a control population of healthy individuals). As predictors, sMRI features including grey and white matter voxel-based morphometry (VBM) are being utilized. This study also provides an enlightening comparative analysis with previous efforts to provide discriminative models for the analogous patient population. Particular reference is made to the importance of methodological and research parameter issues such as the initial sample size, sample balancing techniques, independence between training and test datasets, etc. Interestingly enough, this analysis contains a reference to a study (Brouwer et al., 2014), which reported classification accuracy of 88%, but when its fitted classifiers were applied to external data, the accuracy descended to 65%.

THE REAL-WORLD APPROACH

There are many useful insights one can obtain by studying the academic work on ML applications in the medical field:

- The accumulated research experience shows, without a doubt, that there is excellent potential in implementing ML solutions and has proved the feasibility of developing accurate and useful models using ML methods.
- There is no universal solution, one technique/model/approach "to rule them all" and most of the times, the research and development team must resort to an extensive toolset of algorithms, methods, and data handling approaches
- In many cases, we observe an overestimation of the explanatory and predictive power of the models developed "in vitro" when applied to real-world scenarios. One can state that a 65% accuracy score is significant; however, a drop from 88% to 65% arguably crosses the virtual "line" of practical usefulness and/or production readiness.

This last finding holds great importance, as it adds to the main concern of this article, the limited result reproducibility and efficient exploitation of the research body due to the lack of real-world implementation.

Quite recently, when the author submitted "Machine Learning in Healthcare" as a topic for a speech in an eHealth Forum in Athens, Greece, he found out that few of his peers had any clue. This should really be no surprise, as (not only in Greece) engagement with Machine Learning seems limited to university research groups, international IT corporations (Google, Microsoft, IBM, etc.) with prominent Research Departments and "start-ups" that derive directly (as spin-offs) from the academic community, or have very close bonds with it. Acknowledging the underlying contradiction between the theoretical advancement and the disproportional real-world effect, especially in domains with large software vendor dispersion, like healthcare, there have been emerging voices, which are more or less stating something like this:

Machine learning offers a cornucopia of useful ways to approach problems that otherwise defy manual solution. However, much current ML research suffers from a growing detachment from those real problems. Many investigators withdraw into their private studies with a copy of the data set and work in isolation to perfect algorithmic performance. Publishing results to the ML community is the end of the process. Successes usually are not communicated back to the original problem setting, or not in a form that can be used (Wagstaff, 2012).

Although in the last few years, there has been some progress in that field, in general, the problem still stands, and in order to mitigate the above-mentioned contradiction, actions should be taken in the direction of cultivating extrinsic and intrinsic motivators for more "players" to enter the research and implementation "arena". In the healthcare industry, the crucial role will be played by the Independent Software Vendors of variant size, which should be encouraged and motivated to participate, as they develop and maintain medical software for numerous organizations, affecting indirectly the impact on large patient populations.

In order to provide some case study material, it could be useful mentioning a series of experimentations conducted by the research team of Computer Solutions SA, led by the author, towards:

1. An algorithm that tries to forecast a future number of admissions in a hospital-based on historical data combined with real-time information flow from weather and epidemic awareness data streams, using a Long Short-Term Memory(LSTM) Neural Network (Hochreiter & Schmidhuber, 1997).
2. An algorithm that tries to classify by severity certain types of ultrasound diagnostic reports, based on Natural Language Processing over raw text.
3. An algorithm that tries to assess the possibility of a patient to be readmitted in the next 60 days after the discharge time, using "Support Vector Machine" implementation (Cortes & Vapnik, 1995).

There is a common denominator amongst all these endeavors, which is the effort to come up with solutions that can be easily integrated into products and processes that healthcare organizations are using in their day-to-day reality. The emerging solutions are continuously incorporated into the working software products, and the results are assessed, based on real case comparisons. This approach stems from the belief that there is no way to prove whether the proposed solution can deliver any enhancement to the healthcare process unless it has the opportunity to be applied in real-time to real-world cases.

That is the most important message this article tries to put under the reader's consideration: Machine Learning solutions will get on the path of widespread adoption and seamless integration with already existing technologies, only if they are -by design- crafted with real-world implementation in mind. That is not denying or defying the academic effort and the research process that are essential in the design and implementation of such solutions. There is a good reason for the existence of a saying that they *"come "packaged in a Ph.D."; that is, it requires the sophistication of a graduate student or beyond to successfully deploy ML to solve real problems—and that same Ph.D. is needed to maintain and update the system after its deployment"* (Wagstaff, 2012).

It's just acknowledging the fact that this strategy fulfills the necessary but not always the sufficient conditions of scaling the solution to the goal of widespread impact, as the application of these methods in the real world poses a number of challenges, probably absent in a classical research lab setup, that render any solution unusable until proof of the contrary.

CHALLENGES

Some of the most significant challenges, that, -among others-, affect the implementation of Machine Learning solutions in the healthcare environment, and emerge in almost every related effort, are:

1. **The Algorithms are Not "Plug n' Play."** Although existing implementations targeting on a specific solution to a specific problem most of the times pose significant insights, there is no guarantee that an implementation that worked under certain circumstances will be able to address the same problem elsewhere with the same expected results. Most of the major steps of every model development process (Baer, 2019):
    - Model Design: the overall structure of the model,
    - Data Engineering: the preparation of the data,
    - Model Assembly: the main development process of the algorithm,
    - Model Validation: the review and assertion of the model's fitness for use,
    - Model Implementation: the deployment in actual organizational operations,

are extremely sensitive to the application environment; thus, many critical parameters could (and will) differ. This issue is magnified under the constraint that successful real-world implementations should, many times, work with the input of software systems that are already in production, meaning that there is not always the luxury of pre-defining input parameters according to the specific research needs, which is usually the case in the available research precedents.

2. **Poor Quality of Data**. As mentioned above, having lots of data is of the utmost importance when trying to implement Machine Learning solutions. It is the key element that provides the system with the "experience" to "learn" from.

In the healthcare domain, we have an invaluable treasure in the form of years-and-years of data, collected through the use of medical software systems by medical institutions during their day-to-day operation. However, there is a catch: in most (if not all) of the cases, the provided data sets are "polluted" with large numbers of problematic elements, due to human user error and the design of the software systems in use. Given that the nature of Machine Learning techniques renders them extremely sensitive to the quality of the provided data, extensive, careful, and proficient data preparation procedures must be performed. Some of the most prevalent problems are:

- Missing values. More than often, there will be blanks in the data sets, usually due to the fact that information essential to the research, is not obligatory for the system users to enter in the available software forms. The implementer will have to make per case decisions about ignoring the incomplete data or employing methods of "synthetic" data completion, as every approach has its advantages and disadvantages.
- Outliers. Values that lie way out of the normal ranges can become extremely challenging in their handling. The implementer, based on his domain expertise, must for each case decide whether they are entry errors or valid outstanding cases that should be taken into consideration (as their absence could alter the validity of the calculations)

3. **Adoption "Friction."** In the medical world, there have always been trusting issues, every time technological means and innovations "invaded" fields of the medical practice that the physicians regard as their "inner circle" of expertise and responsibility, with a typical example the diagnosis process.

In this light, one could easily imagine the potential resistance to the broad adoption of these methods, multiplying the regular anticipated inertia with a significant factor deriving from the fact that, more than often, the emerging algorithm can provide no easily interpreted or tangible explanation for the success of its outcome, being most of the times some complex mathematical equation with participating parameters of little logical correlation.

CONCLUSION

There is no doubt that we are witnessing the eve of a new era, driven by the advances in the fields of Machine Learning and Artificial Intelligence. Healthcare, as a process, as a craft, as a scientific discipline and as a social structure, will be heavily involved with this process, due to the nature of its needs. For this advancement to be accelerated and applied to the benefit of large patient populations, there will be a need for multidisciplinary task teams comprising of doctors, health domain experts, mathematicians, computer scientists, software developers, and data experts. Such teams will be able to combine scientific research with the real-world experience and domain expertise towards the ultimate goal of crafting effective solutions in a context where time is of the essence and every life matters.

REFERENCES

Altman, D. G., & Bland, J. M. (1994). Statistics Notes: Diagnostic tests 1: sensitivity and specificity. BMJ (Clinical Research Ed.). doi:10.1136/bmj.308.6943.1552

Arbabshirani, M. R., Plis, S., Sui, J., & Calhoun, V. D. (2017). Single subject prediction of brain disorders in neuroimaging: Promises and pitfalls. [PubMed]. *NeuroImage*, *145*, 137–165. doi:10.1016/j.neuroimage.2016.02.079

Aribisala, B. S., Cowie, C. J. A., He, J., Wood, J., Mendelow, A. D., Mitchell, P., & Blamire, A. M. (2010). Multi-parametric Classification of Traumatic Brain Injury Patients Using Automatic Analysis of Quantitative MRI Scans. Medical Imaging and Augmented Reality: 5th International Workshop, MIAR 2010, Beijing, China, September 19-20, 2010. Proceedings, 51–59. 10.1007/978-3-642-15699-1_6

Baer, T. (2019). *Understand, Manage, and Prevent Algorithmic Bias. Understand, Manage, and Prevent Algorithmic Bias*. Berkeley, CA: Apress; doi:10.1007/978-1-4842-4885-0

Breiman, L., Friedman, J. H., Olshen, R. A., & Stone, C. J. (1984). Classification and Regression Trees. In The Wadsworth statisticsprobability series (Vol. 19). doi:10.1371/journal.pone.0015807

Brouwer, R. M., Schnack, H. G., Nieuwenhuis, M., van Haren, N. E. M., Abramovic, L., Scheewe, T. W., ... Kahn, R. S. (2014). Can structural MRI aid in clinical classification? A machine learning study in two independent samples of patients with schizophrenia, bipolar disorder and healthy subjects. [PubMed]. *NeuroImage*, *84*(January), 299–306. doi:10.1016/j.neuroimage.2013.08.053

Bzdok, D., & Meyer-Lindenberg, A. (2017). Machine learning for precision psychiatry, 1–16. Retrieved from http://arxiv.org/abs/1705.10553

Choi, S., Muizelaar, J., & Barnes, T. (1991). Prediction tree for severely head-injured patients. [PubMed]. *Journalism*, *75*, 251–255. doi:10.3171/jns.1991.75.2.0251

Cortes, C., & Vapnik, V. (1995). Support-vector networks. *Machine Learning*, *20*(3), 273–297. doi:10.1007/BF00994018

Deo, R. C. (2015). Machine Learning in Medicine. [PubMed]. *Circulation*, *132*(20), 1920–1930. doi:10.1161/CIRCULATIONAHA.115.001593

Espino, J. U., Wagner, M. M., Tsui, F.-C., Su, H.-D., Olszewski, R. T., Lie, Z., ... Dara, J. (2004). The RODS Open Source Project: Removing a barrier to syndromic surveillance. *Studies in Health Technology and Informatics*, *107*(Pt 2), 1192–1196.

Galatzer-Levy, I. R., Ma, S., Statnikov, A., Yehuda, R., & Shalev, A. Y. (2017). Utilization of machine learning for prediction of post-traumatic stress: A re-examination of cortisol in the prediction and pathways to non-remitting PTSD. [PubMed]. *Translational Psychiatry*, *7*(3), e0. doi:10.1038/tp.2017.38

Gustavsson, A., Svensson, M., Jacobi, F., Allgulander, C., Alonso, J., Beghi, E., ... Olesen, J. (2011). Cost of disorders of the brain in Europe 2010. [PubMed]. *European Neuropsychopharmacology*, *21*(10), 718–779. doi:10.1016/j.euroneuro.2011.08.008

Hochreiter, S., & Schmidhuber, J. (1997). Long Short-Term Memory. [PubMed]. *Neural Computation*, *9*(8), 1735–1780. doi:10.1162/neco.1997.9.8.1735

Kapur, S., Phillips, A. G., & Insel, T. R. (2012). Why has it taken so long for biological psychiatry to develop clinical tests and what to do about it? [PubMed]. *Molecular Psychiatry*, *17*(12), 1174–1179. doi:10.1038/mp.2012.105

Kavakiotis, I., Tsave, O., Salifoglou, A., Maglaveras, N., Vlahavas, I., & Chouvarda, I. (2017). Machine Learning and Data Mining Methods in Diabetes Research. [PubMed]. *Computational and Structural Biotechnology Journal*, *15*, 104–116. doi:10.1016/j.csbj.2016.12.005

Kourou, K., Exarchos, T. P., Exarchos, K. P., Karamouzis, M. V., & Fotiadis, D. I. (2015). Machine learning applications in cancer prognosis and prediction. [PubMed]. *Computational and Structural Biotechnology Journal*, *13*, 8–17. doi:10.1016/j.csbj.2014.11.005

Liu, Q., Cui, X., Abbod, M. F., Huang, S.-J., Han, Y.-Y., & Shieh, J. (2011). Brain death prediction based on ensembled artificial neural networks in neurosurgical intensive care unit. *Journal of the Taiwan Institute of Chemical Engineers*, *42*(1), 97–107. doi:10.1016/j.jtice.2010.05.006

Low, D., Kuralmani, V., Ng, S. K., Lee, K. K., Ng, I., & Ang, B. T. (2009). Prediction of Outcome Utilizing Both Physiological and Biochemical Parameters in Severe Head Injury. [PubMed]. *Journal of Neurotrauma*, *26*(8), 1177–1182. doi:10.1089/neu.2008.0841

Mack, C. A. (2011). Fifty Years of Moore's Law. *IEEE Transactions on Semiconductor Manufacturing*, *24*(2), 202–207. doi:10.1109/TSM.2010.2096437

Markoff, J., & Lohr, S. (2016). The Race Is On to Control Artificial Intelligence, and Tech's Future. The New York Times. Retrieved April 3, 2017, from https://www.nytimes.com/2016/03/26/technology/the-race-is-on-to-control-artificial-intelligence-and-techs-future.html?_r=0

Mitchell, T. M. (1997). *Machine Learning*. McGraw-Hill.

Moore, G. E. (1965). Cramming More Components Onto Integrated Circuits, Electronics, April 19, 1965. *Electronics (Basel)*, *38*(8), 82–85. doi:10.1109/JPROC.1998.658762

Rosenblatt, F. (1958). The perceptron: A probabilistic model for information storage and organization in the brain. [PubMed]. *Psychological Review*, *65*(6), 386–408. doi:10.1037/h0042519

Rughani, A. I., Dumont, T. M., Lu, Z., Bongard, J., Horgan, M. A., Penar, P. L., ... Object, V. (2010). Use of an artificial neural network to predict head injury outcome. [PubMed]. *Journal of Neurosurgery*, *113*(3), 585–590. doi:10.3171/2009.11.JNS09857

Salvador, R., Radua, J., Canales-Rodrõâguez, E. J., Solanes, A., Sarroa, S., Goikolea, J. M., ... Pomarol-Clote, E. (2017). Evaluation of machine learning algorithms and structural features for optimal MRI-based diagnostic prediction in psychosis. [PubMed]. *PLoS One*, *12*(4), 1–24. doi:10.1371/journal.pone.0175683

Samuel, A. L. (1959). Some Studies in Machine Learning Using the Game of Checkers. *IBM Journal of Research and Development*, *3*(3), 210–229. doi:10.1147/rd.33.0210

Statnikov, A., Aliferis, C. F., Hardin, D. P., & Guyon, I. (2011). A Gentle Introduction To Support Vector Machines. In *Biomedicine*. World Scientific Publishing Co Inc.

Vincent, J. (2017). AI star Andrew Ng announces departure from Chinese tech giant Baidu - The Verge. The Verge. Retrieved from http://www.theverge.com/2017/3/22/15020064/baidu-ai-andrew-ng-resigns

Wagstaff, K. (2012). Machine Learning that Matters. *Journal of the American Medical Informatics Association, 14*(5), 574–580. Retrieved from http://arxiv.org/abs/1206.4656

Waldrop, M. M. (2016). The chips are down for Moore's law. [PubMed]. *Nature, 530*(7589), 144–147. doi:10.1038/530144a

ADDITIONAL READING

Alanazi, H. O., Abdullah, A. H., & Qureshi, K. N. (2017). A Critical Review for Developing Accurate and Dynamic Predictive Models Using Machine Learning Methods in Medicine and Health Care. [PubMed]. *Journal of Medical Systems, 41*(4), 69. doi:10.100710916-017-0715-6

Anastasiou, A., Pitoglou, S., Androutsou, T., Kostalas, E., Matsopoulos, G., & Koutsouris, D. (2019). MODELHealth: An Innovative Software Platform for Machine Learning in Healthcare Leveraging Indoor Localization Services. In 2019 20th IEEE International Conference on Mobile Data Management (MDM) (pp. 443–446). IEEE. 10.1109/MDM.2019.000-5

Baer, T. (2019). *Understand, Manage, and Prevent Algorithmic Bias. Understand, Manage, and Prevent Algorithmic Bias*. Berkeley, CA: Apress; doi:10.1007/978-1-4842-4885-0

Beam, A. A. L., & Kohane, I. S. (2016). Translating Artificial Intelligence Into Clinical Care. [PubMed]. *Journal of the American Medical Association, 316*(22), 2368. doi:10.1001/jama.2016.17217

Beam, A. L., & Kohane, I. S. (2018). Big Data and Machine Learning in Health Care. [PubMed]. *Journal of the American Medical Association, 319*(13), 1317. doi:10.1001/jama.2017.18391

Bruffaerts, R. (2018). Machine learning in neurology: What neurologists can learn from machines and vice versa. [PubMed]. *Journal of Neurology, 265*(11), 2745–2748. doi:10.100700415-018-8990-9

Chen, J. H., & Asch, S. M. (2017). Machine Learning and Prediction in Medicine—Beyond the Peak of Inflated Expectations. [PubMed]. *The New England Journal of Medicine*, *376*(26), 2507–2509. doi:10.1056/NEJMp1702071

Cleophas, T. J., & Zwinderman, A. H. (2014). *Machine Learning in Medicine - Cookbook Two* (Vol. 49). Cham: Springer International Publishing; doi:10.1007/978-3-319-07413-9

Contreras, I., & Vehi, J. (2018). Artificial intelligence for diabetes management and decision support: Literature review. [PubMed]. *Journal of Medical Internet Research*, *20*(5), 1–21. doi:10.2196/10775

Darcy, A. M., Louie, A. K., & Roberts, L. W. (2016). Machine Learning and the Profession of Medicine. [PubMed]. *Journal of the American Medical Association*, *315*(6), 551–552. doi:10.1001/jama.2015.18421

De Bruijne, M. (2016). Machine learning approaches in medical image analysis: From detection to diagnosis. [PubMed]. *Medical Image Analysis*, *33*, 94–97. doi:10.1016/j.media.2016.06.032

Editorial. (2018). AI diagnostics need attention. Nature 555, 285. doi:10.1038/d41586-018-03067-x

Esteva, A., Kuprel, B., Novoa, R. A., Ko, J., Swetter, S. M., Blau, H. M., & Thrun, S. (2017). Dermatologist-level classification of skin cancer with deep neural networks. [PubMed]. *Nature*, *542*(7639), 115–118. doi:10.1038/nature21056

Forsting, M. (2017). Machine Learning Will Change Medicine. [PubMed]. *Journal of Nuclear Medicine*, *58*(3), 357–358. doi:10.2967/jnumed.117.190397

Futoma, J., Morris, J., & Lucas, J. (2015). A comparison of models for predicting early hospital readmissions. [PubMed]. *Journal of Biomedical Informatics*, *56*, 229–238. doi:10.1016/j.jbi.2015.05.016

Leung, M. K. K., Delong, A., Alipanahi, B., & Frey, B. J. (2016). Machine learning in genomic medicine: A review of computational problems and data sets. *Proceedings of the IEEE*. doi:10.1109/JPROC.2015.2494198

Mortazavi, B. J., Downing, N. S., Bucholz, E. M., Dharmarajan, K., Manhapra, A., Li, S. X., ... Krumholz, H. M. (2016). Analysis of Machine Learning Techniques for Heart Failure Readmissions. [PubMed]. *Circulation: Cardiovascular Quality and Outcomes*, *9*(6), 629–640. doi:10.1161/CIRCOUTCOMES.116.003039

Moumtzoglou, A. (2007). The future healthcare and quality. *International Journal of Health Care Quality Assurance*, *20*(4), 277–280. doi:10.1108/09526860710754343

Osuszek, L., Stanek, S., & Twardowski, Z. (2016). Leverage big data analytics for dynamic informed decisions with advanced case management. Journal of Decision Systems, 25(sup1), 436–449. doi:10.1080/12460125.2016.1187401

Pitoglou, S., Koumpouros, Y., & Anastasiou, A. (2019). Using Electronic Health Records and Machine Learning to Make Medical-Related Predictions from Non-Medical Data. *2018 International Conference on Machine Learning and Data Engineering (ICMLDE)*, 56–60. 10.1109/icmlde.2018.00021

Prosperi, M., Min, J. S., Bian, J., & Modave, F. (2018). Big data hurdles in precision medicine and precision public health. [PubMed]. *BMC Medical Informatics and Decision Making*, *18*(1), 1–15. doi:10.118612911-018-0719-2

Ravi, D., Wong, C., Deligianni, F., Berthelot, M., Andreu-Perez, J., Lo, B., ... Lo, B. (2017). Deep Learning for Health Informatics. [PubMed]. *IEEE Journal of Biomedical and Health Informatics*, *21*(1), 4–21. doi:10.1109/JBHI.2016.2636665

Semigran, H. L., Levine, D. M., Nundy, S., & Mehrotra, A. (2016). Comparison of Physician and Computer Diagnostic Accuracy. [PubMed]. *JAMA Internal Medicine*, *176*(12), 1860. doi:10.1001/jamainternmed.2016.6001

Shickel, B., Tighe, P. J., Bihorac, A., & Rashidi, P. (2017). Deep EHR: A Survey of Recent Advances in Deep Learning Techniques for Electronic Health Record (EHR) Analysis. [PubMed]. *IEEE Journal of Biomedical and Health Informatics*, *2194*(c), 1–17. doi:10.1109/JBHI.2017.2767063

Tripoliti, E. E., Papadopoulos, T. G., Karanasiou, G. S., Naka, K. K., & Fotiadis, D. I. (2017). Heart Failure: Diagnosis, Severity Estimation and Prediction of Adverse Events Through Machine Learning Techniques. [PubMed]. *Computational and Structural Biotechnology Journal*, *15*, 26–47. doi:10.1016/j.csbj.2016.11.001

Van Ginneken, B. (2017). Fifty years of computer analysis in chest imaging: Rule-based, machine learning, deep learning. [PubMed]. *Radiological Physics and Technology*, *10*(1), 23–32. doi:10.100712194-017-0394-5

Yao, Y., Sun, R., Poggio, T., Liu, J., Zhong, N., & Huang, J. (Eds.). (1999). Artificial Intelligence in Medicine. In Joint European Conference on Artificial Intelligence in Medicine and Medical Decision Making, AIMDM'99 Aalborg, Denmark, June 20-24, 1999 Proceedings. Aalborg, Denmark: Springer Berlin Heidelberg. 10.1007/978-3-642-15314-3

KEY TERMS AND DEFINITIONS

Artificial Neural Network (ANN): An artificial neuron network (ANN) is a nonlinear statistical data process inspired by the structure and functions of biological neurons, used for pattern recognition and modeling of complex input-output relationships. An ANN "learns" (adjusts its computational parameters) as information "flows" through its node layers, based on that input and output.

Big Data: Big data is an "umbrella term" that describes data processing approaches in situations where enormous and/or unstructured datasets cannot be efficiently manipulated via traditional handling techniques (e.g., relational databases).

Moore's Law: In 1965, Intel co-founder Gordon E. Moore observed that the number of transistors placed on an integrated circuit (IC) doubles approximately every two years. As this observation has been proven repeatedly, it became known as Moore's law.

Natural Language Processing (NLP): Natural language processing is an interdisciplinary field of computer science, artificial intelligence, and computational linguistics and deals with the interactions between computers and human (natural) languages. As a consequence, NLP is closely linked to human-computer interaction. Challenges in the NLP include understanding natural language, that is, trying to make computers capable of extracting meanings from human linguistic data, as well as producing natural language.

Chapter 5
Artificial Intelligence and Image Analysis for the Identification of Endometrial Malignancies:
A Comparative Study

Abraham Pouliakis
https://orcid.org/0000-0002-0074-3619
Second Department of Pathology, National and Kapodistrian University of Athens, Greece

Vasileia Damaskou
https://orcid.org/0000-0002-6584-8833
School of Medicine, Attikon University Hospital, Greece

Niki Margari
https://orcid.org/0000-0003-4975-8616
Independent Researcher, Greece

Efrossyni Karakitsou
Department of Biology, University of Barcelona, Spain

Vasilios Pergialiotis
Third Department of Obstetrics and Gynaecology, National and Kapodistrian University of Athens, Greece

George Valasoulis
https://orcid.org/0000-0003-4444-3711
Department of Obstetrics and Gynaecology, IASO Thessaly Hospital, Larissa, Greece

George Michail
Department of Obstetrics and Gynaecology, Patras University Medical School, Greece

Charalampos Chrelias
Third Department of Obstetrics and Gynaecology, National and Kapodistrian University of Athens, Greece

DOI: 10.4018/978-1-7998-2390-2.ch005

George Chrelias
Third Department of Obstetrics and Gynaecology, National and Kapodistrian University of Athens, Greece

Vasileios Sioulas
Third Department of Obstetrics and Gynaecology, National and Kapodistrian University of Athens, Greece

Alina-Roxani Gouloumi
Second Department of Pathology, National and Kapodistrian University of Athens, Greece

Nektarios Koufopoulos
https://orcid.org/0000-0001-9502-7916
Second Department of Pathology, National and Kapodistrian University of Athens, Greece

Martha Nifora
Second Department of Pathology, National and Kapodistrian University of Athens, Greece

Andriani Zacharatou
Second Department of Pathology, National and Kapodistrian University of Athens, Greece

Sophia Kalantaridou
Third Department of Obstetrics and Gynaecology, National and Kapodistrian University of Athens, Greece

Ioannis G. Panayiotides
Second Department of Pathology, National and Kapodistrian University of Athens, Greece

ABSTRACT

The aim of this study is to compare machine learning algorithms (MLAs) in the discrimination between benign and malignant endometrial nuclei and lesions. Nuclei characteristics are obtained via image analysis and were measured from liquid-based cytology slides. Four hundred sixteen histologically confirmed patients were involved, 168 healthy, and the remaining with pathological endometrium. Fifty percent of the cases were used to three MLAs: a feedforward artificial neural network (ANN) trained by the backpropagation algorithm, a learning vector quantization (LVQ), and a competitive learning ANN. The outcome of this process was the classification of cell nuclei as benign or malignant. Based on the nuclei classification, an algorithm to classify individual patients was constructed. The sensitivity of the MLAs in training set for nuclei classification was in the range of 77%-84%. Patients' classification had sensitivity in the range of 90%-98%. These findings indicate that MLAs have good performance for the classification of endometrial nuclei and lesions.

INTRODUCTION

The endometrium is a human system with inherent complexity because due to the cyclic regeneration during each menstrual cycle under estrogen effects. These effects, as well as, sex steroids, oncogene products, growth factors and peptides (Murphy, Murphy, & Friesen, 1987; Shyamala & Ferenczy, 1981) may cause pre-malignant and malignant transformation of the endometrium. Thus early diagnosis is crucial because it is strongly associated with patient management and on-time therapy. However, and despite the fact that the last decades the incidence of endometrial cancer has increased (Jemal, Siegel, Ward et al., 2006), there is no worldwide and well-established screening method for early detection of endometrial cancer or pre-malignant stages.

The standard procedure for the cytological evaluation of endometrial samples is the cytomorphological evaluation of Papanicolaou-stained direct smears. Despite there is long experience in this technique, there can be errors due to the sampling procedure and due to the remaining cells on the sampling device (Goodman & Hutchinson, 1996) and other errors due to the presence of protein, mucus and blood components (van der Graaf, Vooijs, Gaillard et al., 1987) that may obstruct the cytological view. Such errors can be avoided via liquid-based cytology (LBC). This technique gradually replaces the conventional direct smear preparations. LBC was initially applied for cervical cancer detection and now it is also applied in the assessment of endometrial lesions (Buccoliero, Gheri, Castiglione et al., 2007; Marasinghe, Chintana, Karunananda et al., 2007; Papaefthimiou, Symiakaki, Mentzelopoulou, Tsiveleka et al., 2005). LBC is combined with preparation of single-cell layer slides (mono-layer), thus facilitates the measurement of nuclear features, because cell overlap is reduced in mono-layer specimens. Therefore, an objective cytomorphological discrimination of lesions on the basis of shape and density features is facilitated, especially when such morphological features can be measured by computers.

Machine Learning and in general Artificial Intelligence (AI) techniques are not new in medicine (Almeida & Noble, 2000; Foran, Chen, & Yang, 2011; Grabe, Lahrmann, Pommerencke et al., 2010; Karakitsos, Ioakim-Liossi, Pouliakis et al., 1998; Krzysztof & Krzysztof, 2016; Luo, Ye, Ng et al., 2015; Markopoulos, Karakitsos, Botsoli-Stergiou, Pouliakis, Gogas et al., 1997; Pantazopoulos, Karakitsos, Iokim-Liossi, Pouliakis, Botsoli-Stergiou et al., 1998; Pitoglou, 2018; Salamalekis, Pouliakis, Margari et al., 2019; Seffens, Evans, Minority Health et al., 2015; Siristatidis, Pouliakis, Chrelias et al., 2011; Siristatidis, Vogiatzi, Pouliakis et al., 2016; Su, Xu, He et al., 2016; Vilhena, Vicente, Martins et al., 2017; Vogiatzi, Pouliakis, & Siristatidis, 2019). During the last decades, numerous applications have been reported; these involve either classical statistical models (Cochand-Priollet,

Koutroumbas, Megalopoulou et al., 2006; Georgoulakis, Pouliakis, Koutroumbas et al., 2008; Koutroumbas, Pouliakis, Megalopoulou et al., 2006; Megalopoulou, Koutroumbas, Pouliakis et al., 2006; Tzivras, Megalopoulou, Pouliakis et al., 2008) as well as more advanced techniques, such as neural networks. In the field of, oncology-related medical disciplines, and especially for cytopathology there have been reported numerous efforts (Karakitsos, Cochand-Priollet, Guillausseau et al., 1996; Karakitsos, Cochand-Priollet, Pouliakis et al., 1999; Karakitsos, Megalopoulou, Pouliakis et al., 2004; Karakitsos, Pouliakis, Kordalis et al., 2005; Karakitsos, Pouliakis, Koutroumbas et al., 2000; Karakitsos, Stergiou, Pouliakis et al., 1997; Karakitsos, Stergiou, Pouliakis et al., 1996; Markopoulos, Karakitsos, Botsoli-Stergiou, Pouliakis, Ioakim-Liossi et al., 1997; Pantazopoulos, Karakitsos, Iokim-Liossi, Pouliakis, & Dimopoulos, 1998; Pantazopoulos, Karakitsos, Pouliakis et al., 1998). Despite there is some literature related to endometrial cytological material evaluation by MLAs (Karakitsos, Kyroudes, Pouliakis et al., 2002; Pergialiotis, Pouliakis, Parthenis et al., 2018; Abraham Pouliakis, Margari, Margari et al., 2014; A. Pouliakis, Margari, Karakitsou et al., 2018; A. Pouliakis, Margari, Karakitsou et al., 2019; Zygouris, Pouliakis, Margari et al., 2014), to the authors' knowledge, up to date, publications reporting the comparison of MLAs' performance is rather poor. This is a well-known issue since there is no common method to report results and moreover the measurements used for the classifications are different.

In this report is presented a methodology aiming at the classification of endometrial lesions, this is based on cell nuclei morphometry data and AI. Initially, are presented the morphometrical features and their biological relation subsequently is presented the construction of machine learning systems classifying individual nuclei. According to these cell-nuclei classification results, there are constructed second stage classifiers that aim to classify individual cases (i.e. the patients). The validation is based on the histological result (golden standard), actually all patients that participate in the study had a histologically confirmed diagnosis that was concordant with the cytological result, moreover, a cytological LBC slide should was available in order to perform the image analysis and morphometry. There were selected three different Machine Learning Algorithms (MLAs), the feed-forward Artificial Neural Network (ANN) trained via the backpropagation algorithm, because solves classification problems via function approximation, the Learning Vector Quantizer (LVQ) ANN because by design provides solutions by creation of clusters and the competitive learning ANN because has a clustering approach, however, and in contrast to the two other MLAs is unsupervised. Finally, the applied classifiers are compared according to their performance and technical characteristics.

MATERIALS AND METHODS

Sample Collection and Processing

In this study, there were involved 416 patients, specifically women from which a cytological sample was taken from the endometrial cavity. The biological material was taken by the EndoGyn® Sampler (Biogyn S.n.c., Mirandola, Italy). The device was inserted in the endometrial cavity until the uterus fundus without the use of general anesthesia, and then it was rotated at least 4 times in order to extract cells and small tissue fragments. Subsequently, the sampling device was withdrawn, the material was immersed into a vial containing CytoLyt® solution (Cytyc Corporation). CytoLyt® solution is capable for proteinolysis, mucolysis and hemolysis, thus facilitates the material collection from the sampler and moreover provides the optimal environment to preserve the collected cells at temperatures from 4°C up to room temperature, for up to 7 days until the cells next step of the process, i.e. fixation (J. P. Baak, Kurver, Overdiep et al., 1981). Additionally, CytoLyt® reduces artifacts by removing all the unnecessary material collected during sampling (mainly mucus and blood). The use of this methodology (i.e. LBC) for material collection and preservation is very important, because, not only facilitates the cytological diagnosis through the microscope but provides a clear material for subsequent image analysis, as required by this study.

Subsequently, the vial with the biological material was sent to the cytopathology laboratory, where it was used to prepare a single cytological slide via an automated slide processor (ThinPrep® TP2000, Cytyc Corporation). This device prepares a smear in a 2 cm diameter area containing cell in a single layer with almost no overlap, the time for the slide preparation is 90 seconds. Subsequently, each slide was stained with Papanicolaou stain, using an automated staining machine (Varistain® 24-3 Thermo Electron Corporation [formerly Shandon], Runcorn, U.K.). The application of the slide processor and the procedure in general has many advantages: 1) leads to a representative smear of the collected biological material, 2) cells are mostly arranged in a mono-layer structure, which facilitates both the cytological diagnosis and the image analysis, since there is no cell overlapping, in contrast to conventional slides and 3) the area that requires microscopic examination is less that 50% (it is a 2cm circle) compared to the area of a conventional slide, therefore microscopic examination is faster.

Diagnosis

For every patient there were available the cytological and histological examination results, the second was obtained from biological material obtained via endometrial curettage and/or surgical specimen. To have such consistency, women without histological or cytological examination results were excluded from the study. Histological confirmation is important, as it is the golden standard and without this is not possible to have an accurate (i.e. acceptable by all medical community members) final diagnosis and therefore evaluate the results and performance of the proposed methodology.

The cytological diagnosis was based on the Fox (Fox, 1984) scheme and the histological diagnosis was according to the classification established by the International Society of Gynecological Pathology (Blaustein & Kurman, 2011) classification. In Table 1 is presented the histological outcome of the study cases, along with the total number of measured nuclei. We have involved cases that the cytological result was in agreement with the histological conclusion; otherwise, they were excluded from the study because the aim was to measure cell nuclei that have a confirmed histological agreement. The mean number of measured cell-nuclei from the total of the cytological slides (i.e. patients) in this study was 92.1±24.4.

Workflow of the Systems

The process applied for the classification of patients is depicted in Figure 1. The work-flow starts with the patient's cytological slide, this is analyzed via the image analysis workstation (see next section). Following the identification of individual nuclei and their measurement, is applied the MLA on the measurements; the MLA

Table 1. Histological classification of the studied cases along with the number of measured nuclei

	Histological Diagnosis	Number of cases	Number of nuclei measured
Benign	Proliferative	72	6,849
	Secretory	44	4,590
	Atrophy	48	4,317
	Disorder	4	361
	Polyp	24	2,310
	Hyperplasia without atypia	52	5,097
Malignant	Hyperplasia with atypia	20	1,643
	Endometrioid carcinoma	124	10,594
	Serous carcinoma	10	824
	Adenocarcinoma	18	1,741
	Total	**416**	**38,326**

outcome is the classification of every identified cell-nucleus in the slide in a bi-level approach, i.e. benign or malignant. The next stage is the workflow is a second classifier; this characterizes the patient to be into the benign or malignant category on the basis of the classification results for the nuclei after their measurement and subsequent classification by the MLA. Despite a more detailed classification of patients would be of interest, this approach clinically is very important as can serve as an alert for further patient management.

Image Analysis System, Measurements, and Their Biological Relation

Image analysis was performed on a workstation composed of a computer, equipped with a frame grabber and a digital camera (SONY DFW-X700, Sony Corporation, Tokyo, Japan). The microscope (Leica Microsystems GmbH, Wetzlar, Germany) had attached a color camera, all images were captured via a 40x objective lens. Images were digitized to 1024x768 pixels with 24 bits depth (8 bits for each color: red green and blue). Characteristic images with the segmented and subsequently measured nuclei are presented in Figure 2.

Two software packages were employed for the image analysis: PathSight version 4.3 (Medical Solutions PLC, UK) was used for image acquisition and light calibration and ImagePro Plus (Media Cybernetics, Inc. Bethesda, MD, USA) was used for nuclei segmentation and measurement. Light adjustment/calibration was made in the PathSight software environment, specifically the glass slide placed on the microscope was positioned to an empty field (i.e. without cells or background), subsequently the light intensity and the color look-up tables were adjusted in order to obtain mean value for the three color planes (red, green and blue) equal to standardized predefined values, this process was applied for every slide that was measured.

Background correction was performed with the ImagePro Plus software. This correction is required to remove noise due to remaining dust in the light path optical components and to correct non-uniformities of the lighting source. For this purpose an image of an empty field was captured, subsequently, this image was subtracted from every captured image containing the cells. Therefore, the effects of artifacts in the light path and the digitized image were alleviated.

Figure 1. Workflow for the classification of patients.

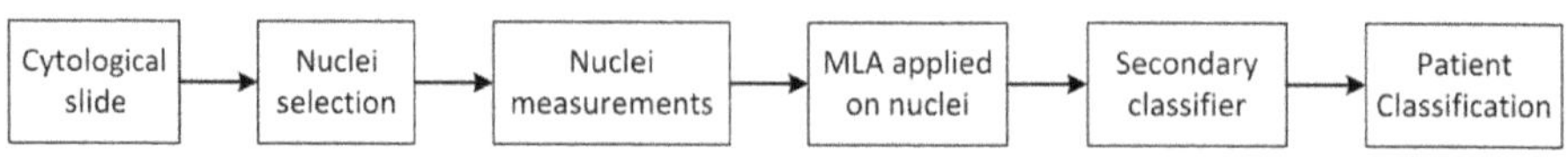

Figure 2. Cytological images from endometrial LBC samples with isolated nuclei left: image with benign (secretory endometrium) nuclei and right: image with endometrioid carcinoma nuclei.

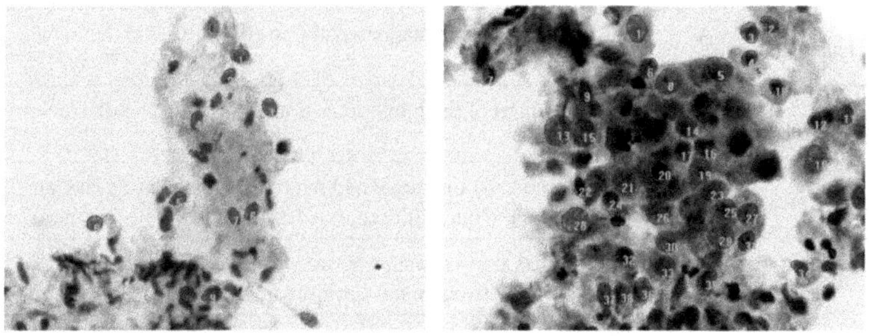

From each slide there we selected about 100 representative nuclei via a manual selection/segmentation process; this requires about 10 - 20 minutes, in practice, this is a process of definition of nuclei borderline. The characteristics measurement time following nuclei selection is negligible and was performed massively through software built in the programming language of ImagePro Plus. In total there were measured were 38,326 nuclei (Table 1) from the 416 slides. The features are summarized in Table 2 and details for the applied algorithms can be found in the literature. (J. P. A. Baak, 1991; Abraham Pouliakis, Margari, Margari, Chrelias, Zygouris, Meristoudis, Panayiotides, & Karakitsos, 2014; Russ, 1995; Sonka, Hlavac, & Boyle, 1993; Varlatzidou, Pouliakis, Stamataki et al., 2011)

There were two main categories of features: related to a) nucleus shape and b) nucleus density (i.e. pixel values) (Baxes, 1994; Bibbo, Bartels, Galera-Davidson et al., 1986; Haralick, Shanmugam, & Dinstein, 1973; Jain, 1989; Pitas, 2000; Sonka, Hlavac, & Boyle, 1993). Shape features are calculated from the nucleus boundary and are related to nucleus outline and size. In malignant cases and during carcinogenesis the nucleus skeleton, as well as, the cytoplasm skeleton are destroyed, therefore their shape is not similar to the healthy nuclei. The shape characteristics can reflect this nuclear alteration due to carcinogenesis or precancerous effects. The second group (density related characteristics) is relevant to the DNA quantity and status; these are measured from the pixels of each nucleus. Measurements of the nucleus color and texture on the basis on nucleus pixels may reflect the DNA amount and distribution; these are expressed via nuclear color characteristics, the optical density and textural characteristics (i.e. margination and heterogeneity).

These features were selected because they are related to the characteristics that cytopathologists examine during the routine microscopic examination. Specifically, cytopathologists during slide screening examine the nuclear size, boundary abnormalities, elongation of nuclei, and other shape-based characteristics of the

Table 2. Nuclear morphometry features involved in the study

	Feature	Description
Nucleus shape characteristics (boundary based)	Nucleus area	The area occupied by a nucleus expressed in square μm
	Nucleus major axis	The length of the major axis of an ellipse fitted o the nucleus (expressed in μm)
	Nucleus minor axis	The length of the minor axis of an ellipse fitted o the nucleus (expressed in μm)
	Aspect ratio	The ration of the major and minor axis considering that an ellipse is fitted to the nucleus (expressed as a number without units)
	Maximum caliper	The maximum distance between two perimeter points while the nucleus is between two parallel lines (expressed in μm)
	Minimum caliper	The minimum distance between two perimeter points while the nucleus is between two parallel lines (expressed in μm)
	Average value of caliper	The mean value of the distances measured between two perimeter points while the nucleus is between two parallel lines (expressed in μm)
	Maximum nucleus radius	The maximum distance between the nucleus centroid and the nucleus outline (the nucleus centroid is the center of nucleus mass when considering that the nucleus is uniform) (expressed in μm)
	Minimum nucleus radius	The minimum distance between the nucleus centroid and the nucleus outline (expressed in μm)
	Radius ratio	The ratio between the maximum and minimum radius (expressed as a number without units)
	Nucleus perimeter	The length of the nucleus boundary (expressed in μm)
	Nucleus roundness	Defined by the formula (Perimeter*Perimeter)/(4π*Area), it is an indication of the nucleus circularity, a perfectly circular nucleus has roundness equal to 1 while anything not perfectly circular has higher roundness, for example, the roundness of a square is 4/π=1.27 (expressed as a number without units)
	Fractal dimension	The fractal dimension of the nucleus boundary is an indication of repetitive patterns in the nucleus outline (Mandelbrot, 1983)

continues on following page

nuclei. Moreover, nucleus density (i.e. darkness), the distribution of DNA in the nucleus center or membrane as well as the texture caused by chromatin distribution (i.e. the existence of coarse or fine dots of chromatin in the nucleus) are important diagnostic characteristics. (Margari, Pouliakis, Anoinos et al., 2016)

Classification Targets

The primary target during diagnosis both in cytological and histological material is to discriminate between benign and malignant cases. Thus, the data were categorized into these two major categories: a) benign cases: i.e. histologically normal cases

Table 2. Continued

	Feature	Description
Nucleus density characteristics (pixel based)	Integrated optical density	The sum of the pixel values of the nucleus (when color is not considered) if the nucleus intensity is light and the area is large then integrated optical density becomes higher. Can be calculated the formula (Area)*(Mean optical density)
	Mean value of the nucleus red color	The average value of the nucleus pixels values of the red color plane, it is a number between 0 and 255
	Mean value of nucleus green color	The average value of the nucleus pixels values of the green color plane, it is a number between 0 and 255
	Mean value of nucleus blue color	The average value of the nucleus pixels values of the blue color plane, it is a number between 0 and 255
	Mean value of optical density	The average value of the nucleus pixels when color is not considered, it is a number between 0 and 255
	The maximum value of optical density	The maximum value that have the pixels inside the nucleus, it is a number between 0 and 255
	The minimum value of optical density	The minimum value that have pixels inside the nucleus, it is a number between 0 and 255
	The standard deviation of optical density	The standard deviation of the nucleus pixels when no color is considered, it is an indication of the range of gray values that has the nucleus
	Margination	The percentage of nucleus pixels that deviate more than 10% of the mean value of the nucleus density
	Heterogeneity	An index of homogeneity between the center of the nucleus and the borders, a homogeneous nucleus (i.e. all nuclei pixels have the same value) has heterogeneity = 0.33 while nuclei with the brighter center have higher heterogeneity. Heterogeneity is indicative of the distribution of DNA in the center of the nucleus membrane

including atrophy, secretory and proliferative endometrium, disordered endometrium, polyps and hyperplasias without atypia, and b) the group of malignant cases composed of the hyperplasias with atypia and the carcinomas (endometrioid, serous and adenocarcinomas) (Table 1).

Training and Test Sets

In order to respect the distribution of data to the relevant histological categories, 50% of the patients/cases (along with their nuclei) were randomly selected and were used as training set; the remaining nuclei (from the rest 50% of the cases) formed the test set. The distribution of the cases and the nuclei into the two sets are presented in Table 3. By this methodology was ensured that a) representative nuclei obtained via cytological material from all histological groups were included in both sets b) there was no mixing of patients' nuclei between the training set and test set and c) there was a balance between the training and test set.

Table 3. Distribution of the cases and the related cell nuclei into the training and test sets

		Number of cases (patients)			Number of cell nuclei		
	Histological Diagnosis	**Training set**	**Test set**	**Total**	**Training set**	**Test set**	**Total**
Benign	Proliferative	36	36	72	3,256	3,593	6,849
	Secretory	22	22	44	2,194	2,396	4,590
	Atrophy	24	24	48	2,081	2,236	4,317
	Disorder	2	2	4	181	180	361
	Polyp	12	12	24	1,214	1,096	2,310
	Hyperplasia without atypia	26	26	52	2,577	2,520	5,097
Malignant	Hyperplasia with atypia	10	10	20	773	870	1,643
	Endometrioid carcinoma	62	62	124	5,503	5,091	10,594
	Serous carcinoma	5	5	10	367	457	824
	Adenocarcinoma	9	9	18	792	949	1,741
	Total	**208**	**208**	**416**	**18,938**	**19,388**	**38,326**

Machine Learning and Tools

It was tested the performance of three different classifiers:

1. A multilayer feed-forward ANN (Haykin, 1999) trained by the backpropagation algorithm
2. The Learning Vector Quantization (LVQ) classifier (Teuvo Kohonen, 1989) and
3. A competitive learning ANN (Haykin, 1999; Rumelhart, McClelland, & University of California San Diego. PDP Research Group., 1986)

All these ML tools were implemented within the MATLAB environment and the available programming language (The MathWorks, Inc. Natick, Massachusetts, U.S.A.).

ANNs are complex mathematical models inspired by the human brain structure, they are capable of learning and pattern recognition. (Duda, Hart, & Stork, 2001; Theodoridis & Koutroumbas, 2009) This capability is suitable for classification and prediction tasks in numerous practical situations. The basic component of ANNs is artificial neuron (Figure 3). Neurons are inspired and have similarities with brain dendrite cells, where each neuron cell is interconnected with other neurons through

Figure 3. A typical model of an artificial neuron, inputs (I_1- I_n) are multiplied by weights (W_1- W_n), subsequently the products are summarized (block Σ) and finally the output is produced as the response of the non-linear function.

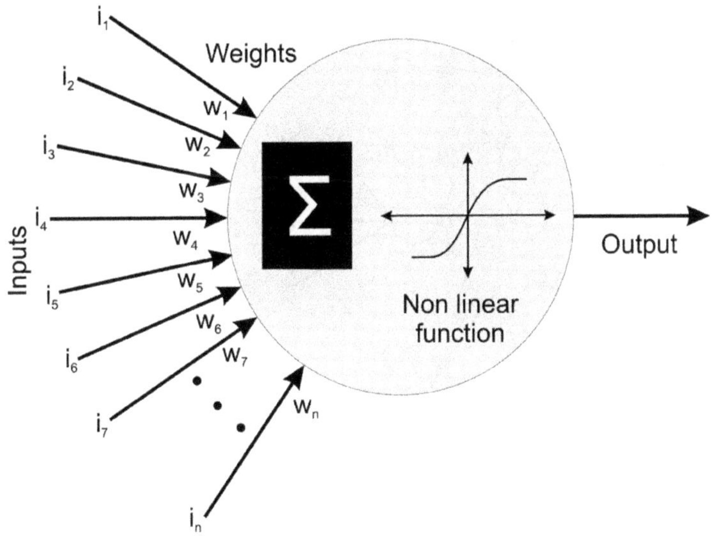

synapses. In ANNs neurons perform a relatively simple task: the inputs (i_1- i_N) are multiplied one by one by synaptic weight (ω_1- ω_N), the products are added, and the result is passed via a non-linear function which represents the artificial neuron output.

The capability of the ANNs to learn is due to the neurons' weights and the capability to address complex problems is due to the nonlinear function and architectures that interconnect many neurons together in several layers and the use of training (learning) algorithms.

The Multilayer Feed Forward ANN

A typical architecture of a multilayer feed-forward ANN is depicted in Figure 4. The data measurements form the inputs of the first layer of neurons (the input layer) where processing is performed, the outputs of the first layer, serve as inputs of the second layer (hidden layer), similarly, data are propagated and processed from layer to layer until they become inputs of the output layer. The results of this last layer are the ANN outputs.

Due to their design multilayer feed-forward, ANNs are ideal for function approximation, i.e. they create a function (through the weights, the non-linear component of the neurons as well as their interconnections) that maps the inputs to the outputs.

Figure 4. Multilayer architecture of a feed-forward ANN with two hidden layers, one input layer and one output layer.

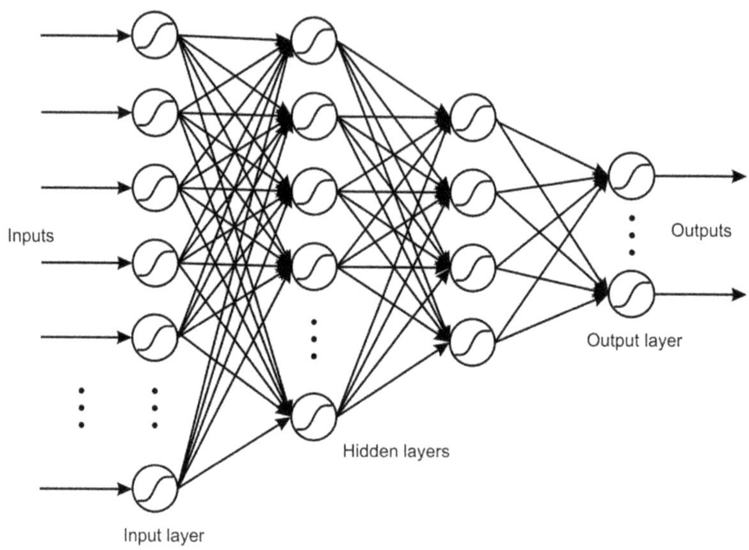

The LVQ Classifier

The LVQ is a supervised classifier, during the training phase LVQ creates partitions of the feature space, each partition is characterized by a vector in the center of the partition being called codebook vector; the class of the codebook vector characterizes the class of the complete partition. During training the codebook vectors are modified to represent the complete feature space; passing of all the training vectors to the classifier several times and by the application of a training algorithm LVQ based MLAs store the knowledge in the network components (i.e. in the codebook vectors). (Teuvo Kohonen, 1989; T. Kohonen, Kangas, Laaksonen et al., 1992)

During a test or operational phase, unknown vectors are presented to the LVQ, the class of each unknown vector is determined to be the same to the class of the partition that the unknown vector resides. This class is determined by identifying the codebook vector that is nearest to the unknown vector.

The Competitive Learning ANN

Competitive learning ANNs (Rumelhart, McClelland, & University of California San Diego. PDP Research Group., 1986) are unsupervised networks, their neurons compete to gain the right to respond for parts of the input data, this is performed by specialization of the nodes during training. These ANNs employ competition mechanisms that specific neurons have the right to respond for specific data subsets, in a way that only one output neuron responds each time in a "winner-take-all" manner.

These three different ANNs were selected to be evaluated on the data of the training set because they have different characteristics: the first ANN has the capability to map the problem through a function, the second as a clustering problem; while the third is capable to solve clustering problems, but in contrast to the first two ANNs this is unsupervised.

Cases Classification

We constructed case classifiers based on the result of nuclei classification by the MLAs using a method similar to a system proposed in the past for the classification of thyroid and endometrial lesions (Abraham Pouliakis, Margari, Margari, Chrelias, Zygouris, Meristoudis, Panayiotides, & Karakitsos, 2014; Varlatzidou, Pouliakis, Stamataki, Meristoudis, Margari, Peros, Panayiotides, & Karakitsos, 2011). This second stage classifiers are built on the basis of the percentage of nuclei classified as malignant from the MLAs. During the training of second stage classifiers, the aim is to find a threshold that optimizes patients' classification based on the training data. For this purpose we evaluated the case classification results for a broad range of thresholds; starting from 0% and increasing up to 100% (indicating the percentage of the patient's malignant nuclei as assigned by the MLA) the increment step was 0.1%. For each threshold value was calculated the number of cases that were true positive, true negative and false positive or false negative, thus it was possible to calculate the various performance indexes: sensitivity, specificity, Positive Predictive Value (PPV), Negative Predictive Value (NPV), False Positive Rate (FPR), False Negative Rate (FNR), Overall Accuracy (OA), odds ratio and Yuden's index. As an optimum threshold was selected the threshold that maximized the overall accuracy on the training cases. The software for the logic of the cases classifiers and the performance indices was implemented within the MATLAB environment.

RESULTS

Results are reported in two levels: a) the nuclei classification level where the MLAs were trained by the measurements obtained from the 18,938 nuclei of the training set (208 cases) and tested on the nuclei from the remaining 208 cases (19,388 measured nuclei) and b) the case classification level where the thresholds for the case classifiers were found on the basis of the training results obtained from the MLAs and subsequently tested on the rest of the cases.

Performance on Nuclei Classification

In terms of architectural characteristics the multilayer feed-forward ANN had 23 input neurons (equal to the number of measured nuclei features), 10 neurons in a single hidden layer and 1 neuron at the output layer, the output was set to 0.1 for the benign cases and to 0.9 for the malignant cases. It was employed the Levenberg-Marquardt back-propagation algorithm and 36 iterations over the training set were adequate to achieve a drop of the mean square error down to 0.087. In relation to the LVQ ANN the number of the nodes (codebook vectors) representing the number of clusters used to separate the data was 300, the results of the clusters' layer were fed to a second layer with 2 nodes in order to discriminate into the two target categories (benign and malignant), the number of iterations on the training data set was only 3. As training algorithm was used the LVQ.1 algorithm (T. Kohonen, Kangas, Laaksonen, & Torkkola, 1992). The training procedure for the LVQ ANN required much more computational resources than the feed-forward ANN. Finally the Competitive layer ANN was configured to separate data into two classes. All ANNs were trained and evaluated on the training set and subsequently evaluated on the test set and on the complete data set. The performance of all three ANNs is presented in Table 4.

Table 4. Performance of the Feed Forward, LVQ and Competitive Learning ANNs in nuclei classification for the training and test sets

	Feedforward ANN		LVQ		Competitive Learning	
	Training set	Test set	Training set	Test set	Training set	Test set
Sensitivity	78.58%	80.85%	74.05%	77.95%	81.79%	84.35%
Specificity	82.03%	88.86%	74.31%	73.93%	70.01%	69.07%
PPV	68.31%	67.14%	49.59%	50.50%	33.28%	33.50%
NPV	88.59%	89.72%	89.35%	90.77%	95.46%	95.98%
FPR	17.97%	19.14%	25.69%	26.06%	29.99%	30.93%
FNR	21.42%	19.14%	25.95%	22.05%	18.21%	15.65%
OA	80.86%	80.86%	74.24%	74.96%	71.83%	71.45%
Odds Ratio	16.75	17.84	8.25	10.03	10.48	12.04
Youden Index	60.61%	61.72%	48.36%	51.89%	51.80%	53.43%

Case Classification Results Analysis and Performance Metrics

For the case classification system based on the feed-forward ANN training results, the threshold that maximized the overall accuracy was 35% (i.e. if a case had more than 35% of the measured nuclei classified by the feed-forward ANN as malignant, then it was assigned to the malignant group). The sensitivity, specificity, PPV, and NPV were respectively 98.84%, 92.62%, 90.43% and 99.12% on the test set. The performance metrics for this case classifier appear in Table 5 for the training and test set separately. In detail this classifier predicted correctly 228 benign cases (115 in the training set and 113 in the test set) and missed 16 cases by classifying them as malignant (see Table 6), from the histologically malignant cases; 169 cases were classified correctly and 3 cases were misclassified.

Out of the 16 benign misclassified cases 3 were histologically polyps, 2 atrophy, 6 proliferative, 2 disordered and 3 hyperplasias without atypia; out of these cases only the 2 atrophy cases and the 6 proliferative cases may be considered as normal endometrium while the remaining 8 cases indicate an endometrial issue, especially the three cases of hyperplasia without atypia may pose diagnostic dilemmas during the cytological examination. Out of the three misclassified malignant cases, one was hyperplasia with atypia and two endometrioid carcinomas, as in the case of hyperplasia without atypia, hyperplasias with atypia are difficult to diagnose in cytology. Moreover, the percentage of nuclei classified as malignant for these cases

Table 5. Performance indices of the cases classifier on the basis of the MLP and LVQ outcomes (training and test sets)

	Case classifier based on the Feedforward ANN results		**Case classifier based on LVQ classifier results**		**Case classifier based on the competitive layer ANN results**	
	Training set	**Test set**	**Training set**	**Test set**	**Training set**	**Test set**
Sensitivity	97.67%	98.84%	93.02%	90.70%	94.19%	93.02%
Specificity	94.26%	92.62%	86.89%	82.79%	87.70%	80.33%
PPV	92.31%	90.43%	83.33%	78.79%	84.38%	76.92%
NPV	98.29%	99.12%	94.64%	92.66%	95.54%	94.23%
FPR	5.74%	7.38%	13.11%	17.21%	12.30%	19.67%
FNR	2.33%	1.16%	6.98%	9.30%	5.81%	6.98%
OA	96.67%	95.19%	89.42%	86.06%	90.38%	85.58%
Odds Ratio	690.00	1067.22	88.33	46.89	115.56	54.44
Youden Index	91.94%	91.46%	79.91%	73.48%	81.89%	73.35%

by the feed-forward ANN was 30.77%, 28.42%, and 33.67% respectively; these percentages are near the identified threshold (35%), thus the use of a safety area around the identified threshold, whereas cases falling in this area are marked as uncertain, maybe of some value.

The case classifier based on the results on the LVQ outcome missed 14 malignant cases and 37 benign cases (Table 6) resulting in a sensitivity and specificity on the test set equal to 90.70% and 82.79% respectively (Table 5). Finally, the case classifier that was based the competitive learning ANN results, had a sensitivity and specificity on the test set equal 93.02% and 80.33% respectively (Table 5) and missed 11 malignant cases and 39 benign (Table 6).

Table 6. Cross-tabulation of the assignment of the cases for the three tested classifiers according to the histological group. Results are presented separately for the training and test sets

		Assigned Category		
	Case classifier based on the feed-forward ANN			
Histological result		**Benign**	**Malignant**	**Grand Total**
Training set	Benign	115	7	122
	Malignant	2	84	86
Test Set	Benign	113	9	122
	Malignant	1	85	86
	Grand total	231	185	416
	Case classifier based on the LVQ ANN			
Histological result		**Benign**	**Malignant**	**Grand Total**
Training set	Benign	106	16	122
	Malignant	6	80	86
Test Set	Benign	101	21	122
	Malignant	8	78	86
	Grand total	221	195	416
	Case classifier based on the Competitive learning ANN			
Histological result		**Benign**	**Malignant**	**Grand Total**
Training set	Benign	107	15	122
	Malignant	5	81	86
Test Set	Benign	98	24	122
	Malignant	6	80	86
	Grand total	216	200	416

Definitely, the feed-forward based classifier had better performance than LVQ and the competitive layer ANN. Thus a solution based on a function approximation seems to fit better on the nuclei and cases classification problem. It is worth noting that from the 19 cases missed by the feed-forward based case classifier, 15 cases were missed by the LVQ based classifier and the 13 by the competitive learning classifier. Specifically, the LVQ identified correctly two atrophy cases, one polyp, and one endometrioid carcinoma while misclassified the remaining 15 cases that misclassified the feed-forward ANN. Similarly, the competitive learning ANN identified correctly two more cases (one endometrioid carcinoma and one proliferative) and misclassified the same 13 cases that were misclassified both by the feed-forward ANN and the LVQ. This fact indicates that all three classifiers have many similarities and tend to misclassify the same specific cases. Furthermore from the 51 cases missed by the LVQ based case classifier and the 51 cases missed by the competitive learning, based classifier 42 were in common.

Role of Nuclei Features

In order to investigate the role of the selected nuclei features, it was performed the analysis of effects by the Fisher scoring method (Longford, 1987) on the training set measurements, in this test the most influential features for discrimination have the highest score (chi-square) while the statistical significance is indicated by the p-value. The ranked results are presented in *Table 7*, the 8 most important features are related to shape characteristics while density characteristics are ranked after the 9th position.

In order to highlight the role of features in the two major histological groups, the mean value and standard deviation of each feature for the histologically benign and malignant nuclei was calculated (using the combined data of the training and test set). The t-test indicates that there are statistically significant differences between the two groups for all features, the examination of the mean values and standard deviation indicates that there is overlap for feature values (Table 8) and that malignant nuclei are in general larger (mean value of area 41.61 μm2) than the benign nuclei (mean value of area 21.94 μm2) however their size has a higher variation, as the standard deviation (24.30) is more than two times the standard deviation of the benign nuclei (9.99). Similar variations do exist in almost all nuclei characteristics.

DISCUSSION

Endometrial carcinoma is the most common malignancy of the female genital tract (Papaefthimiou, Symiakaki, Mentzelopoulou, Tsiveleka, Kyroudes, Voulgaris,

Table 7. Analysis of effects via Fisher scoring

Rank order	Effect	Score (Chi-Square)	p
1	Average value of caliper	5619.60	<.0001
2	Nucleus perimeter	5375.47	<.0001
3	Maximum caliper	5294.80	<.0001
4	Nucleus major axis	5239.83	<.0001
5	Maximum nucleus radius	5212.34	<.0001
6	Nucleus area	4830.90	<.0001
7	Minimum caliper	4712.01	<.0001
8	Nucleus minor axis	4640.54	<.0001
9	Integrated optical density	4209.97	<.0001
10	Minimum nucleus radius	4068.65	<.0001
11	Margination	1351.83	<.0001
12	Mean value of nucleus blue color	1168.46	<.0001
13	Maximum value of optical density	1154.24	<.0001
14	Mean value of nucleus red color	920.16	<.0001
15	Mean value of optical density	877.48	<.0001
16	Heterogeneity	772.50	<.0001
17	Standard deviation of optical density	742.70	<.0001
18	Mean value of nucleus green color	425.12	<.0001
19	Fractal dimension	202.65	<.0001
20	Aspect ratio	201.60	<.0001
21	The minimum value of optical density	110.28	<.0001
22	Radius ratio	71.05	<.0001
23	Nucleus roundness	56.20	<.0001

Tzonou, & Karakitsos, 2005; Parazzini, La Vecchia, Bocciolone et al., 1991), it affects women at reproductive age and after menopause as well. Mean age of diagnosis in the USA is 60 years,(American Cancer Society, 2005) in the UK is 61 years(Soliman, Oh, Schmeler et al., 2005) and in European countries is 63. (Colombo, Preti, Landoni et al., 2013) The probability of carcinoma is as follows: 0% for women younger than 20, 1.6% for women between 20–34 years, 6.1% for women between 35–44 years, 19.2% for women aged 45–54, 31.8% for women between 55–64 years, 22.1% for women between 65–74, 14.2% for women aged 75–84 and 4.8% for women older than 84. (Howlader, Noone, Krapcho et al., 2011) The most frequent symptom of endometrial carcinoma is postmenopausal bleeding;(ACOG, 2005) but, only 10% of the women with postmenopausal bleeding have endometrial

Table 8. Mean value, standard deviation and t-test results for the nuclei feature for the histologically benign and malignant cases

	Histologically benign nuclei		Histologically malignant nuclei			
Feature	**Mean value**	**Standard deviation**	**Mean value**	**Standard deviation**	**t-test**	**p**
Nucleus area	21.94	9.99	41.61	24.30	-110.22	<.0001
Nucleus major axis	6.07	1.49	8.46	2.57	-114.92	<.0001
Nucleus minor axis	4.46	1.02	5.94	1.71	-106.41	<.0001
Aspect ratio	1.39	0.31	1.46	0.37	-20.10	<.0001
Maximum caliper	6.05	1.49	8.42	2.54	-115.49	<.0001
Minimum caliper	4.37	1.02	5.87	1.71	-107.29	<.0001
Average value of caliper	5.29	1.18	7.27	2.04	-120.41	<.0001
Maximum nucleus radius	3.11	0.77	4.34	1.33	-114.15	<.0001
Minimum nucleus radius	2.01	0.50	2.68	0.84	-97.86	<.0001
Radius ratio	1.61	1.33	1.85	2.92	-10.65	<.0001
Nucleus perimeter	16.57	3.78	22.94	6.85	-117.14	<.0001
Nucleus roundness	1.12	0.15	1.14	0.15	-10.97	<.0001
Fractal dimension	1.06	0.01	1.06	0.03	12.81	<.0001
Integrated optical density	1891.10	1176.98	4052.27	3015.11	-98.64	<.0001
Mean value of nucleus red color	71.90	23.78	81.85	24.65	-39.31	<.0001
Mean value of nucleus green color	68.72	25.83	75.53	23.47	-26.01	<.0001
Mean value of nucleus blue color	112.35	26.12	124.62	27.31	-44.00	<.0001
Mean value of optical density	84.32	24.26	94.00	24.37	-37.95	<.0001
Maximum value of optical density	135.16	33.27	150.69	36.37	-42.93	<.0001
Minimum value of optical density	64.20	21.85	66.83	19.28	-11.99	<.0001
Standard deviation of optical density	12.85	5.26	14.68	5.34	-33.01	<.0001
Margination	0.37	0.02	0.36	0.02	53.44	<.0001
Heterogeneity	0.06	0.07	0.08	0.09	-33.46	<.0001

carcinoma,(Iatrakis, Diakakis, Kourounis et al., 1997; Taskin, Bozaci, Seval et al., 2006) moreover 5-10% of endometrial carcinoma cases are asymptomatic. (Smith-Bindman, Kerlikowske, Feldstein et al., 1998) In an autopsy study, the rate of undetected endometrial carcinomas was 26.6 per 10,000. (Horwitz, Feinstein, Horwitz et al., 1981) According to the American National Institute of Health (NIH), and specifically the Surveillance, Epidemiology and End Result (SEER) program, the number of new cases of endometrial cancer for 2016 is estimated to be 60,050 with 10,470 deaths. The age-adjusted rates based on 2009-2013 data; was 25.4 endometrial cancers per 100,000 women per year. The number of deaths is 4.5 per 100,000 women per year. Moreover the lifetime riskof developing endometrial cancer is approximately 2.8% of women will be diagnosed with endometrial cancer at some point during their lifetime (based on 2011-2013 data). In 2013, there was estimated that 635,437 women were living with endometrial cancer in the United States. According to the World Health Organization, there are worldwide 188,000 new endometrial carcinomas every year. According to GLOBOCAN, the endometrial cancer age-standardized rate for 2012 is 8.2 per 100,000 for the world and for Japan (a sole country that is applied endometrial cancer screening) the incidence is significantly reduced to 3.9 per 100,000.

The cytological examination of the endometrium by cytopathology experts can be a very subjective process, at first there is no measurement procedure; instead, cellular morphology and cell formations are evaluated by the eye according to the cytopathologists' experience, this process is very dependent on the training and the skills of the cytopathologists. Second, the criteria to conclude towards a diagnosis are complex and sometimes overlapping thus making the diagnosis process extremely difficult. Therefore, endometrial cytology is not the standard and worldwide accepted method for the investigation of endometrial malignancies. (Kaur, Chahal, Bandlish et al., 2014; Papaefthimiou, Symiakaki, Mentzelopoulou, Tsiveleka, Kyroudes, Voulgaris, Tzonou, & Karakitsos, 2005; Reagan, 1980; Tezuka, Namiki, & Higashiiwai, 1992) As a consequence, there are new proposed classification systems/reporting systems (Fulciniti, Yanoh, Karakitsos et al., 2018; J. A. Maksem, Meiers, & Robboy, 2007; Margari, Pouliakis, Anoinos, Terzakis, Koureas, Chrelias, Marios Makris, Pappas, Bilirakis, Goudeli, Damaskou, Papantoniou, Panayiotides, & Karakitsos, 2016) and not consistent management of patients. (Ferenczy & Bergeron, 1992).

During the last decade, cytopathology was suggested by many researchers as an alternative or ancillary to Dilatation and Curettage (D&C) diagnostic tool,(Buccoliero, Castiglione, Gheri et al., 2007; Fambrini, Buccoliero, Bargelli et al., 2008; Garcia, Barker, Davis et al., 2003; Kipp, Medeiros, Campion et al., 2008; Kyroudi, Paefthimiou, Symiakaki et al., 2006; Papaefthimiou, Symiakaki, Mentzelopoulou, Giahnaki et al., 2005; Papaefthimiou, Symiakaki, Mentzelopoulou,

Tsiveleka, Kyroudes, Voulgaris, Tzonou, & Karakitsos, 2005; Sams, Currens, & Raab, 2012) being nowadays the standard procedure. According to various studies (Karakitsos, Kyroudes, Pouliakis, Stergiou, Voulgaris, & Kittas, 2002; Papaefthimiou, Symiakaki, Mentzelopoulou, Giahnaki, Voulgaris, Diakomanolis, Kyroudes, & Karakitsos, 2005; Papaefthimiou, Symiakaki, Mentzelopoulou, Tsiveleka, Kyroudes, Voulgaris, Tzonou, & Karakitsos, 2005) morphological characteristics of nuclei have an important role in endometrial cytology diagnosis irrelevant of the technique (conventional or LBC); in addition characteristics of structures formed by the observed cells (contextual characteristics) are important as well. The application of LBC is in line with the objectivity requirements, as advantages of LBC are related to common diagnostic approach, because there is standardized procedure related to fixation, transfer, and cyto-preparation of the biological material; additionally observed cellular overlap is related to the real 3 dimensional structures and not due to the slide preparation methods, finally the cells are layered in non-overlapping sheets, a fact that facilitates their measurement. The proposed methodology introduces additional objectivity in two levels: first cell nuclei are measured in a reproducible manner (a procedure facilitated by LBC) and secondly, these characteristics are evaluated via computerized algorithms.

According to the results, all three tested ANN-based classifiers gave promising results, the classifier that solved the problem via a function approximation gave better results than the two classifiers that had a clustering approach, whilst the two clustering classifiers had similar performance. Moreover, it seems that all classifiers have the tendency to misclassify the same cases.

Obviously, the performance of the three MLAs on nuclei classification is worse than the performance of the complete system for the classification of cases. For instance, the sensitivity on the test set for nuclei classification ranges from 77.95% to 84.35%, and the PPV is within the range 33.50% - 67.14%, depending on the MLP (*Table 4*), while the sensitivity of the complete system on case classification is between 90.70% and 98.84% and the PPV between 76.92% and 90.43% (*Table 5*). This performance improvement is due to the second stage classification system and the application of the optimal threshold that maximizes the overall accuracy (on the training set).

In the literature the reported performance of endometrial cytology is different, according to Maksem et.al.,(J.A. Maksem, Robboy, Bishop et al., 2009) endometrial cytology without the aid of cell block or immunocytochemistry and using hysterectomy as golden standard; has sensitivity 88%, specificity 92%, PPV 79%, and NPV 95% (2,133 cases). The addition of cell block examination is reported to increase the overall accuracy for benign/atrophic endometrium and adenocarcinoma discrimination to 96% and 100% respectively. According to Norimatsu et.al, (Norimatsu, Yanoh, & Kobayashi, 2013), the use of LBC yielded human-based sensitivity and specificity equal to 96.4 and 100%, respectively, with PPV and NPV 100 and 98.9%, respectively (118 cases). The sensitivity of the proposed classifiers on the test set (208 cases) was 98.84%, 90.70%, and 93.02% and the specificity 92.62%, 82.79% and 80.33% for the forward ANN, LVQ and competitive layer ANN respectively (see table 5).

Artificial intelligence has been widely applied in medicine and leads to new methods in aiding towards a more accurate and specific manner and making the proper decision. (Adams, Bello, & Dumancas, 2015; Cruz & Wishart, 2006; Darcy, Louie, & Roberts, 2016; Giacomini, Ruggiero, Calegari et al., 2000; Karar & El-Brawany, 2011; Mouwen, Capita, Alonso-Calleja et al., 2006; A. Pouliakis, Karakitsou, Margari et al., 2016) This application of endometrial cytological diagnosis may help to overcome the subjective nature of the standard evaluation, being related to the lack of consensus in a measuring process and common diagnostic criteria. These may result in poor reproducibility, and significant interobserver and intraobserver variability. (Reagan, 1980; Tezuka, Namiki, & Higashiiwai, 1992) The presented results may be inscribed in the wider context of encouraging findings of the performance of cytology in the diagnosis of endometrial cancer. (Papaefthimiou, Symiakaki, Mentzelopoulou, Giahnaki, Voulgaris, Diakomanolis, Kyroudes, & Karakitsos, 2005; Sams, Currens, & Raab, 2012; Yanoh, Norimatsu, Hirai et al., 2009) Nuclear morphological characteristics seem to play a central role in this context, a finding which has been observed in previous studies as well. (Karakitsos, Kyroudes, Pouliakis, Stergiou, Voulgaris, & Kittas, 2002; Papaefthimiou, Symiakaki, Mentzelopoulou, Giahnaki, Voulgaris, Diakomanolis, Kyroudes, & Karakitsos, 2005; Papaefthimiou, Symiakaki, Mentzelopoulou, Tsiveleka, Kyroudes, Voulgaris, Tzonou, & Karakitsos, 2005; Abraham Pouliakis, Margari, Margari, Chrelias, Zygouris, Meristoudis, Panayiotides, & Karakitsos, 2014) The rationale behind this is the fact that carcinogenesis causes destruction of the cellular structure and especially the nucleoskeleton thus resulting in nuclear deformations. Shape characteristics reflect such changes, while the second group of density characteristics reflects nucleus DNA changes. Despite nuclear morphological characteristics can be evaluated both by conventional and liquid-based cytology; the latter contributes towards standardization due to lysis of mucus and blood using a standardized procedure, standardized fixation, transfer and cytological preparation of the biological material and in this study by improving image analysis due to the reduction of cell overlapping.

FUTURE RESEARCH DIRECTIONS AND STUDY LIMITATIONS

The nuclei selection/segmentation process applied in this study is manual, specifically two experienced cytopathologist have chosen the nuclei that will be measured and moreover defined the nuclei boundaries. This process may be prone to errors both for nuclei selection as well as for nuclei segmentation. To alleviate the nuclei selection issues there were selected nuclei that both cytopathologists agreed on their nature (i.e. they were either benign or malignant), moreover, both cytopathologists agreed that nuclei borders were correctly defined. The time to manually select about 100 nuclei from a slide ranges from 10-20 minutes, while the time required for the microscopic examination is in the range of 5–10 minutes. However for non-experienced cytopathologists, the time for diagnosis may be much higher than 10 minutes and eventually, a second opinion may be requested.

Random selection of nuclei in this non-automated process is not expected to improve the results, as for the malignant cases the cytological slides contain benign and malignant cells. Specifically, the percentage of benign nuclei is by far higher than the percentage of malignant. This should not be an issue in fully automated systems where all nuclei of a slide would be classified one by one.

Note that aim of this paper is not to propose a fully automated system being capable to 1) scan a cytological slide, 2) detect nuclei, 3) measure them and finally 4) classify the slide (i.e. patient) as benign or malignant. Our aim is to compare classifiers when nuclei measurements are already available, thus we propose a subsystem that has the potential to be a part of a completed automated system.

Automated systems, especially for cervical cytopathology, have been proposed (Mellors & Silver, 1951) just a decade after test Papanicolaou appearance (Diamantis, Magiorkinis, & Koutselini, 2014; Papanicolaou & Traut, 1941), since then, various system generations have been evolved, this offer increased automation (Bengtsson & Malm, 2014). To the authors' knowledge, there are no such systems for the evaluation of endometrial cytological slides, moreover, systems targeting cervical material cannot be applied in endometrial images, because cell characteristics and appearance are so different in cervical and endometrial cell images.

A solution towards a fully automated system could be the application of deep ANNs. Recently, algorithms based on deep learning have shown impressive performance in machine vision applications including medical image processing and histopathology image analysis (Chen & Chefd'hotel, 2014; Ciresan, Giusti, Gambardella et al., 2013; Sirinukunwattana, Raza, Tsang et al., 2016). Deep learning ANNs have the same architecture as feed-forward ANNs (see Figure 4), but in contrast to classical feed-forward ANNs the number of hidden layers is greater than the standard than one or at most two hidden layers are incorporated. Their main advantage is that they do not need predefined features; as they can learn features from the data; therefore, perform well in image recognition and classification tasks (Chen & Chefd'hotel, 2014; Ciresan, Giusti, Gambardella, & Schmidhuber, 2013; Lai, 2015; Sirinukunwattana, Raza, Tsang, Snead, Cree, & Rajpoot, 2016) directly from image pixels. To the authors' knowledge, deep ANNs have not been applied yet in cytopathology images, however, their performance in histological images indicate that their potential is very promising in cytology as well (A. Pouliakis, Karakitsou, Margari, Bountris, Haritou, Panayiotides, Koutsouris, & Karakitsos, 2016), moreover software systems have been designed and proposed to serve such medical facilities (Perroti, Pouliakis, Margari et al., 2018; Siristatidis, Vogiatzi, Pouliakis, Trivella, Papantoniou, & Bettocchi, 2016).

After slide preparation the remaining genetic material in the LBC vial can be used to assess genetic or molecular markers by the use of medical analyzers; for example through human or viral DNA / mRNA detection. Recently, has been reported that image features can be related to such markers; for example morphologic characteristics of histological slides could be correlated to BRAF gene mutations in papillary thyroid carcinomas,(Finkelstein, Levy, Hui et al., 2012; Virk, Theoharis, Prasad et al., 2014; Virk, Van Dyke, Finkelstein et al., 2013) in cytological images there is just one study reporting similar (Margari, Pouliakis, Spathis et al., 2015). However, there is no report correlating image features and molecular markers for endometrial cytological images.

CONCLUSION

Concluding, the proposed objective approach using ANNs, gave promising results in the discrimination between malignant and benign endometrial cases, one MLA had very good performance and two other MLAs showed encouraging results, the integration of this technique in the laboratory routine may become a useful adjunct in the future leading towards a more objective diagnosis of endometrial malignancies.

REFERENCES

ACOG. (2005). ACOG practice bulletin, clinical management guidelines for obstetrician-gynecologists, number 65, August 2005: Management of endometrial cancer. *Obstetrics and Gynecology*, *106*(2), 413–425. PMID:16055605

Adams, L. J., Bello, G., & Dumancas, G. G. (2015). Development and Application of a Genetic Algorithm for Variable Optimization and Predictive Modeling of Five-Year Mortality Using Questionnaire Data. *Bioinformatics and Biology Insights*, *9*(Suppl 3), 31–41. doi:10.4137/BBI.S29469 PMID:26604716

Almeida, J. S., & Noble, P. A. (2000). Neural computing in microbiology. *Journal of Microbiological Methods*, *43*(1), 1–2. doi:10.1016/S0167-7012(00)00200-1 PMID:11084224

American Cancer Society. (2005). *Detailed Guide: Endometrial Cancer: What are the Risk Factors for Endometrial Cancer?* Retrieved 20 March 2015, 2015, from http://www.cancer.org/cancer/endometrialcancer/detailedguide/endometrial-uterine-cancer-risk-factors

Baak, J. P., Kurver, P. H., Overdiep, S. H., Delemarre, J. F., Boon, M. E., Lindeman, J., & Diegenbach, P. C. (1981). Quantitative, microscopical, computer-aided diagnosis of endometrial hyperplasia or carcinoma in individual patients. *Histopathology, 5*(6), 689–695. doi:10.1111/j.1365-2559.1981.tb01835.x PMID:7033100

Baak, J. P. A. (1991). *Manual of quantitative pathology in cancer diagnosis and prognosis*. Berlin: Springer-Verlag.

Baxes, G. A. (1994). *Digital image processing: principles and applications* (1st ed.). New York: Wiley.

Bengtsson, E., & Malm, P. (2014). Screening for Cervical Cancer Using Automated Analysis of PAP-Smears. *Computational and Mathematical Methods in Medicine, 12*. doi:10.1155/2014/842037 PMID:24772188

Bibbo, M., Bartels, P. H., Galera-Davidson, H., Dytch, H. E., & Wied, G. L. (1986). Markers for malignancy in the nuclear texture of histologically normal tissue from patients with thyroid tumors. *Analytical and Quantitative Cytology and Histology, 8*(2), 168–176. PMID:2425826

Blaustein, A., & Kurman, R. J. (2011). *Blaustein's pathology of the female genital tract* (6th ed.). New York, NY: Springer.

Buccoliero, A. M., Castiglione, F., Gheri, C. F., Garbini, F., Fambrini, M., Bargelli, G., ... Taddei, G. L. (2007). Liquid-based endometrial cytology: Its possible value in postmenopausal asymptomatic women. *International Journal of Gynecological Cancer, 17*(1), 182–187. doi:10.1111/j.1525-1438.2006.00757.x PMID:17291251

Buccoliero, A. M., Gheri, C. F., Castiglione, F., Garbini, F., Barbetti, A., Fambrini, M., ... Taddei, G. L. (2007). Liquid-based endometrial cytology: Cyto-histological correlation in a population of 917 women. *Cytopathology, 18*(4), 241–249. doi:10.1111/j.1365-2303.2007.00463.x PMID:17559564

Chen, T., & Chefd'hotel, C. (2014). Deep Learning Based Automatic Immune Cell Detection for Immunohistochemistry Images. In G. Wu, D. Zhang, & L. Zhou (Eds.), *Machine Learning in Medical Imaging* (Vol. 8679, pp. 17–24). Springer International Publishing. doi:10.1007/978-3-319-10581-9_3

Ciresan, D. C., Giusti, A., Gambardella, L. M., & Schmidhuber, J. (2013). Mitosis detection in breast cancer histology images with deep neural networks. *Med Image Comput Comput Assist Interv*, *16*(Pt 2), 411–418. PMID:24579167

Cochand-Priollet, B., Koutroumbas, K., Megalopoulou, T. M., Pouliakis, A., Sivolapenko, G., & Karakitsos, P. (2006). Discriminating benign from malignant thyroid lesions using artificial intelligence and statistical selection of morphometric features. *Oncology Reports*, *15*(Spec no), 1023–1026. PMID:16525694

Colombo, N., Preti, E., Landoni, F., Carinelli, S., Colombo, A., Marini, C., & Sessa, C. (2013). Endometrial cancer: ESMO Clinical Practice Guidelines for diagnosis, treatment and follow-up. *Annals of Oncology: Official Journal of the European Society for Medical Oncology*, *24*(Suppl 6), vi33–vi38. doi:10.1093/annonc/mdt353 PMID:24078661

Cruz, J. A., & Wishart, D. S. (2006). Applications of machine learning in cancer prediction and prognosis. *Cancer Informatics*, *2*, 59–77. doi:10.1177/117693510600200030 PMID:19458758

Darcy, A. M., Louie, A. K., & Roberts, L. W. (2016). Machine Learning and the Profession of Medicine. *Journal of the American Medical Association*, *315*(6), 551–552. doi:10.1001/jama.2015.18421 PMID:26864406

Diamantis, A., Magiorkinis, E., & Koutselini, H. (2014). 50 years after the death of George Nicholas Papanicolaou (1883-1962): Evaluation of his scientific work. *Acta Medico-Historica Adriatica: AMHA*, *12*(1), 181–188. PMID:25310617

Duda, R. O., Hart, P. E., & Stork, D. G. (2001). *Pattern classification* (2nd ed.). New York: Wiley.

Fambrini, M., Buccoliero, A. M., Bargelli, G., Cioni, R., Piciocchi, L., Pieralli, A., ... Marchionni, M. (2008). Clinical utility of liquid-based cytology for the characterization and management of endometrial polyps in postmenopausal age. *International Journal of Gynecological Cancer*, *18*(2), 306–311. doi:10.1111/j.1525-1438.2007.01019.x PMID:17624992

Ferenczy, A., & Bergeron, C. (1992). Endometrial hyperplasia. In D. Lowe & H. Fox (Eds.), *Advances in Gynaecological Pathology* (pp. 207–234). Edinburgh, UK: Churchill Livingstone.

Finkelstein, A., Levy, G. H., Hui, P., Prasad, A., Virk, R., Chhieng, D. C., ... Prasad, M. L. (2012). Papillary thyroid carcinomas with and without BRAF V600E mutations are morphologically distinct. *Histopathology*, *60*(7), 1052–1059. doi:10.1111/j.1365-2559.2011.04149.x PMID:22335197

Foran, D. J., Chen, W., & Yang, L. (2011). Automated image interpretation computer-assisted diagnostics. *Analytical Cellular Pathology (Amsterdam)*, *34*(6), 279–300. doi:10.1155/2011/239761 PMID:22082571

Fox, H. (1984). The endometrial hyperplasias. *Obstetrics and Gynecology Annual*, *13*, 197–209. PMID:6371615

Fulciniti, F., Yanoh, K., Karakitsos, P., Watanabe, J., Di Lorito, A., Margari, N., ... Hirai, Y. (2018). The Yokohama system for reporting directly sampled endometrial cytology: The quest to develop a standardized terminology. *Diagnostic Cytopathology*, *46*(5), 400–412. doi:10.1002/dc.23916 PMID:29479846

Garcia, F., Barker, B., Davis, J., Shelton, T., Harrigill, K., Schalk, N., ... Hatch, K. (2003). Thin-layer cytology and histopathology in the evaluation of abnormal uterine bleeding. *The Journal of Reproductive Medicine*, *48*(11), 882–888. PMID:14686021

Georgoulakis, J., Pouliakis, A., Koutroumbas, K., Megalopoulou, T. M., Archontakis, S., Kataitianos, I. G., ... Karakitsos, P. (2008). Discrimination of benign from malignant breast lesions using statistical clasifiers. *Archives of the Balkan Medical Union*, *43*(3), 149–153.

Giacomini, M., Ruggiero, C., Calegari, L., & Bertone, S. (2000). Artificial neural network based identification of environmental bacteria by gas-chromatographic and electrophoretic data. *Journal of Microbiological Methods*, *43*(1), 45–54. doi:10.1016/S0167-7012(00)00203-7 PMID:11084227

Goodman, A., & Hutchinson, M. L. (1996). Cell surplus on sampling devices after routine cervical cytologic smears. A study of residual cell populations. *The Journal of Reproductive Medicine*, *41*(4), 239–241. PMID:8728075

Grabe, N., Lahrmann, B., Pommerencke, T., von Knebel Doeberitz, M., Reuschenbach, M., & Wentzensen, N. (2010). A virtual microscopy system to scan, evaluate and archive biomarker enhanced cervical cytology slides. *Cellular Oncology*, *32*(1-2), 109–119. doi:10.3233/CLO-2009-0508 PMID:20208139

Haralick, R. M., Shanmugam, K., & Dinstein, I. H. (1973). Textural Features for Image Classification. *Systems, Man and Cybernetics. IEEE Transactions on*, *3*(6), 610–621.

Haykin, S. S. (1999). *Neural networks: a comprehensive foundation* (2nd ed.). Upper Saddle River, NJ: Prentice Hall.

Horwitz, R. I., Feinstein, A. R., Horwitz, S. M., & Robboy, S. J. (1981). Necropsy diagnosis of endometrial cancer and detection-bias in case/control studies. *Lancet*, *2*(8237), 66–68. doi:10.1016/S0140-6736(81)90412-8 PMID:6113441

Howlader, N., Noone, A. M., Krapcho, M., Neyman, N., Aminou, R., Waldron, W., … Edwards, B. K. (2011). *SEER Cancer Statistics Review, 1975-2008*. Retrieved 10 January 2015, 2015, from http://seer.cancer.gov/archive/csr/1975_2008/

Iatrakis, G., Diakakis, I., Kourounis, G., Sakellaropoulos, G., Rammos, G., Ladopoulos, J., ... Tzingounis, V. (1997). Postmenopausal uterine bleeding. *Clinical and Experimental Obstetrics & Gynecology*, *24*(3), 157. PMID:9478305

Jain, A. K. (1989). *Fundamentals of digital image processing* (1st ed.). Englewood Cliffs, NJ: Prentice Hall.

Jemal, A., Siegel, R., Ward, E., Murray, T., Xu, J., Smigal, C., & Thun, M. J. (2006). Cancer statistics, 2006. *CA: a Cancer Journal for Clinicians*, *56*(2), 106–130. doi:10.3322/canjclin.56.2.106 PMID:16514137

Karakitsos, P., Cochand-Priollet, B., Guillausseau, P. J., & Pouliakis, A. (1996). Potential of the back propagation neural network in the morphologic examination of thyroid lesions. *Analytical and Quantitative Cytology and Histology*, *18*(6), 494–500. PMID:8978873

Karakitsos, P., Cochand-Priollet, B., Pouliakis, A., Guillausseau, P. J., & Ioakim-Liossi, A. (1999). Learning vector quantizer in the investigation of thyroid lesions. *Analytical and Quantitative Cytology and Histology*, *21*(3), 201–208. PMID:10560492

Karakitsos, P., Ioakim-Liossi, A., Pouliakis, A., Botsoli-Stergiou, E. M., Tzivras, M., Archimandritis, A., & Kyrkou, K. (1998). A comparative study of three variations of the learning vector quantizer in the discrimination of benign from malignant gastric cells. *Cytopathology*, *9*(2), 114–125. doi:10.1046/j.1365-2303.1998.00063.x PMID:9577738

Karakitsos, P., Kyroudes, A., Pouliakis, A., Stergiou, E. B., Voulgaris, Z., & Kittas, C. (2002). Potential of the learning vector quantizer in the cell classification of endometrial lesions in postmenopausal women. *Analytical and Quantitative Cytology and Histology*, *24*(1), 30–38. PMID:11865947

Karakitsos, P., Megalopoulou, T. M., Pouliakis, A., Tzivras, M., Archimandritis, A., & Kyroudes, A. (2004). Application of discriminant analysis and quantitative cytologic examination to gastric lesions. *Analytical and Quantitative Cytology and Histology*, *26*(6), 314–322. PMID:15678613

Karakitsos, P., Pouliakis, A., Kordalis, G., Georgoulakis, J., Kittas, C., & Kyroudes, A. (2005). Potential of radial basis function neural networks in discriminating benign from malignant lesions of the lower urinary tract. *Analytical and Quantitative Cytology and Histology*, *27*(1), 35–42. PMID:15794450

Karakitsos, P., Pouliakis, A., Koutroumbas, K., Stergiou, E. B., Tzivras, M., Archimandritis, A., & Liossi, A. I. (2000). Neural network application in the discrimination of benign from malignant gastric cells. *Analytical and Quantitative Cytology and Histology*, *22*(1), 63–69. PMID:10696462

Karakitsos, P., Stergiou, E. B., Pouliakis, A., Tzivras, M., Archimandritis, A., Liossi, A., & Kyrkou, K. (1997). Comparative study of artificial neural networks in the discrimination between benign from malignant gastric cells. *Analytical and Quantitative Cytology and Histology*, *19*(2), 145–152. PMID:9113307

Karakitsos, P., Stergiou, E. B., Pouliakis, A., Tzivras, M., Archimandritis, A., Liossi, A. I., & Kyrkou, K. (1996). Potential of the back propagation neural network in the discrimination of benign from malignant gastric cells. *Analytical and Quantitative Cytology and Histology*, *18*(3), 245–250. PMID:8790840

Karar, M. E., & El-Brawany, M. A. (2011). Automated Cardiac Drug Infusion System Using Adaptive Fuzzy Neural Networks Controller. *Biomedical Engineering and Computational Biology*, *3*, 1-11. doi:10.4137/BECB.S6495

Kaur, N., Chahal, J. S., Bandlish, U., Kaul, R., Mardi, K., & Kaur, H. (2014). Correlation between cytological and histopathological examination of the endometrium in abnormal uterine bleeding. *Journal of Cytology / Indian Academy of Cytologists*, *31*(3), 144–148. doi:10.4103/0970-9371.145645 PMID:25538383

Kipp, B. R., Medeiros, F., Campion, M. B., Distad, T. J., Peterson, L. M., Keeney, G. L., ... Clayton, A. C. (2008). Direct uterine sampling with the Tao brush sampler using a liquid-based preparation method for the detection of endometrial cancer and atypical hyperplasia: A feasibility study. *Cancer*, *114*(4), 228–235. doi:10.1002/cncr.23636 PMID:18548528

Kohonen, T. (1989). *Self-organization and associative memory* (3rd ed.). Berlin: Springer-Verlag. doi:10.1007/978-3-642-88163-3

Kohonen, T., Kangas, J., Laaksonen, J., & Torkkola, K. (1992). *LVQPAK: A software package for the correct application of Learning Vector Quantization algorithms.* Paper presented at the Neural Networks, 1992. IJCNN., International Joint Conference on.

Koutroumbas, K., Pouliakis, A., Megalopoulou, T., Georgoulakis, J., Giachnaki, A.-E., & Karakitsos, P. (2006). Discrimination of Benign from Malignant Breast Lesions Using Statistical Classifiers. In G. Antoniou, G. Potamias, C. Spyropoulos, & D. Plexousakis (Eds.), *Advances in Artificial Intelligence* (Vol. 3955, pp. 543–546). Springer Berlin Heidelberg. doi:10.1007/11752912_64

Krzysztof, W., & Krzysztof, P. M. (2016). Translation of Medical Texts using Neural Networks. *International Journal of Reliable and Quality E-Healthcare*, *5*(4), 51–66. doi:10.4018/IJRQEH.2016100104

Kyroudi, A., Paefthimiou, M., Symiakaki, H., Mentzelopoulou, P., Voulgaris, Z., & Karakitsos, P. (2006). Increasing diagnostic accuracy with a cell block preparation from thin-layer endometrial cytology: A feasibility study. *Acta Cytologica*, *50*(1), 63–69. doi:10.1159/000325896 PMID:16514842

Lai, M. (2015). *Deep Learning for Medical Image Segmentation.* preprint arXiv, arXiv:1505.02000.

Longford, N. T. (1987). A fast scoring algorithm for maximum likelihood estimation in unbalanced mixed models with nested random effects. *Biometrika*, *74*(4), 817–827. doi:10.1093/biomet/74.4.817

Luo, H., Ye, H., Ng, H. W., Shi, L., Tong, W., Mendrick, D. L., & Hong, H. (2015). Machine Learning Methods for Predicting HLA-Peptide Binding Activity. *Bioinformatics and Biology Insights*, *9*(Suppl 3), 21–29. doi:10.4137/BBI.S29466 PMID:26512199

Maksem, J. A., Meiers, I., & Robboy, S. J. (2007). A primer of endometrial cytology with histological correlation. *Diagnostic Cytopathology*, *35*(12), 817–844. doi:10.1002/dc.20745 PMID:18008351

Maksem, J. A., Robboy, S. J., Bishop, J. W., & Meiers, I. (2009). *Endometrial Cytology with Tissue Correlations*. New York: Springer US.

Mandelbrot, B. B. (1983). The fractal geometry of nature (Updated and augm. ed.). New York: W.H. Freeman.

Marasinghe, J. P., Chintana, H. D., Karunananda, S. A., & Amarasinghe, A. A. (2007). Liquid-based endometrial cytology: its possible value in postmenopausal asymptomatic women. *Int J Gynecol Cancer, 17*(4), 934; author reply 935. doi:10.1111/j.1525-1438.2007.00918.x

Margari, N., Pouliakis, A., Anoinos, D., Terzakis, E., Koureas, N., Chrelias, C., ... Karakitsos, P. (2016). A reporting system for endometrial cytology: Cytomorphologic criteria-Implied risk of malignancy. *Diagnostic Cytopathology*, *44*(11), 888–901. doi:10.1002/dc.23605 PMID:27653446

Margari, N., Pouliakis, A., Spathis, A., Mastorakis, E., Karakostas, E. S. S., Panayiotides, I., & Karakitsos, P. (2015). Quality Control and Telemedicine for BRAF V600E Mutations in Papillary Thyroid Carcinomas: Image Analysis and Classification and Regression Trees. *International Journal of Reliable and Quality E-Healthcare*, *4*(2), 12–30. doi:10.4018/IJRQEH.2015040102

Markopoulos, C., Karakitsos, P., Botsoli-Stergiou, E., Pouliakis, A., Gogas, J., Ioakim-Liossi, A., & Kyrkou, K. (1997). Application of back propagation to the diagnosis of breast lesions by fine needle aspiration. *The Breast*, *6*(5), 293–298. doi:10.1016/S0960-9776(97)90008-4

Markopoulos, C., Karakitsos, P., Botsoli-Stergiou, E., Pouliakis, A., Ioakim-Liossi, A., Kyrkou, K., & Gogas, J. (1997). Application of the learning vector quantizer to the classification of breast lesions. *Analytical and Quantitative Cytology and Histology*, *19*(5), 453–460. PMID:9349906

Megalopoulou, T. M., Koutroumbas, K., Pouliakis, A., Sivolapenko, G., & Karakitsos, P. (2006). The potential of feature selection by statistical techniques and the use of statistical classifiers in the discrimination of benign from malignant gastric lesions. *Oncology Reports*, *15*(Spec no), 1033–1036. PMID:16525696

Mellors, R. C., & Silver, R. (1951). A micro-fluorometric scanner for the differential detection of cells; application of exfoliative cytology. *Science*, *114*(2962), 356–360. doi:10.1126cience.114.2962.356 PMID:14883859

Mouwen, D. J., Capita, R., Alonso-Calleja, C., Prieto-Gomez, J., & Prieto, M. (2006). Artificial neural network based identification of Campylobacter species by Fourier transform infrared spectroscopy. *Journal of Microbiological Methods*, *67*(1), 131–140. doi:10.1016/j.mimet.2006.03.012 PMID:16632003

Murphy, L. J., Murphy, L. C., & Friesen, H. G. (1987). Estrogen induces insulin-like growth factor-I expression in the rat uterus. *Molecular Endocrinology (Baltimore, Md.)*, *1*(7), 445–450. doi:10.1210/mend-1-7-445 PMID:2484720

Norimatsu, Y., Yanoh, K., & Kobayashi, T. K. (2013). The role of liquid-based preparation in the evaluation of endometrial cytology. *Acta Cytologica*, *57*(5), 423–435. doi:10.1159/000353148 PMID:24021666

Pantazopoulos, D., Karakitsos, P., Iokim-Liossi, A., Pouliakis, A., Botsoli-Stergiou, E., & Dimopoulos, C. (1998). Back propagation neural network in the discrimination of benign from malignant lower urinary tract lesions. *The Journal of Urology*, *159*(5), 1619–1623. doi:10.1097/00005392-199805000-00057 PMID:9554366

Pantazopoulos, D., Karakitsos, P., Iokim-Liossi, A., Pouliakis, A., & Dimopoulos, K. (1998). Comparing neural networks in the discrimination of benign from malignant lower urinary tract lesions. *British Journal of Urology*, *81*(4), 574–579. doi:10.1046/j.1464-410x.1998.00587.x PMID:9598630

Pantazopoulos, D., Karakitsos, P., Pouliakis, A., Iokim-Liossi, A., & Dimopoulos, M. A. (1998). Static cytometry and neural networks in the discrimination of lower urinary system lesions. *Urology*, *51*(6), 946–950. doi:10.1016/S0090-4295(98)00024-7 PMID:9609631

Papaefthimiou, M., Symiakaki, H., Mentzelopoulou, P., Giahnaki, A. E., Voulgaris, Z., Diakomanolis, E., ... Karakitsos, P. (2005). The role of liquid-based cytology associated with curettage in the investigation of endometrial lesions from postmenopausal women. *Cytopathology*, *16*(1), 32–39. doi:10.1111/j.1365-2303.2004.00224.x PMID:15859313

Papaefthimiou, M., Symiakaki, H., Mentzelopoulou, P., Tsiveleka, A., Kyroudes, A., Voulgaris, Z., ... Karakitsos, P. (2005). Study on the morphology and reproducibility of the diagnosis of endometrial lesions utilizing liquid-based cytology. *Cancer*, *105*(2), 56–64. doi:10.1002/cncr.21025 PMID:15751019

Papanicolaou, G., & Traut, H. (1941). The diagnostic value of vaginal smears in carcinoma of the uterus. *American Journal of Obstetrics and Gynecology*, *42*(2), 193–206. doi:10.1016/S0002-9378(16)40621-6

Parazzini, F., La Vecchia, C., Bocciolone, L., & Franceschi, S. (1991). The epidemiology of endometrial cancer. *Gynecologic Oncology*, *41*(1), 1–16. doi:10.1016/0090-8258(91)90246-2 PMID:2026352

Pergialiotis, V., Pouliakis, A., Parthenis, C., Damaskou, V., Chrelias, C., Papantoniou, N., & Panayiotides, I. (2018). The utility of artificial neural networks and classification and regression trees for the prediction of endometrial cancer in postmenopausal women. *Public Health*, *164*, 1–6. doi:10.1016/j.puhe.2018.07.012 PMID:30149185

Perroti, R., Pouliakis, A., Margari, N., Panopoulou, E., Karakitsou, E., Iliopoulou, D., ... Koutsouris, D. D. (2018). CytoNet, A Versatile Web-Based System for Accessing Advisory Cytology Services: Application of Artificial Intelligence. *International Journal of Reliable and Quality E-Healthcare*, *7*(3), 37–56. doi:10.4018/IJRQEH.2018070103

Pitas, I. (2000). *Digital image processing algorithms and applications* (1st ed.). New York: Wiley.

Pitoglou, S. (2018). Machine Learning in Healthcare, Introduction and Real World Application Considerations. *International Journal of Reliable and Quality E-Healthcare*, *7*(2), 27–36. doi:10.4018/IJRQEH.2018040102

Pouliakis, A., Karakitsou, E., Margari, N., Bountris, P., Haritou, M., Panayiotides, J., ... Karakitsos, P. (2016). Artificial Neural Networks as Decision Support Tools in Cytopathology: Past, Present, and Future. *Biomedical Engineering and Computational Biology*, *7*, 1–18. doi:10.4137/BECB.S31601 PMID:26917984

Pouliakis, A., Margari, C., Margari, N., Chrelias, C., Zygouris, D., Meristoudis, C., ... Karakitsos, P. (2014). Using classification and regression trees, liquid-based cytology and nuclear morphometry for the discrimination of endometrial lesions. *Diagnostic Cytopathology*, *42*(7), 582–591. doi:10.1002/dc.23077 PMID:24273089

Pouliakis, A., Margari, N., Karakitsou, E., Alamanou, E., Koureas, N., Chrelias, G., ... Karakitsos, P. (2018). Artificial Intelligence for the Identification of Endometrial Malignancies: Application of the Learning Vector Quantizer. *International Journal of Reliable and Quality E-Healthcare*, *7*(2), 37–50. doi:10.4018/IJRQEH.2018040103

Pouliakis, A., Margari, N., Karakitsou, E., Valasoulis, G., Koufopoulos, N., Koureas, N., ... Panayiotides, I. G. (2019). Artificial Intelligence via Competitive Learning and Image Analysis for Endometrial Malignancies: Discriminating Endometrial Cells and Lesions. *International Journal of Reliable and Quality E-Healthcare*, *8*(4), 38–54. doi:10.4018/IJRQEH.2019100102

Reagan, J. W. (1980). Can screening for endometrial cancer be justified? *Acta Cytologica*, *24*(2), 87–89. PMID:6768202

Rumelhart, D. E., McClelland, J. L., & University of California San Diego. PDP Research Group. (1986). *Parallel distributed processing: explorations in the microstructure of cognition*. Cambridge, MA: MIT Press.

Russ, J. C. (1995). *The image processing handbook* (2nd ed.). Boca Raton, FL: CRC Press.

Salamalekis, E., Pouliakis, A., Margari, N., Kottaridi, C., Spathis, A., Karakitsou, E., ... Chrelias, C. (2019). An Artificial Intelligence Approach for the Detection of Cervical Abnormalities: Application of the Self Organizing Map. *International Journal of Reliable and Quality E-Healthcare*, *8*(2), 15–35. doi:10.4018/IJRQEH.2019040102

Sams, S. B., Currens, H. S., & Raab, S. S. (2012). Liquid-based Papanicolaou tests in endometrial carcinoma diagnosis. Performance, error root cause analysis, and quality improvement. *American Journal of Clinical Pathology*, *137*(2), 248–254. doi:10.1309/AJCPLFBK1A2XJDQI PMID:22261450

Seffens, W., Evans, C., Minority Health, G. N., & Taylor, H. (2015). Machine Learning Data Imputation and Classification in a Multicohort Hypertension Clinical Study. *Bioinformatics and Biology Insights*, *9*(Suppl 3), 43–54. doi:10.4137/BBI.S29473 PMID:27199552

Shyamala, G., & Ferenczy, A. (1981). The effect of sodium molybdate on the cytoplasmic estrogen and progesterone receptors in human endometrial tissues. *Diagnostic Gynecology and Obstetrics*, *3*(4), 277–282. PMID:7200003

Sirinukunwattana, K., Raza, S., Tsang, Y. W., Snead, D., Cree, I., & Rajpoot, N. (2016). Locality Sensitive Deep Learning for Detection and Classification of Nuclei in Routine Colon Cancer Histology Images. *IEEE Transactions on Medical Imaging*, *35*(5), 1196–1206. doi:10.1109/TMI.2016.2525803 PMID:26863654

Siristatidis, C., Pouliakis, A., Chrelias, C., & Kassanos, D. (2011). Artificial intelligence in IVF: A need. *Systems Biology in Reproductive Medicine*, *57*(4), 179–185. doi:10.3109/19396368.2011.558607 PMID:21375363

Siristatidis, C., Vogiatzi, P., Pouliakis, A., Trivella, M., Papantoniou, N., & Bettocchi, S. (2016). Predicting IVF Outcome: A Proposed Web-based System Using Artificial Intelligence. *In Vivo (Athens, Greece)*, *30*(4), 507–512. PMID:27381616

Smith-Bindman, R., Kerlikowske, K., Feldstein, V. A., Subak, L., Scheidler, J., Segal, M., ... Grady, D. (1998). Endovaginal ultrasound to exclude endometrial cancer and other endometrial abnormalities. *Journal of the American Medical Association*, *280*(17), 1510–1517. doi:10.1001/jama.280.17.1510 PMID:9809732

Soliman, P. T., Oh, J. C., Schmeler, K. M., Sun, C. C., Slomovitz, B. M., Gershenson, D. M., ... Lu, K. H. (2005). Risk factors for young premenopausal women with endometrial cancer. *Obstetrics and Gynecology*, *105*(3), 575–580. doi:10.1097/01.AOG.0000154151.14516.f7 PMID:15738027

Sonka, M., Hlavac, V., & Boyle, R. (1993). *Image processing, analysis, and machine vision* (1st ed.). London: Chapman & Hall Computing. doi:10.1007/978-1-4899-3216-7

Su, J., Xu, X., He, Y., & Song, J. (2016). Automatic Detection of Cervical Cancer Cells by a Two-Level Cascade Classification System. *Analytical Cellular Pathology (Amsterdam)*, *9535027*. doi:10.1155/2016/9535027 PMID:27298758

Taskin, S., Bozaci, E. A., Seval, M. M., & Unlu, C. (2006). Transvaginal sonographic assessment of endometrial thickness and endometrial morphology in postmenopausal bleeding. *International Journal of Gynaecology and Obstetrics: the Official Organ of the International Federation of Gynaecology and Obstetrics*, *92*(2), 155–156. doi:10.1016/j.ijgo.2005.10.023 PMID:16360156

Tezuka, F., Namiki, T., & Higashiiwai, H. (1992). Observer variability in endometrial cytology using kappa statistics. *Journal of Clinical Pathology*, *45*(4), 292–294. doi:10.1136/jcp.45.4.292 PMID:1577966

Theodoridis, S., & Koutroumbas, K. (2009). *Pattern recognition* (4th ed.). London: Academic Press.

Tzivras, M., Megalopoulou, T. M., Pouliakis, A., Giahnaki, A. E., Karaitianos, I. G., Archondakis, S., ... Karakitsos, P. (2008). The potential of tree classifiers on the cytological examination of gastric lesions. *Archives of the Balkan Medical Union*, *43*(4), 239–244.

van der Graaf, Y., Vooijs, G. P., Gaillard, H. L., & Go, D. M. (1987). Screening errors in cervical cytologic screening. *Acta Cytologica*, *31*(4), 434–438. PMID:3604538

Varlatzidou, A., Pouliakis, A., Stamataki, M., Meristoudis, C., Margari, N., Peros, G., ... Karakitsos, P. (2011). Cascaded learning vector quantizer neural networks for the discrimination of thyroid lesions. *Analytical and Quantitative Cytology and Histology*, *33*(6), 323–334. PMID:22590810

Vilhena, J., Vicente, H., Martins, M. R., Grañeda, J., Caldeira, F., Gusmão, R., ... Neves, J. I. (2017). An Artificial Intelligence Approach to Thrombophilia Risk. *International Journal of Reliable and Quality E-Healthcare*, *6*(2), 49–69. doi:10.4018/IJRQEH.2017040105

Virk, R. K., Theoharis, C. G., Prasad, A., Chhieng, D., & Prasad, M. L. (2014). Morphology predicts BRAF (V600E) mutation in papillary thyroid carcinoma: An interobserver reproducibility study. *Virchows Archiv*, *464*(4), 435–442. doi:10.100700428-014-1552-3 PMID:24549591

Virk, R. K., Van Dyke, A. L., Finkelstein, A., Prasad, A., Gibson, J., Hui, P., ... Prasad, M. L. (2013). BRAFV600E mutation in papillary thyroid microcarcinoma: A genotype-phenotype correlation. *Modern Pathology*, *26*(1), 62–70. doi:10.1038/modpathol.2012.152 PMID:22918165

Vogiatzi, P., Pouliakis, A., & Siristatidis, C. (2019). An artificial neural network for the prediction of assisted reproduction outcome. *Journal of Assisted Reproduction and Genetics*, *36*(7), 1441–1448. doi:10.100710815-019-01498-7 PMID:31218565

Yanoh, K., Norimatsu, Y., Hirai, Y., Takeshima, N., Kamimori, A., Nakamura, Y., ... Shiraishi, T. (2009). New diagnostic reporting format for endometrial cytology based on cytoarchitectural criteria. *Cytopathology*, *20*(6), 388–394. doi:10.1111/j.1365-2303.2008.00581.x PMID:18657157

Zygouris, D., Pouliakis, A., Margari, N., Chrelias, C., Terzakis, E., Koureas, N., ... Karakitsos, P. (2014). Classification of endometrial lesions by nuclear morphometry features extracted from liquid-based cytology samples: A system based on logistic regression model. *Analytical and Quantitative Cytopathology and Histopathology*, *36*(4), 189–198. PMID:25291856

KEY TERMS AND DEFINITIONS

Artificial Intelligence (AI): It is also called machine intelligence. The term is used often to for machines (i.e., computers) that can mimic some cognitive functions of humans, for example learning/recognizing or solving problems.

Artificial Neural Networks (ANNs): They are complex computational models inspired by the human brain nervous system, capable of learning and pattern recognition (an AI-related branch).

Cytopathology: A specialty of medicine relevant to the study and diagnosis of diseases by the examination of cells.

Learning Vector Quantizer (LVQ): Is a pattern-based artificial neural network that belongs to the supervised networks family. A winner-take-all learning approach is applied.

Machine Learning (ML): It is a subset of artificial intelligence. The main characteristic of this discipline is related to the study of algorithms (including statistical models) that can be used by computerized systems in order to perform learning and recognition tasks however without using extensive and explicit instructions, instead learning of patterns and inference is used.

Chapter 6
Personalized Nutrition Recommendations in Food Services

Katerina Giazitzi
School of Health Science and Education, Department of Nutrition-Dietetics, Harokopio University of Athens, Greece

Vaios T. Karathanos
Harokopion University, Greece

George Boskou
Department of Nutrition-Dietetics, Harokopio University, Greece

ABSTRACT

The nutritional information on food services could be part of a public health policy against the increasing rate of obesity. The aim of this work is to present the state of art for the nutritional information on food services and the mHealth application usage, worldwide. A particular case study is presented that refers to an Electronic Intelligent System of Personalized Dietary Advice (DISYS) for tablets and smartphones. This application provides nutritional analysis of menu items and personalized suggestions according to the nutritional demands of each customer. The application was characterized as an easy-to-use, comprehensive, and useful tool. Volunteers considered that this application contributes to overall health by enabling the modulation of body weight throughout healthier choices, reduction of calorie intake, and self-monitoring. mHealth applications designed to provide nutritional information seem to be useful for customers as they recommend appropriate nutritional options. They are an effective tool for caterers and nutritionists, who can provide value-added services.

DOI: 10.4018/978-1-7998-2390-2.ch006

INTRODUCTION

Obesity and nutrition-related diseases are a major public health problem. According to the World Health Organization (WHO), it is estimated that over 1.9 billion people aged 18 years are overweight worldwide, and over 650 million are obese. Additionally, in 2016, over 41 million children under the age of 5 years and over 340 million children and adolescents aged 5-19 were overweight or obese. Obesity rates have tripled from 1975 to 2018 (WHO, 2018). This global epidemic is not only limited to developed countries but also developing countries. In particular, according to a World Health Organization report, in Africa since 2000, there has been a 50% increase in overweight children under five years of age. It is estimated that by 2030, 51% of the world's population will be obese (Finkelstein et al., 2012).

At the same time, as food consumption outside the home is constantly increased, and the consumption of nutritious, healthy meals is reduced. Many studies has addressed this issue and have shown that eating out is associated with increased energy intake and reduced intake of micronutrients in Europe (Orphanos et al., 2007), in the USA (Bowman & Vinyard, 2004; Kant et al., 2004) and Australia (Burns et al., 2001). Based on the findings of a systematic study, there is a positive correlation between eating habits away from the home environment and the increase in body weight (Bezerra et al., 2012). In addition, a study published in the British Journal of Nutrition (2007) showed that increased fast-food consumption is linked to healthy eating and adversely affects the body weight of people, leading to the risk of obesity (Schroder et al., 2007).

BACKGROUND

Nutritional Information in Food Services

The increasing consumption of food away-from-home has contributed to the rise in the prevalence of obesity. Initiatives, such as nutritional information on food services, can be a health policy for the management of obesity (WHO, 2015; Orfanos et al., 2007). This type of policy has been adopted by the USA and the Australian government. The relevant legislation states that the menu labeling (calorie posting on menus) is obligatory to restaurants and similar retail food establishments if they are part of a chain of 20 or more locations (FDA, 2018). As far as Europe is concerned, Ireland has begun to implement the calorie posting on certain food services since 2015 (Health Service Executive, 2015).

According to the US Food and Drug Administration (FDA), all US states will follow a common nutrition labeling regulation that will remove the local regulations currently in force. Since 2018, the calorie content will be displayed next to the food, mandatory in all US states, not only in restaurants but also in vending machines as well as in fast food chains with more than 20 branches. Food labeling regulations will not cover smaller chain restaurants, schools, and means of transport such as trains and airplanes. The nutrition information of the food will appear clearly in order to be understood by all consumers. Together with the caloric value, there must be a statement "consumption of 2,000 calories a day is a general nutritional assumption, the daily energy needs vary according to the individual". However, because adults and children have quite different nutritional needs, the statement says "consumption of 1200 to 1400 calories a day for children aged 4 to 8 is a general nutritional assumption, the daily needs of children in energy vary according to the individual ". In restaurants, the calorie value of the food will be next to the name and price of each food or drink on the menu or food tables. In the case of self-service restaurants, the caloric value will be at some point near the food.

With regard to vending machines, the caloric value will be in the electronic or digital form next to each food item. Calorie labeling will concern:

- Meals or snacks in restaurants, fast food, cafes, bakeries, ice cream shops.
- Food purchased by car from fast-food windows.
- Food distributed by fast-food employees at home, such as pizza.
- Products at a grocery store (delicatessen).
- Foods like popcorn consumed in entertainment venues such as cinema.
- Alcoholic beverages and cocktails.

In addition to the labeling of the caloric value of food, additional information on its nutritional value will be provided. This information should be written and include most of the food information provided on labels of packaged food (FDA, 2018).

As far as Australia is concerned, the legislation was applied in February 2011, with a 12-month compliance period, to all fast-food chains with more than 20 restaurants in the state or over 50 nationally. These businesses must indicate the kilojoules in the menus, as well as the following statement: "The average daily intake of energy for adults is 8700 Kj." Nutritional information should be located next to the price of the product in the directories and on the websites for online orders. The Food Regulation Committee has developed guidelines to help develop nationally consistent guidelines for product labeling in the menus. Since then, Australian states such as Victoria, Queensland, South Australia and the Australian Capital Territory have followed the Obesity Policy Coalition (2018).

In the European Union, the issue of nutritional information on the menu of restaurants and fast food is at an early stage. Time-to time, small initiatives are taken to inform governments and consumers about the nutrition information of the menus, but there is a lack of training on this issue.

As far as Greece is concerned, nutrition analysis is not mandatory and therefore the Greek population, both consumers and caterers is not very mobilized. For this reason, the number of restaurants or fast food outlets that provide nutritional information is small compared to what is happening in the US.

Updating menus for the presence of allergens or components associated with intolerances is an important element of nutrition information. According to the article 44 of the EU regulation 1169/2011, all ingredients that may cause allergies or intolerance, in foods that are not packed, must be communicated to the customers since December the 13th 2014 (EU regulation 1169/2011). The communication means are not specified, but any kind of effective information is acceptable.

Apart from numeric information, there are other types of nutritional information. For example, in the United States of America, due to mandatory nutrition labeling in food services, there are various certification standards that certify healthy meals in restaurants.

The "American Heart Association" (AHA) with the "Heart Check" program has created the nutritional requirements that a restaurant can follow to ensure that its meals are nutritionally certified and carry the following label "Heart-Check Mark". The nutritional requirements are based on AHA's scientific research on nutritional recommendations, including nutrients and food categories that are consistent with healthy eating. The majority of dietary requirements refer to the portion of the food under consideration (Table 1).

Table 1. Nutrition requirements for certified meals (AHA, 2018)

Energy and nutrients	**Per 100g**	**Per meal**
energy		Up to 700 Kcal
fat	Up to 3g	Up to 26g and up to 30% of the energy provided from fats
saturates	Up to 1g	Up to 5g and up to 10% of the energy provided from saturates
cholesterol	Up to 20 mg	Up to 105 mg
trans fats		Up to 0,5 mg
sodium		Up to 960 mg
vitamin A,C, calcium,iron,edible fiber and proteins		At least 10% coverage of Daily Values (DV)

All the above, of course, create the demand for the development of information technology that will be used to make a reliable nutritional analysis of menus and to provide comprehensive information to the customers of food services.

Nutrition and Diet Apps

The rapid development of technological devices provides customers with great opportunities in the framework of nutritional information and guidance (Bennett et al., 2013; Pelletier, 2012). In particular, applications designed for use on mobile technologies, i.e., smartphones and tablets, known as mHealth applications or mHealth "apps" can be used in large-scale interventions providing health care information (Morris and Aguilera, 2012; Dennison et al., 2013; Drosos et al., 2015; Kumar et al., 2013). The available mHealth apps were approximately 325,000 at the end of 2017 (Pohl, 2017). The nutrition apps may influence customers to make informed and healthier choices when they order food on food services. (Okumus et al., 2018). Furthermore, technological solutions offered by mHealth can constitute a challenging field of interaction and communication amongst customers and caterers for healthier choices (Handel, 2011).

Most of the diet/ nutrition apps allow users to add the food items they consume on a daily basis. The apps convert food consumption (24h recall into nutrition intake (compare energy expenditure with energy consumption) and compare them with the daily nutritional goal. Moreover, they offer nutrition and dieting advices (Jospe et al., 2015).

These applications offer the potential for active management and participation of consumers in the process of improving their diet and health outcomes. Technological solutions offered by mHealth can constitute a challenging field of interaction and communication among consumers and caterers for healthier choices. Since technological gadgets are part of our everyday life, development of applications provides fertile ground for real-time behavior change interventions (Garcia-Gomez et al., 2014; Ventola, 2014). Consumers can be informed and educated through electronic applications at restaurants. They will probably make healthier choices when they are informed by a smart application (Okumus & Bilgihan, 2014). Concerning the characteristics of the consumers that use diet applications, those with a sense of personal innovativeness think that these apps are easier to use (Lu et al., 2005; Okumus et al., 2016; Nollen et al., 2014). Their intention to use a diet app is negatively influenced by technical barriers, and on the other hand, their perception that the app is easy-to-use positively affects their intention.

Moreover the applications should be understandable and convenient. It would be useful if they allow users to add their data as far as food intake, medical history, and exercise habits in order to receive personalized recommendations. A list with very healthy foods ("superfoods") or a personalized reminder for regular drinking water may be very interesting for the end-user (Okumus et al., 2016).

The use of diet apps seems to influence the health-consciousness, self-education upon nutrition and physical activity and the social life of users. They help the maintenance of a healthy diet (Wang et al., 2016). There is a great interest for electronic applications for self-monitoring of an everyday diet and dietary recommendations. This type of applications collects dietary intake by using nutrition assessment method such as food diary record. However, none of the apps had the capability to provide personalized dietary advice (Franco et al., 2016; Wang et al., 2016).

THE CASE OF DISYS

In the above framework, an Electronic Intelligent System of Personalized Dietary Advice called "DISYS" (http://www.disys.gr) was developed and evaluated (Figure 1). This application, suggests healthy choices in restaurant menus by evaluating personal nutritional profile and health factors, i.e., body weight, blood sugar, arterial pressure etc.. In a more technical sense, it runs sophisticated algorithms that analyze

Figure 1. Logo of DISYS, an electronic intelligent system of personalized dietary advice

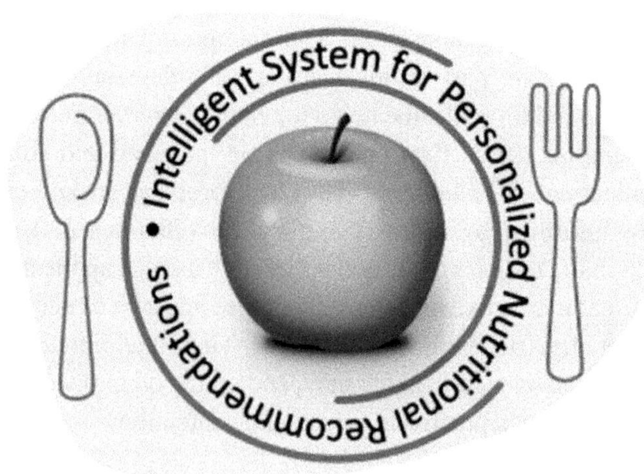

the nutritional value of each meal as well as the impact on consumers' health. In contrast to the available apps, this is an innovative Greek application as it permits an active interaction among consumers and restaurant owners.

The aim of the following study was to evaluate the pilot operation of the "DISYS" application by the consumers. In the assessment, factors such as technical features, taste satisfaction, the information provided, as well as the effect on nutrition and health, are included.

A tailor-made questionnaire (ANNEX I) with 15 questions was developed in order to evaluate DISYS app. Questions were either closed or in 5 grade likert scale, i.e., Not at all, A little, Moderate, Enough, Very much. The questionnaire as an electronic form was incorporated into the app, and it had to be answered after the end of its first use. End-users had access to the "DISYS" features either via a web-browser or an application on a smart-phone or tablet running on the android platform (Figure 1).Figure 1 Example of the web-based interface for the caterer to feed in the recipes for the menu. (the language is in Greek since it is service-oriented to the Greek market)

Hotels, restaurants and catering units (Ho.Re.Ca.) participated in the pilot application and trusted their recipes to researchers. Menus and nutritional information were uploaded on the online platform to be available for potential customers. Pilot testing was performed with real customers (Dimitriou et al., 2017).

The chefs were responsible for feeding information about the menus in the system, according to the guidance of dietitians. Pilot application, and collection of questionnaires took place in July-August 2015, with 75 customers (end- users). Brochures and promotional banners were used in order to promote this initiative at the points of interest. End-users (chefs and customers) could have access to 'DISYS, either via a web-browser or via an application on a smartphone or tablet running on android platform. Customers had to download the app and insert their personal medical and nutritional information (24-h recall). After data processing by the app, each user could receive personalized recommendations based on the restaurants' menu. After using the app for the very first time, users filled in the questionnaire for evaluation.

Data collected all by the online questionnaire was delivered in a comma-delimited format by the IT company distributing the "DISYS" app. The data were incorporated into spreadsheets of LibreOffice Calc and were analyzed for frequencies (Dimitriou et al., 2017). The Statistica 8.0. was applied to produce association rules (Palisidis et al., 2016). The results of the statistical analysis are presented below.

The application was evaluated regarding its meal recommendation. At least 36% of the customers find the suggestions tasty enough and 21% very tasty. As far as, those customers that are not satisfied with the proposed meals, most of them reported that they do not like a particular component of the recipe (Figure 1).

Figure 2. "How satisfying did you find the recommended choices, according to your food preferences?"

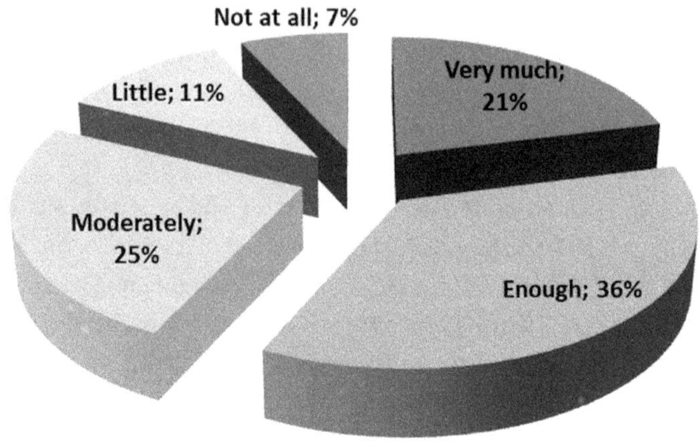

The customers referred that the proposed choices correspond very well to their dietary needs (20%), while 23% of the responders answered that the meals moderately covered their dietary needs (Figure 2). The customers believed that the meal proposal helps enough the improvement of their body weight (41%) (Figure 3).

A quarter of customers respond that they would use the app for self-monitoring in order to lose weight, whereas 28% of them believe that application could help them choose healthier meals. The rest of them mentioned that the app would be used for self-monitoring BMI or selecting restaurants with good quality meals (Figure 4). Customers considered that this mHealth app would help to improve their quality of

Figure 3. "Do you believe that the received proposals meet your nutritional needs?"

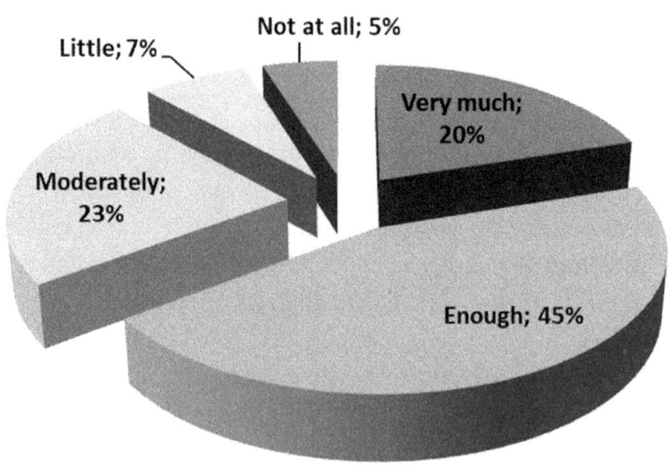

Figure 4. "Do you believe that the proposals that were made, can improve your body weight and other health factors and well-being?"

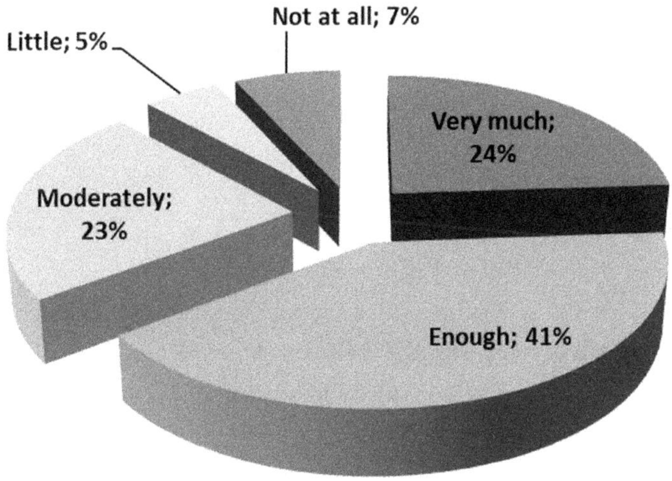

diet and their dietary habits in various ways. Actually, it can contribute to increase micro-nutrient intake (12%), reduce calorie intake (19%), to plan healthier meals (12%), to promote healthy choices away-from-home and healthier meals (Figure 5)

Concerning the ease of use for the application, one-third of the customers mentioned that the app has a friendly environment (33%). Another third found that the app has a pleasant design (32%). The rest of them described the application as fast and comprehensive in use (Figure 6). Moreover, they commented that the app was useful (22%), pleasant (10%) and effective (18%).

Figure 5. "How would you use the app to improve your weight?"

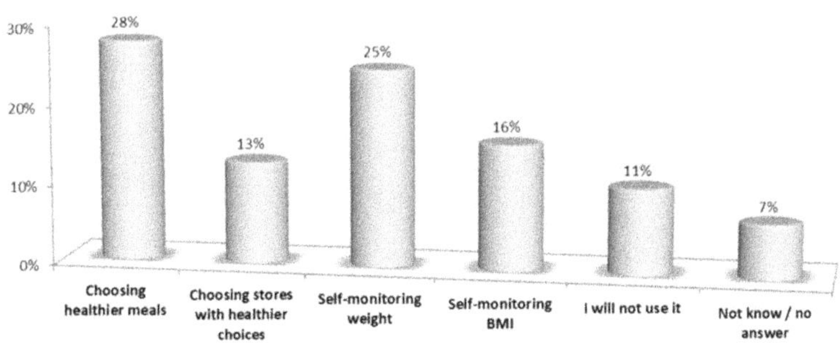

Figure 6. "How does the app contribute to the improvement of your diet?"

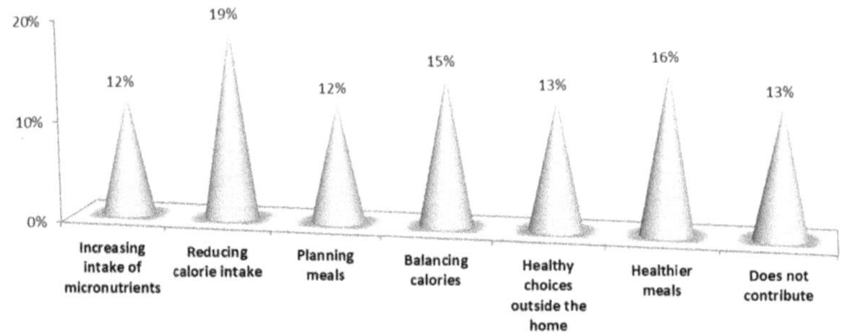

When the customers were asked if the information received was adequate, at least half of them replied that there is no information missing. The others proposed some improvements, as shown in Figure 7. In general, the customers seemed satisfied by the app as 26% of them were willing to use it most of the week days (Figure 8). Three-quarters of volunteers would suggest the app to some friends or relatives.

Most of the customers (35,3%) would not pay to use it, and 24% would pay up to 0.99€ if there were a trial period. In general, the percentage of willingness to pay was higher if the trial period was included (Figure 9). Finally, "NutriPlan" was one out of the seven proposed brand names that seems to be more favorable (34.7%) and the next one was "NutriPal" (18.7%).

With the use of the 'a priori' algorithm, some association rules were detected. This algorithm runs through the data to find frequent items and item sets (cases and case combinations). For the function of association rules with Statistica, the parameters set were: minimum support 20% and minimum confidence 80%. The

Figure 7. "How easy-to use is this application?"

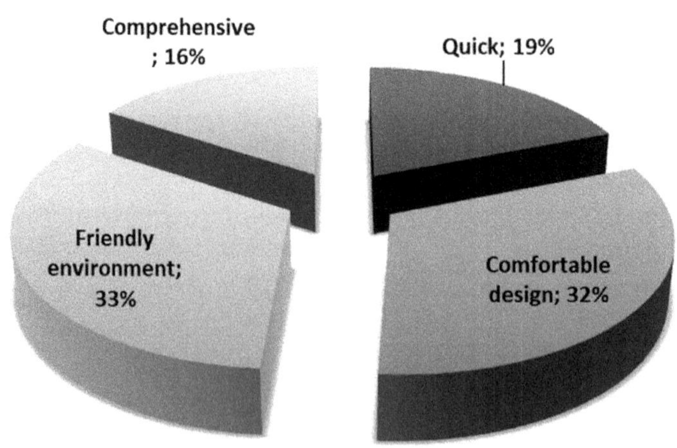

Figure 8. "At what point does the information received lack?"

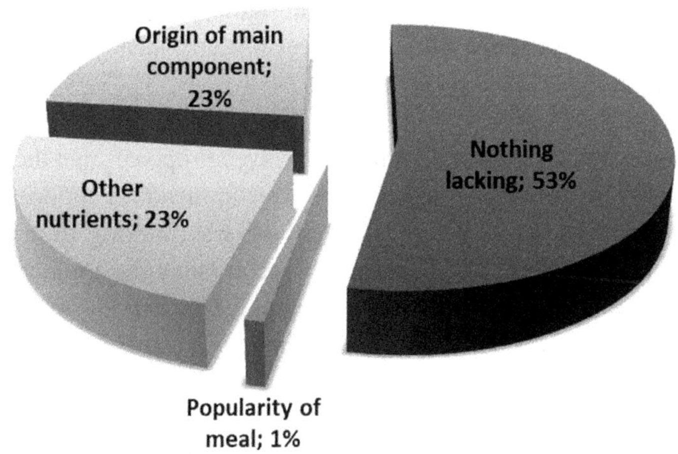

Figure 9. "How often could you use the app?"

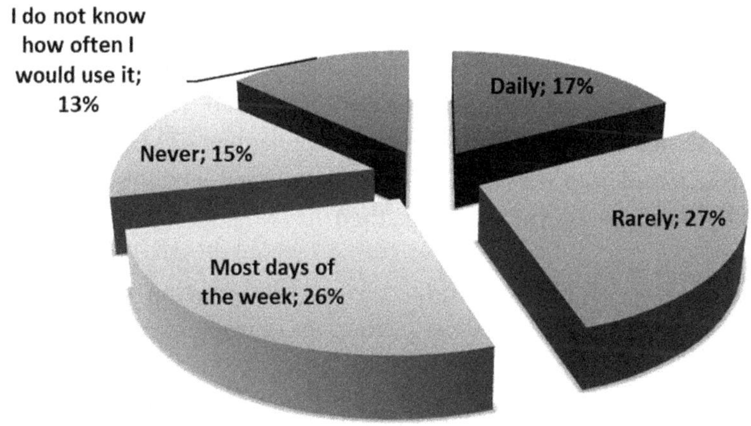

Figure 10. "How much would you pay for this app?"

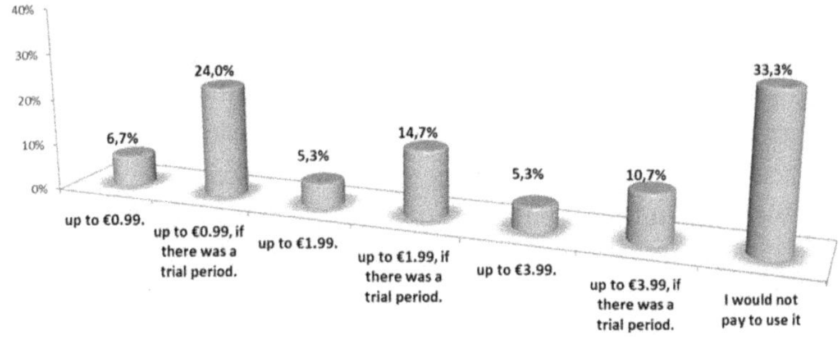

association rules presented below are the ones with 100% confidence. The logical operators are marked in bold letters, and the figure in parenthesis represents the percentage of cases that support the rule with 100% confidence. The overall results of the association rules are presented on ANNEX II.

1. **If** the food was tasty enough, **and** the received proposals met their nutritional needs enough, **then** the customers would recommend the application (29.3%).
2. **If** the food was tasty enough **and** nothing was missing from the received information, **then** the customers would recommend the application (25.3%).
3. **If** the proposals that were made can improve their body weight **and** other health factors **and** well-being enough, **then** the customers would recommend the application (24%).
4. **If** the food was tasty enough **and**, according to their food preferences, costumers found the recommended choices satisfying enough; **then** they would recommend the application (22.6%).
5. **If** the food was tasty enough **and** the proposals that were made can improve their body weight **and** other health factors **and** enough well-being, **then** the customers would recommend the application (22.6%).
6. **If** according to their food preferences, customers found the recommended choices satisfying enough, **and** the customers used 'DISYS' most days of the week, **then** they would recommend the application (22.6%).
7. **If** the received proposals met their nutritional needs enough **and** the customers used DISYS' most days of the week, **then** they would recommend the application (22.6%).
8. **If** nothing was missing from the received information **and** the application was characterized comprehensive, **then** the customers would recommend the application (21.3%).
9. **If** the food was tasty enough **and**, according to costumers' food preferences, customers found the recommended choices satisfying enough, **and** the received proposals met their nutritional needs enough, **then** they would recommend the application (21.3%).
10. **If** the food was tasty enough **and** nothing was missing from the received information, **and** the received proposals met customers' nutritional needs enough, **then** they would recommend the application (21.3%).
11. **If** the proposals that were made can improve customers' body weight **and** other health factors **and** well-being enough and they used DISYS most days of the week, **then** they would recommend the application (20%).

In general, electronic tools that provide nutritional information in food services have a great scientific interest as part of public health policy. It seems that labeling could be associated with various health parameters and affects many health indicators. The increasing use of technology products ("gadgets") could facilitate access to more information, some of which could be about meals and food prepared outside the home (Hebden et al., 2012).

Some studies have shown that preserving healthy metabolism, by nutrition, eating patterns or physical activity, is in many cases as much important as having a normal weight. Therefore, giving the opportunity to improve health and well-being factors as deemed by the app users provides great benefits to the overall health. The app helps people improve their dietary habits by making small changes every day, such as to organize their meals, choose healthier meals or visit restaurants with more healthy dishes etc. It is well established that making small changes leads to the adoption of healthier habits, gradual weight loss and weight maintenance. A scientific review aroused 193 scientific articles related to the use of smartphone applications for promoting healthy diet and nutrition. The main result of the review was that there should be more studies in this topic, with the need for culturally appropriate, tailored health messages to increase knowledge and awareness of health behaviors such as healthy eating. Smartphone apps are likely to be a useful and low-cost intervention for improving diet and nutrition and addressing obesity in the general population (Coughlin et al., 2015).

Moreover, it is really important that users have the opportunity to self-monitor their weight and their diet (Sama et al., 2014). Frequent body weight measurement is associated with greater weight loss as it increases participants' awareness and commitment. Food recording gives a feedback to users so that they can observe closely their nutrient intake and balance calories consumption. Feedback is also received through dietary analysis of suggested menu items at certain restaurants after processing personal medical and dietary patterns. Personalized recommendations are given to customers to guide them towards healthier choices, help them obtain valuable education out of the experience and build a strong motivation for trying more. These nutritional advices are the ultimate goal of our application contributing to the organization "eating out" and modification of the eating behavior.

Although, mHealth apps for mobile and tablets are available for years and widespread among health care professionals, there is still a lack of data on how to evaluate these apps and how to properly use them. Our study contributes positively to this problem by presenting a thorough pilot evaluation of an innovative designed application.

From the current study, DISYS seemed to be useful in promoting dietary and health information. This fact has been confirmed in previous studies not only in the case of public restaurants but also in hospital settings. It seems that it is able to satisfy restaurant clients and to promote healthy eating, in the framework of weight management and improvement of health factors.

Comparing the results of relevant studies, the main conclusion is that populations from various studies show interest in the use of advanced technologies to improve their health and wellness. A similar research project held in the United Kingdom examined the relevance of a focus-group consisted of 19 students, in terms of their receptiveness to the use of a mobile application, as a mean of improving their health quality and promoting a healthy lifestyle. The findings showed that young and healthy adults have significant interest in such applications. Accuracy, legality, safety, the effort required and their disposal are major influences on the use of the application (Dennison et al., 2013). The present study shows similar results; 75% of the subjects would propose the use of this application. Their intention to propose the application was associated with the proposal of the app. If its meal proposal was tasty or it could improve their weight and overall health, then customers had the intention to propose the app to someone else. Balasubramanian et al. (2015) evaluated another perspective of this issue. They evaluated a similar to DISYS application as an advertising tool of a restaurant. There was a positive correlation between the existence of the app and the satisfaction of customers and their preference for a restaurant with this service (Balasubramanian et al., 2015).

The limitations of this study have to do with the sample size, which was small. The results would be more reliable, and the conclusions would be safer if more volunteers had been included. Also, this was a pilot study and the first attempt to evaluate an app with such a potential, in the Greek market. It will be possible to generalize the findings in a future and larger study. Possible further research on this topic would be important. Apart from a big sample, correlations could be done between questionnaires' results and other factors of the subjects, such as age, body mass index and gender. Furthermore, similar research could be conducted in more regions of Greece, such as smaller touristic cities and towns. This would help to generalize the findings.

CONCLUSION

This study indicates that there is an important interest from consumers to use this type of app. Moreover, DISYS is an effective tool for the management of a nutritional plan and for the restaurant owners, who provide value-added services. Finally, this study could trigger the research interest on this topic, not only of the evaluation of similar application as an effective tool, but also the best possible and most desirable characteristics of this tool in order to educate in the topic of nutrition and to be an effective tool for dietary interventions and healthy lifestyles.

In conclusion, the provision of personalized nutritional recommendations on food service outlets through mHealth applications could be a new public health policy aimed at improving out-of-home meals' choices. The personalized nutritional advice may contribute to the modification of the eating behavior on food service outlets. On the framework of an initiative like this, issues like inaccurate nutritional information, recipe or portions raise. It is important for the proper implementation of the action to standardize the procedure and cooperate with the chefs, and nutritionists. The standardization of the procedure, the nutritional analysis, the recipes and the portion sizes would lead to the minimization of food waste. This reduction will have a positive effect on the economy and well-functioning of food service outlets. The communication of all the above aspects could be facilitated from the use of mHealth applications.

ACKNOWLEDGMENT

This research is co-financed by Greece and the European Union (European Social Fund- ESF) through the Operational Programme Human Resources Development, Education and Lifelong Learning in the context of the project "Strengthening Human Resources Research Potential via Doctorate Research" (MIS-5000432), implemented by the State Scholarships Foundation (IKY).

We would like also to thank the dietitians Dimitriou Maria and Stavidi Eva for the support to carry out the project.

REFERENCES

AHA (American Heart Association). (2018). *Heart-Check Meal Certification Program Nutrition Requirements.* Retrieved May 1, 2008, from: https://www.heart.org/en/healthy-living/company-collaboration/heart-check-certification/heart-check-meal-certification-program-foodservice/heart-check-meal-certification-program-nutrition-requirements

Balasubramanian, K., Balraj, A., Kumar, J., & Jaykumar. (2015). Customer Preferences to Select a Restaurant Through Smart Phone Applications: An Exploratory Study. *Advanced Science Letters*, *21*(5), 1489–1493. doi:10.1166/asl.2015.6081

Bennett, G. G., Steinberg, D. M., Lanpher, M. G., Askew, S., Lane, I. B., Levine, E. L., ... Foley, P. B. (2013). Availability of and ease of access to calorie information on restaurant websites. *PLoS One*, *8*(8), e72009. doi:10.1371/journal.pone.0072009 PMID:23977193

Bezerra, I. N., Curioni, C., & Sichieri, R. (2012). Association between eating out of home and body weight. *Nutrition Reviews, 70*(2), 65–79. doi:10.1111/j.1753-4887.2011.00459.x PMID:22300594

Bowman, S. A., & Vinyard, B. T. (2004). Fast Food Consumption of U.S. Adults: Impact on Energy and Nutrient Intakes and Overweight Status. *Journal of the American College of Nutrition, 23*(2), 163–168. doi:10.1080/07315724.2004.10719357 PMID:15047683

Coughlin, S., Whitehead, M., Sheats, J., Mastromonico, J., Hardy, D., & Smith, S. (2015). Smartphone Applications for Promoting Healthy Diet and Nutrition: A Literature Review. *Jacobs Journal of Food and Nutrition, 2*(3), 21.

Dennison, L., Morrison, L., Conway, G., & Yardley, L. (2013). Opportunities and challenges for smartphone applications in supporting health behavior change: Qualitative study. *Journal of Medical Internet Research, 15*(4), e86. doi:10.2196/jmir.2583 PMID:23598614

Dimitriou, M., Giazitzi, K., Stavridi, E., Palisidis, G., Karathanos, V., & Boskou, G. (2017). Evaluation of an Electronic Application for Nutritional Information in Food Service Outlets: A Pilot mHealth Application. *International Journal of Reliable and Quality E-Healthcare, 6*(1), 46–58. doi:10.4018/IJRQEH.2017010104

Drosos, D., Tsotsolas, N., Chalikias, M., Skordoulis, M., & Koniordos, M. (2015). A survey on the use of social networking sites in Greece. In A. Kravets, M. Shcherbakov, M. Kultsova, & O. Shabalina (Eds.), *Creativity in Intelligent, Technologies and Data Science, Communications in Computer and Information Science* (pp. 556–570). Cham, Switzerland: Springer.

FDA (Food and Drug Administration). (2018). *Menu Labeling Requirements.* Retrieved August 13, 2019, from: https://www.fda.gov/food/food-labeling-nutrition/menu-labeling-requirements

Finkelstein, E. A., Khavjou, O. A., Thompson, H., Trogdon, J. G., Pan, L., Sherry, B., & Dietz, W. (2011). Obesity and severe obesity forecasts through 2030. *American Journal of Preventive Medicine, 42*(6), 563–570. doi:10.1016/j.amepre.2011.10.026 PMID:22608371

Franco, R. Z., Fallaize, R., Lovegrove, J. A., & Hwang, F. (2016). Popular Nutrition-Related Mobile Apps: A Feature Assessment. *JMIR mHealth and uHealth, 4*(3), e85. doi:10.2196/mhealth.5846 PMID:27480144

Garcia-Gomez, J. M., de la Torre-Diez, I., Vicente, J., Robles, M., Lopez-Coronado, M., & Rodrigues, J. J. (2014). Analysis of mobile health applications for a broad spectrum of consumers: A user experience approach. *Health Informatics Journal*, *20*(1), 74–84. doi:10.1177/1460458213479598 PMID:24550566

Handel, M. J. (2011). mHealth (mobile health)-using Apps for health and wellness. *Explore (New York, N.Y.)*, *7*(4), 256–261. doi:10.1016/j.explore.2011.04.011 PMID:21724160

Health Service Executive. (2015). *Guidance for calorie posting implementation*. Retrieved from: https://www.hse.ie/eng/health/hl/calorieposting/

Hebden, L., Cook, A., Van der Ploeg, H., & Allman-Farinelli, M. (2012). Development of Smartphone Applications for Nutrition and Physical Activity Behavior Change. *JMIR Research Protocols, 1(2), e9*. doi:10.2196/resprot.2205

Jospe, M. R., Fairbairn, K. A., Green, P., & Perry, T. L. (2015). Diet app use by sports dietitians: A survey in five countries. *JMIR mHealth and uHealth*, *3*(1), e7. doi:10.2196/mhealth.3345 PMID:25616274

Kant, A. K., & Graubard, B. I. (2004). Eating out in America, 1987-2000: Trends and nutritional correlates. *Preventive Medicine*, *38*(2), 243–249. doi:10.1016/j.ypmed.2003.10.004 PMID:14715218

Kumar, S., Nilsen, W. J., Abernethy, A., Atienza, A., Patrick, K., Pavel, M., ... Swendeman, D. (2013). Mobile health technology evaluation: The mHealth evidence workshop. *American Journal of Preventive Medicine*, *45*(2), 228–236. doi:10.1016/j.amepre.2013.03.017 PMID:23867031

Lu, J., Yao, J. E., & Yu, C.-S. (2005). Personal innovativeness, social influences and adoption of wireless Internet services via mobile technology. *The Journal of Strategic Information Systems*, *14*(3), 245–268. doi:10.1016/j.jsis.2005.07.003

Morris, M. E., & Aguilera, A. (2012). Mobile, Social, and Wearable Computing and the Evolution of Psychological Practice. *Professional Psychology, Research and Practice*, *43*(6), 622–626. doi:10.1037/a0029041 PMID:25587207

Nollen, N. L., Mayo, M. S., Carlson, S. E., Rapoff, M. A., Goggin, K. J., & Ellerbeck, E. F. (2014). Mobile technology for obesity prevention: A randomized pilot study in racial- and ethnic-minority girls. *American Journal of Preventive Medicine*, *46*(4), 404–408. doi:10.1016/j.amepre.2013.12.011 PMID:24650843

Obesity Policy Coalition. (2018). *Policy brief: Menu kilojoule labelling in chain food outlets in Australia.* Retrieved January, 2018 from: http://www.opc.org.au/downloads/policy-briefs/menu-kj-labelling-in-chain-food-outlets-in-australia.pdf

Okumus, B., Ali, F., Bilgihan, A., & Ozturk, A. B. (2018). Psychological factors influencing customers' acceptance of smartphone diet apps when ordering food at restaurants. *International Journal of Hospitality Management, 72*, 67–77. doi:10.1016/j.ijhm.2018.01.001

Okumus, B., & Bilgihan, A. (2014). Proposing a model to test smartphone users' intention to use smart applications when ordering food in restaurants. *Journal of Hospitality and Tourism Technology, 5*(1), 31–49. doi:10.1108/JHTT-01-2013-0003

Okumus, B., Bilgihan, A., & Ozturk, A. B. (2016). Factors Affecting the Acceptance of Smartphone Diet Applications. *Journal of Hospitality Marketing & Management, 25*(6), 726–747. doi:10.1080/19368623.2016.1082454

Orfanos, P., Naska, A., Trichopoulos, D., Slimani, N., Ferrari, P., van Bakel, M., ... Trichopoulou, A. (2007). Eating out of home and its correlates in 10 European countries. The European Prospective Investigation into Cancer and Nutrition (EPIC) study. *Public Health Nutrition, 10*(12), 1515–1525. doi:10.1017/S1368980007000171 PMID:17582244

Palisidis, G., Giazitzi, K., Karathanos, V. T., & Boskou, G. (2016). Nutritional application software for restaurants: The tool of customer satisfaction and behavior. *International Journal of Electronic Customer Relationship Management, 10*(2-4).

Pelletier, S. (2012). *Explosive growth in health care apps raises oversight questions.* Retrieved October, 2012, from: http://www.aamc.org/newsroom/reporter/october2012/308516/health-care-apps.html

Pohl, M. (2017). *325,000 mobile health apps available in 2017, Android now the leading mHealth platform.* Retrieved from: Research 2 Guidance https://research2guidance.com/325000-mobile-health-apps-available-in-2017/

EU Regulation No 1169/2011 of the European Parliament and of the Council of 25 October 2011 on the provision of food information to consumers, OJ L 304 22.11.2011

Sama, P. R., Eapen, Z. J., Weinfurt, K. P., Shah, B. R., & Schulman, K. A. (2014). An evaluation of mobile health application tools. *JMIR mHealth and uHealth, 2*(2), e19. doi:10.2196/mhealth.3088 PMID:25099179

Schroder, H., Fıto, M., & Covas, M. I. (2007). Association of fast food consumption with energy intake, diet quality, body mass index and the risk of obesity in a representative Mediterranean population. *British Journal of Nutrition, 98*(6), 1274–1280. doi:10.1017/S0007114507781436 PMID:17625027

Ventola, C. L. (2014). Mobile devices and apps for health care professionals: Uses and benefits. *P&T, 39*(5), 356–364. PMID:24883008

Wang, Q., Egelandsdal, B., Amdam, G. V., Almli, V. L., & Oostindjer, M. (2016). Diet and Physical Activity Apps: Perceived Effectiveness by App Users. *JMIR mHealth and uHealth, 4*(2), e33. doi:10.2196/mhealth.5114 PMID:27056639

WHO. (2015). *Healthy diet.* Retrieved from: http://www.who.int/mediacentre/factsheets/fs394/en/

WHO. (2018). *Obesity and overweight.* Retrieved from: http://www.who.int/en/news-room/fact-sheets/detail/obesity-and-overweight

KEY TERMS AND DEFINITIONS

Calorie Posting: Information concerning the calories of a meal within a food service outlet.

Food Service: Restaurants, catering, and other establishments where the food is prepared and served.

Nutritional Analysis: The process of estimating the output of a meal in calories, macronutrients and micronutrients.

Nutritional Certification: Procedures to certify that a restaurant is providing nutritional information and/ or nutritionally balanced meals.

Nutritional Information: Information concerning the calories, the macronutrients and the micronutrients of a meal.

Nutritional Information Applications: Applications that provide nutritional information for meals in food services.

Nutritionally Balanced: A meal under certain restrictions for calories or specific macronutrients.

APPENDIX

Table 2. Questionnaire for evaluation that was incorporated within the application

Q1: How tasty did you find the recommended choices?						
Very much	Enough	Moderately	Little	Not at all		
Q2:If you find moderately/ little/ not at all tasty the recommended choices, select the reasons why you were not satisfied.						
I do not like a particular component of the recipe	Did not match the time of day	It was too salty or too sweet for me	In general, I do not like this recipe			
Q3: How satisfying did you find the recommended choices, according to your food preferences?						
Very much	Enough	Moderately	Little	Not at all		
Q4: How can the received proposals be improved?						
More outlets	More proposals	I could categorize / filter results	I do not think that received proposals can be improved	More widely type stores (restaurants, fast food etc.)	Searching meals based on principal component	
Q5: Is there anything missing from the received information?						
Other nutrients	The popularity of meal	Origin of main components (meat, fish, vegetable)	Nothing is missing			
Q6: How does the app contribute to the improvement of your diet?						
Increasing intake of micronutrients	Reducing calorie intake	Planning meals	Balancing calories	Healthy choices outside the home	Healthier meals	Does not contribute
Q7: Do you believe that the received proposals meet your nutritional needs?						
Very much	Enough	Moderately	Little	Not at all		
Q8:Do you believe that the proposals that were made can improve your body weight and other health factors and wellbeing?						
Very much	Enough	Moderately	Little	Not at all		
Q9: How would you use the app to improve your weight?						
Choosing healthier meals	Choosing stores with healthier choices	Self-monitoring weight	Self-monitoring BMI	I will not use it	Not know / no answer	
Q10: How easy to use is this application?						
Quick	Comfortable design	Friendly environment	Comprehensive			

continues on following page

Table 2. Continued

Q11: How often could you use "DISYS"?						
Daily	Most days of the week	Some days of the week	rarely	I do not know how often I would use it		
Q12: How much do you pay to use "DISYS"?						
I would pay up to €0.99.	I would pay up to €0.99, if there was a trial period.	I would pay up to €1.99.	I would pay up to €1.99, if there was a trial period.	I would pay up to €3.99.	I would pay up to €3.99, if there was a trial period.	I would not pay to use it
Q13: Which of the following names seems more appropriate for the application's trademark?						
NutriPlan	HealthyOut	NutriPal	My dietitian	Healthily	Health & Nutrition	Nutrily
Q14: How would you characterize it?						
Effective	Useful	Rapid	Pleasant	Promoting overall health	Promoting healthy diet	Without any problem
Q15: Would you recommend "DISYS" to someone else?						
Yes	No	Not sure				

Table 3. Association rules with Min. support = 20% and Min. confidence = 80% as produced by the "a priori" algorithm

IF	THEN	Support%	Confidence%
the food was enough tasty	the customers would recommend the application	36	100
the food was enough tasty, and the received proposals met their nutritional needs enough	the customers would recommend the application	29.3	100
the customers used "DISYS" most days of the week	they would recommend it	28	100
the food was enough tasty, and nothing was missing from the received information	the customers would recommend the application	25.3	100
the proposals that were made can improve their body weight and other health factors and wellbeing enough	the customers would recommend the application	24	100
the food was enough tasty and, according to their food preferences, costumers found the recommended choices enough satisfying	they would recommend the application	22.6	100
the food was enough tasty and the proposals that were made can improve their body weight and other health factors and wellbeing enough	the customers would recommend the application	22.6	100
according to their food preferences, customers found the recommended choices enough satisfying, and the customers used "DISYS" most days of the week	they would recommend the application	22.6	100
the received proposals met their nutritional needs enough, the customers used "DISYS" most days of the week	they would recommend the application	22.6	100

continues on following page

Table 3. Continued

IF	THEN	Support%	Confidence%
nothing was missing from the received information, and the application was characterized comprehensive	the customers would recommend the application	21.3	100
the food was enough tasty and, according to costumers' food preferences, costumers found the recommended choices enough satisfying, and the received proposals met their nutritional needs enough	they would recommend the application	21.3	100
the food was enough tasty, and nothing was missing from the received information, and the received proposals met customers' nutritional needs enough	they would recommend the application	21.3	100
the proposals that were made can improve customers' body weight and other health factors and wellbeing enough, and they used "DISYS" most days of the week	they would recommend the application	20	100
nothing was missing from the received information, and the received proposals met customers' nutritional needs enough	they would recommend the application	30.6	95.8
according to their food preferences, customers found the recommended choices enough satisfying	they would recommend the application	25.3	95
the received proposals met customers' nutritional needs enough	they would recommend the application	42.6	94.1
the food was enough tasty and, according to customers' food preferences, they found the recommended choices enough satisfying	the received proposals would meet customers' nutritional needs enough, and they would recommend the application	21.3	94.1
the food was enough tasty and, according to their food preferences, customers found the recommended choices enough satisfying	the received proposals would meet customers' nutritional needs enough	21.3	94.1
the food was enough tasty and, according to their food preferences, customers found the recommended choices enough satisfying, and they recommended the application	the received proposals would meet customers' nutritional needs enough	21.3	94.1
the food was very tasty	the customers would recommend the application	20	93.7
according to their food preferences, customers found the recommended choices enough satisfying, and nothing was missing from the received information	they would recommend the application	20	93.7
nothing was missing from the received information, and customers used the app to self-monitor their weight to improve it	they would recommend the application	20	93.7
according to their food preferences, customers found the recommended choices enough satisfying, and the received proposals met their nutritional needs enough	they would recommend the application	28	91.3
the received proposals met customers' nutritional needs enough, and the proposals that were made can improve their body weight and other health factors and wellbeing enough	they would recommend the application	26.6	90.9

continues on following page

Table 3. Continued

IF	THEN	Support%	Confidence%
Customers used the app to choose healthier meals to improve their weight	the customers would recommend the application	25.3	90.4
nothing was missing from the received information, and the proposals that were made can improve customers' body weight and other health factors and wellbeing enough	they would recommend the application	25.3	90.4
the proposals that were made can improve customers' body weight and other health factors and wellbeing enough	they would recommend the application	37.3	90.3
according to their food preferences, customers found the recommended choices enough satisfying	They would recommend the application	34.6	89.6
according to their food preferences, customers found the recommended choices enough satisfying, and the proposals that were made can improve their body weight and other health factors and wellbeing enough	the received proposals would meet customers' nutritional needs enough	22.6	89.4
customers used the app to self-monitor their weight to improve it	they would recommend the application	22.6	89.4
according to their food preferences, customers found the recommended choices enough satisfying, and the proposals that were made can improve their body weight and other health factors and wellbeing enough	the customers would recommend the application	22.6	89.4
"NutriPlan" seems more appropriate for the application's trademark	the customers would recommend the application	30.6	88.4
according to their food preferences, customers found the recommended choices enough satisfying, and the proposals that were made can improve their body weight and other health factors and wellbeing enough, and the customers recommended the application	the received proposals would meet customers' nutritional needs enough	20	88.2
customers used the app to self-monitor their weight to improve it, and the customers recommended the application	nothing would be missing from the received information	20	88.2
nothing was missing from the received information	the customers would recommend the application	46.67	87.5
the food was enough tasty, and nothing was missing from the received information	the customers would recommend the application	21.3	84.2
the food was enough tasty, and nothing was missing from the received information	the received proposals would meet customers' nutritional needs enough	21.3	84.2
the food was enough tasty, and nothing was missing from the received information, and the customers recommended the application	the received proposals would meet customers' nutritional needs enough	21.3	84.2
customers used the app to self-monitor their weight to improve it	nothing would be missing from the received information	21.3	84.2
the food was enough tasty	the customers would recommend the application	29.3	81.4

continues on following page

Table 3. Continued

IF	THEN	Support%	Confidence%
the food was enough tasty	the received proposals would meet customers' nutritional needs enough	29.3	81.4
the food was enough tasty, and the customers recommended the application	the received proposals would meet customers' nutritional needs enough	29.3	81.4
the customers used "DISYS" most days of the week	according to their food preferences, customers would find the recommended choices enough satisfying, and the customers would recommend the application	22.6	80.9
the customers used "DISYS" most days of the week	according to their food preferences, customers would find the recommended choices enough satisfying	22.6	80.9
the customers recommended the application, and they used "DISYS" most days of the week	according to their food preferences, customers would find the recommended choices enough satisfying	22.6	80.9
the customers used "DISYS" most days of the week	the received proposals would meet customers' nutritional needs enough, and they would recommend the application	22.6	80.9
the customers used "DISYS" most days of the week	the received proposals would meet customers' nutritional needs enough	22.6	80.9
the customers recommended the application, and they used "DISYS" most days of the week	the received proposals would meet customers' nutritional needs enough	22.6	80.9
according to their food preferences, customers found the recommended choices enough satisfying, and the customers would recommend the application	the received proposals would meet customers' nutritional needs enough	28	80.7
the application was characterized comprehensive, and the customers would recommend the application	nothing was missing from the received information	21.3	80
the application was characterized comprehensive	the customers would recommend the application	26.6	80

Chapter 7
Major Metrics, Concerns, and Assessment Strategy for Mobility Assistive Devices

Yiannis Koumpouros
University of West Attica, Greece

ABSTRACT

The ageing of the population is one of the major societal and financial problems. The prevalence of disability increases dramatically by age. The loss of mobility can be devastating to the elderly. Mobility aids are a one-way street to maintain independent mobility. The performance of daily activities is restrained by a series of factors related to the assistive device limitations, or the ones emerged from environmental causes. A literature review reveals minimal tools for assessing mobility assistive devices able to capture users' satisfaction. The chapter presents an assessment methodology in order to investigate assistive mobility devices' limitations, dissatisfaction reasons, and identifies the most appropriate tools to study such limitations and conclude in valid outcomes. One of the valuable characteristics of the study presented in its generalizability since it is not disease oriented. A summary of the results from both the literature review and the real case study on a mixed group of end users are presented in the chapter.

INTRODUCTION

Between 2015 and 2050, the proportion of the world's population over 60 years will nearly double from 12% to 22% (WHO, 2019). The ageing of the population is one of the major problems faced by the society causing significant problems (healthcare expenditure, social care, etc.) since the prevalence of disability increases dramatically

DOI: 10.4018/978-1-7998-2390-2.ch007

by age. To this end, elderly people are often assumed to be frail or dependent and a burden to society. The healthcare systems around the globe should prepare to address the various concerns of older people. Healthy ageing is the target of most countries nowadays. The leading causes of disability globally among aged 60 years or over, according to WHO estimates for 2012 are: unipolar depressive disorders, hearing loss, back and neck pain, Alzheimer's disease and other dementias, and osteoarthritis. Falls is also a major cause of disability among older persons globally (United Nations, 2015). The main geriatric syndromes include frailty, urinary incontinence, falls, delirium and pressure ulcers (WHO, 2019).

The loss of mobility, which is a widespread occurrence, can be devastating to the elderly and seniors. The Census Bureau of the USA reports that mobility problems are the most common disability among the elderly (United States Census Bureau, 2019). Mobility loss is also highly interconnected with depression. Mobility aids have been used to maintain independent mobility. Studies have argued that use of the devices may actually increase risk of falling by causing tripping or by disrupting balance control through other mechanisms (Walsh et al., 2009; Charron, Kirby & MacLeod, 1995; Roman de Mettelinge & Cambier, 2015). Although many studies have reported that mobility aids and/or environmental obstacles are associated with falls, the possible link between these two risk factors has not been studied.

The use of gait assistive devices, although can provide precious help for the elderly (Cetin, Muzembo, Pardessus, Puisieux & Thevenon, 2010) or the mobility-impaired, can also have limitations or adverse consequences. Studies show that 30% to 50% of people prescribed with a gait assistive device abandon their device soon after receiving it, mainly because they do not meet the needs of individuals. In one survey, almost half of the reported problems were associated with the difficulty or risk to use the prescribed device (Bateni & Maki, 2005). Another study reveals that 58.3% of knee osteoarthritis patients abandon the mobility aid due to adverse outcome and feeling of stigmatization (Akinbo, Sokunbi & Ogunbameru, 2008). According to (Lezzoni, Rao & Kinkel, 2009) the vast majority of persons with multiple sclerosis (MS) own more than one type of mobility aids. Persons with MS appear to "mix and match" different devices to suit their specific mobility needs. Canes and crutches are prescribed for people with moderate levels of mobility impairment, and walkers are prescribed for people with generalized weakness, poor lower-limb weight-bearing, debilitating conditions, or poor balance control, while wheeled walkers are favored for patients with Parkinson disease (Minor & Minor, 2013).

Some of the most commonly mentioned assistive device limitations or dissatisfaction reasons, as mentioned by users and health scientists, are: (i) handling the rollator gait assistive device (Brandt, Iwarsson & Ståhl, 2003; Hallén, Orrenius & Rose, 2006), (ii) the weight of the device (Brandt, Iwarsson & Ståhl, 2003; Hallén, Orrenius & Rose, 2006; Hill, Goldstein, Gartner & Brooks, 2008), (iii) the brake-use of rollator devices (Thomas et al., 2010), (iv) users are prone to falling because of the dependence on memory to activate the rollator's parking mechanism, (v) the inability of the current rollator to effectively park when the braking mechanism is engaged (Siu et al., 2008), (vi) social stigmatizing (association with aging and physical decline) (Hallén, Orrenius & Rose, 2006) (Hill, Goldstein, Gartner & Brooks, 2008; Thomas et al., 2010; Resnik, Allen, Isenstadt, Wasserman & Iezzoni, 2009), and (vii) upper-extremity pathologies because of the extended use of walking aids (i.e. tendonitis, osteoarthritis, and carpal tunnel syndrome) (Bateni & Maki, 2005).

It is evident from the above that the performance of daily activities by device-assisted walkers is partially restrained by a series of factors having to do with the assistive device limitations or/and the limitations emerged from environmental causes. Nowadays, there is no valid and reliable assessment tool able to identify and classify the limitations of walking aids or users' satisfaction. One of the most common instruments used in the bibliography is the Quebec User Evaluation of Satisfaction with assistive Technology - QUEST 2.0. QUEST 2.0 was designed to measure the level of satisfaction attribute to assistive technologies. It does so by using variables that are scored in terms of perceived importance and satisfaction (Demers, Weiss-Lambrou & Ska, 2000; Demers, Monette, LaPierre, Arnold & Wolfson, 2002; Koumpouros, Karavasili, Papageorgiou & Siavelis, 2016). However, being a generic assessment tool, some potential items, relevant to specific pieces of technology or delivery systems, are absent. For example, for gait assistive devices, the information extracted is limited to describing the satisfaction level of the user in terms of certain aspects (dimensions, safety feeling, effectiveness, etc.) (Demers, Weiss-Lambrou & Ska, 2000). Thus, it cannot be used to point out specific problems or limitations to be exceeded. In our study, we tried to identify the right tools in order to measure the limitations of the most commonly used mobility aids (rollator, frame walker and crutches) from a user perspective.

METHODOLOGICAL APPROACH

The study was conducted in a Greek rehabilitation hospital, and utilized semistructured individual interviews for data collection, using a combination of already valid and reliable tools.

Patient Selection

In order to understand the user needs of assistive gait devices and get an impression about their limitations, we interviewed 20 people (8 males and 12 females) depended on mobility aids. The participants were grouped in two main categories:

(i) rehabilitation group (the ones that were undertaken rehabilitation at the time of the study), and (ii) the elderly group (the ones aged over 65 years old and did not need rehabilitation). 9 of the participants were currently engaged in rehabilitation and the rest 11 where older adults. According to the inclusion criteria, all subjects should fall under the following categories: (i) being users of a mobility aid for at least four weeks, (ii) had no or moderate mental impairment [scored more than 17/30 at the Mini Mental State Examination - MMSE], and (iii) had a moderate motor impairment [subject is unable to stand up and sit down unassisted on a standard chair (standardised 100% leg length) without problem, 5-chair stand >16,7 sec and gait speed >0.6 m/sec unassisted].

Tools Selection

Since there is no single tool able to capture the desired data of the current research study, we conducted a thorough survey of the literature in order to identify the most proper ones. Three questionnaires (the Impact on Participation and Autonomy - IPA, the EuroQol EQ-5D - EQ5D and the 12-item Short-Form Health Survey - SF-12) were finally chosen from a wide variety of tools, as considered to best match the goals of our research, which are to understand mobility-assistive-device user needs and get an impression about the limitations of their mobility aids. Our choice was based on the fact that the EQ5D and the SF-12 are among the most commonly used and the most widely evaluated measures of Quality of Life (QOL). The IPA questionnaire was mainly chosen because of the extensive variety of the described aspects of daily activities, analyzing not only the mobility dimension but also the whole spectrum and needs of the mobility aid users. The advantage of comments by the user on every separate dimension was also taken into consideration since data that could not have been foreseen were allowed to enter, especially data that could lead to a detailed description of problems/limitations of the used mobility aids. All three questionnaires are generic measurements of health-related quality of life (HRQOL). The main advantage of generic instruments is that they are suitable for use across a broad range of health problems and that they can also be used with healthy populations to generate normative data that can be used to compare different patient groups (University of Oxford) (for example, as in our case, patients undergoing rehabilitation and elderly people). Disease-specific questionnaires were excluded from the beginning since some of the volunteers would be considered a healthy population and the rehabilitation group didn't face with only one specific disease. Apart from the QUEST 2.0 (which does not fulfil the needs of detailed and extended users' evaluation of mobility aids), there is no other valid and reliable assessment tool able to identify and classify the mobility aids' limitations and the user's satisfaction. Moreover, although QUEST 2.0 could provide valuable data, in our case (three different categories of mobility aids used by the volunteers) could probably lead to collecting insufficient data for all categories of mobility aids. Concluding, information on user needs and limitations of the used mobility aids was extracted from a combination of the three questionnaires. EQ5D, SF-12 and IPA (in this order) are of gradually increasing complexity and specification, all including at least one sector referring to mobility issues but without being narrowed to it.

Tools

EQ5D Questionnaire

The EuroQol EQ-5D is a two-part, generic, preference-based measure of Health-related quality of life (HRQOL) developed by a multidisciplinary consortium of investigators from five European countries (EuroQol, 1990). As a generic tool, rather than being aimed at one particular disease or treatment, it is designed for use across a wide range of health interventions (Brooks, 1996). The revised version of the instrument, which has become the most widely used HRQOL instrument for obtaining health state utilities (Whynes, McCahon, Ravenscroft, Hodgkinson, Evley & Hardman, 2013), addresses five domains: mobility, self-care, usual activities, pain/discomfort, and anxiety/depression. Each domain is divided into three severity levels, corresponding to no problem, some problem, and extreme problem. A dimension for which there are no problems is said to be at level 1, while a dimension for which there are extreme problems is said to be at level 3. Combining one level from each domain results in defining 243 different health states, and it is possible to obtain social values for each, thereby generating a tariff of health state valuations. The second part of the EQ-5D consists of a vertical 0 to 100 Visual Analog Scale (VAS), with 0 and 100 representing the worst and best possible health states, respectively. The EQ-5D is a self-report easily completed questionnaire, cognitively undemanding and applicable to a wide range of health conditions and treatments. Stahl et al. showed that only 10-20% of patients with COPD (chronic obstructive pulmonary disease) completing the EQ-5D reported any difficulties with it (Stahl, Jansson, Jonsson, Svensson, Lundback & Andersson, 2003). Also, in a study of 573 patients with various chronic diseases, 60-75% of the respondents found EQ-5D easy to respond to and easy to understand (Nilsson, Wenemark, Bendtsen & Kristenson, 2007). The EQ-5D was originally designed for self-completion by respondents but is also ideally suited for use in face-to-face interviews (EuroQol, 2007). Validity and reliability of the instrument have been tested among the general population and a variety of clinical conditions and for countries inside and outside the European Union. De Smedt et al. (2013) tested EQ-5D for validity and reliability in large European patients' population with coronary heart disease. Findings showed that the EQ-5D is a reliable and valid instrument for use in a stable coronary population, both on aggregate European level and on country-specific level. The overall Cronbach's alpha for the EQ-5D equaled 0.73, indicating an acceptable internal consistency of the measure. As far as the Greek sample is concerned (n=120, age 62.4±9.6 years), the value was 0.75, also indicating acceptable internal reliability. Criterion validity was also confirmed for EQ-5D, and at the same time the EQ-5D and the EQ-VAS showed good correlations with the overall health criterion SF12 (Ware Jr, Kosinski & Keller, 1996). According to the authors, the strong correlation between SF12 and both the EQ-5D and the EQ-VAS confirmed good criterion validity for EQ-5D and EQ-VAS (De Smedt et al., 2013). Tested by Soer et al. (2012) on a population of Dutch patients suffering from low-back pain, the clinimetric values of the EQ-5D were described as follows: although criterion validity was confirmed, responsiveness was found borderline sufficient for both the EQ-5D index (AUC=0.71) and for the EQ-VAS question (AUC=0.70). The authors suggest that in clinical practice, any improvement at the EQ-5D, can be categorized as clinically important (Soer, Reneman, Speijer, Coppes & Vroomen, 2012). Hurst et al. (1997) measuring QOL amongst rheumatoid arthritis (RA) patients, concluded that the EQ-5D has construct validity in RA and it is at least as responsive to self-reported clinical change and as reliable as many of the condition-specific instruments used in RA. Also, the EQ-VAS is reliable and clearly useful for measuring changes in perceived health (Hurst, Kind, Ruta, Hunter & Stubbings, 1997). J. Yfantopoulos conducted a translation process of the EQ-5D questionnaire to the Greek language, according to the EQ-NET guidelines. The translation of the questionnaire to the Greek language was found to be adaptable to the Greek culture, and it was reported from all members of the pilot sample to be easily comprehensive. For the purposes of the specific research, a valuation exercise of the EQ-5D in a sample of 500 individuals in Greece was reported, and Greek values were compared with the corresponding European values using a correlation coefficient matrix and regression charts. A high degree of association was demonstrated between the Greek and the European values. Based on these findings it can be argued that EQ-5D is a reliable and valid instrument which can be used effectively in QOL measurement in Greek clinical trials and population-based exercises (Yfantopoulos, 2001). Kontodimopoulos et al tested the validity of the EQ-5D instrument in a Greek general population (n=1007). The study reports on the first application in a large and representative sample of the Greek population, and the first extensive evaluation of its basic psychometric properties. Initial evidence has been provided on construct and concurrent validity, reliability, and sensitivity of the instrument, supported by self-reported data on sociodemographic and clinical characteristics. This implies that the EQ-5D is potentially suitable for inclusion in large-scale health surveys in Greece, for providing HRQOL data to be used for cross-cultural quality of life comparisons. According to the authors' conclusion, the EQ-5D demonstrated construct validity in a large and representative sample of the Greek general population (Kontodimopoulos, Pappa, Niakas, Yfantopoulos, Dimitrakaki & Tountas, 2008). Besides being tested on the general population, studies using the EQ-5D questionnaire on specific patient categories in Greece already exist: Papadopoulos et al used the EQ-5D in order to assess the HRQOL of Greek Diabetes mellitus type 2 (DM-2) patients (Papadopoulos, Ikonomakis, Kontodimopoulos, Frydas & Niakas, 2007).

The SF-12 Short Form Health Survey

The SF-12 Health Survey (Ware Jr, Kosinski & Keller, 1996) is a multipurpose short-form survey with 12 questions, all selected from the 36-item Short-Form Health Survey (SF-36 Health Survey) (Ware, Snow, Kosinski, Gandek & Institute, 1993). The SF-12 and the original SF-36 health survey have been translated into several languages by the International Quality of Life Assessment Project (IQOLA) (Hoffmann et al., 2005). The SF-12, as a brief and reliable measure of overall health status, is often included in substantial population health surveys (Vilagut et al., 2013). The 12 items instrument is summarized in two indices exploring the physical health (physical component summary - PCS-12) and the mental health (mental component summary - MCS-12) (Pezzilli et al., 2006). The benefit of reduced administration time and the ability to validly measure physical and mental components makes the SF-12 a reliable outcomes tool (Globe, Levin, Chang, Mackenzie & Azen, 2002). The SF-12 is weighted and summed to provide easily interpretable scales for physical and mental health. The data obtained with the SF-12 has been developed, tested and validated by Quality Metric Incorporated (Utah Department of Health, 2001). However, for the purpose of our study, since gait assistive device user needs and an impression about the limitations of their mobility aids are searched for, we focus on the item-by-item qualitative information that can be extracted, rather than the overall scaled data that can only provide general (physical and mental) health status information. Gandek et al (1998) maintained data from general population surveys (n = 1,483 to 9,151) in nine European countries (Denmark, France, Germany, Italy, the Netherlands, Norway, Spain, Sweden, and the United Kingdom) and analyzed them in order to cross-validate the selection of questionnaire items for the SF-12 Health Survey and scoring algorithms for 12-item physical and mental component summary measures. Replication of the 36-item summary measures by the 12-item summary measures was then evaluated through comparison of mean scores and the strength of product-moment correlations. Product-moment correlations between SF-36 summary measures and SF-12 summary measures (standard and country-specific) were very high, ranging from 0.94–0.96 and 0.94–0.97 for the physical and mental summary measures, respectively. Mean 36-item summary measures and comparable 12-item summary measures were within 0.0 to 1.5 points (median = 0.5 points) in each country and were comparable across age groups (Gandek et al., 1998). Another study that evaluated the construct validity of the SF-12 (version 2) in adolescent population was conducted in China by Fong et al. (2010). Although the second version of the SF-12 questionnaire was measured, there are minor differences in terms of wording and scoring between the two versions and the two versions are summed and weighted to be comparable with each other (Utah Department of Health, 2001). The researchers used clinical and psychometric standards to evaluate the construct validity of the standard Chinese SF-12v2 scales in a large sample of Chinese adolescents. The evaluation by clinical criteria generally confirmed the hypothesized relationships used in the previous evaluations of the SF-12 or SF-36. Specifically, the two-component scales of the SF-12v2 discriminated between adolescents with physical and mental health problems and performed well in associating with other clinical criteria (Fong et al., 2010). Kontodimopoulos et al. (2007) provided initial evidence on the construct and concurrent validity of the instrument when applied to a Greek general population sample. Their research showed that the SF-12 is potentially suitable for inclusion in large-scale health surveys in Greece and cross-cultural quality of life comparisons, as a valid alternative to the SF-36. More specifically, SF-12 summary scores distinguished well, and in an expected manner, between groups of respondents on the basis of gender, age, education, socio-economic status, self-reported health problems and health services utilization, thus providing evidence of construct validity. Effect size differences between SF-36 and SF-12 summary scores were generally small (<0.2), supporting concurrent (criterion) validity. Significantly lower mean PCS-12 and MCS-12 scores were observed for respondents reporting chronic conditions compared to those without ($P < 0.001$). Convergent and divergent validity were supported by expected relationships with the EQ-5D questionnaire. Reporting a problem in an EQ dimension was associated with lower SF-12 summary scores, supporting concurrent validity. The sensitivity of the Greek SF-12 and replication of the original measurement and conceptual model were demonstrated. No floor or ceiling effects in the SF-12 scores were observed in this general population sample, indicating the ability of the instrument to capture a full range of health states (Kontodimopoulos N., Pappa, Niakas & Tountas, 2007). De Smedt et al. (2013), confirmed validity and reliability of three commonly used QOL measures (SF-12, EQ5D and HADS) in a large European population of coronary heart disease patients. Overall, favorable results were found, supporting the use of the SF-12 in a European coronary population. Internal consistency was confirmed, with good to excellent Cronbach's alpha values for the PCS-12 scale, and moderate to good values for the MCS-12 scale, across all 22 countries. Good construct validity was shown for SF-12. In addition, high factor loadings were observed, indicating a good correlation between observed variables and extracted components for SF-12.

Discriminative validity for all the QOL measures was confirmed. Convergent validity was supported by the correlations found between the different constructs for which an association was theoretically expected. Also, moderate to strong correlations were observed between the SF-12 constructs and the EQ-5D index and EQ-VAS scores. In conclusion, the results observed in the study confirmed the validity and reliability of the SF-12v2 for use in a stable coronary population, both on aggregate European level and on country-specific level (De Smedt et al., 2013). Globe et (2002) al also confirmed validity of the SF-12 questionnaire in an ophthalmic cohort with retinal disease. On the basis of the findings of their analysis, the SF-12 is a valid measure of general health status for ophthalmic research (Globe, Levin, Chang, Mackenzie & Azen, 2002). Rubenach et al. (2002) reported on the responsiveness of the SF-12 to changes in quality of life following acute myocardial infarction (MI). In conclusion, although their results are generally consistent with previous reports that the SF12 reflects the expected poorer HRQOL following MI, the comparison of the SF-12 summary scores and SF-36 subscales shows that the SF-12 physical score obscured an important association between changed perceptions of general health and participation in usual activities (Rubenach, Shadbolt, McCallum & Nakamura, 2002). The same results and confirmation of the validity of the SF-12 in an Australian heart disease population are also noted by Lim and Fisher (1999). Focusing on the Mental Component of the Short-Form 12, Vilagut et al mention that the SF-12 yielded acceptable results for detecting both active and recent depressive disorders in general population samples, suggesting that the questionnaire could be used as a useful screening tool for monitoring the prevalence of affective disorders and for targeting treatment and prevention (Vilagut et al., 2013).

IPA Questionnaire

The outcome measure "Impact on Participation and Autonomy - IPA" was developed in 1999 by (Cardol, de Haan, van den Bos, de Jong & de Groot, 1999). According to the developers, it is a generic outcome measure that can be used in populations or with individuals with a range of diagnoses. Rather than focusing on ability or capacity, the IPA questionnaire focuses on autonomy and participation of people with chronic disorders. The IPA questionnaire examines autonomy as opposed to dependency by measuring several aspects of participation. Participation, can be defined as "the involvement of an individual in life situations in relation to health conditions, body function and structures, activities and contextual factors" (Cardol, de Jong & Ward, 2001) or as "persons' own lived experiences of their involvement in a life situation" (WHO, 2001). That is a new concept in the context of the World Health Organization's classification of health outcomes and has replaced the concept "handicap" (WHO, 1980). The IPA questionnaire quantifies limitations in participation and autonomy and examines the extent to which these limitations are experienced as "problematic". The IPA has been validated in several cases (Sibley, Kersten, Ward, White, Mehta & George, 2006; Cardol, de Haan, de Jong, van den Bos & de Groot, 2001; Vazirinejad, Lilley & Ward, 2003; Kersten, Cardol, George, Ward, Sibley & White, 2007).

PROCEDURE

The volunteers were officially informed about the purpose and the procedures of the research through a written form and were also asked to sign a consent form. At the next step, they were given the questionnaires above: the IPA, the EQ5D, and the SF-12. The questionnaires were given in random order to prevent any order effect. The subjects completed the forms following the clear guidelines, with the presence and, if required, with the explanations/assistance of a physical therapist. Whenever needed, the assisting physical therapist would either read or explain the questions to the volunteer, avoiding using other phrases than the ones used in the questionnaire. As far as the IPA questionnaire is concerned, wherever the tool foresaw open-ended questions (in the form of comments), the assistant reviewed the previous questions (for which the comments were asked). Maximum completion time of the three questionnaires was approximately 35 minutes.

STATISTICAL ANALYSIS

For the purpose of statistical analysis, the Statistical Package for Social Sciences (SPSS, version 20) was used. The size of the sample (N=20) combined with the uncertainty related to the satisfaction of normal distribution prerequisite, led to use of non-parametric tests such as Wilcoxon–Mann–Whitney and Kruskal-Wallis non-parametric ANOVA in the event of comparison between groups of participants with quantitative measurements.

In cases where values are discretional, for the purpose of patients' groups' comparison Exact (Significance) Tests for Contingency Tables were used. In the event of multiple comparisons, a Z-Test was used for comparing whose results are noted on the respective tables. Statistical significance for all the above tests was determined at $p=0.05$.

RESULTS

The current section presents the results of the measurements that took place in a rehabilitation center in Greece. The five domains of the EQ-5D were answered by the participants regarding the level of significance for each one of them. Figure 1 presents the findings from the EQ-5D questionnaire.

The mean scores of the EQ-5D VAS [Kruskal Wallis chi-square (df=2, N=20)=0.31, p=0.86] are presented in Table 1.

Table 2 presents the category frequencies of the SF-12 items. All participants answered the SF-12 questions taking into account their health status as it was the last 30 days (when supported by the mobility aid).

Table 3 presents detailed data on the category frequencies of SF-12 questions for the two groups of participants (rehabilitation patients group and elderly group) per walking aid. Table 4 presents the analytical findings on the means and standard deviations of IPA subscales for both groups per walking aid.

Figure 1. EQ-5D dimensions

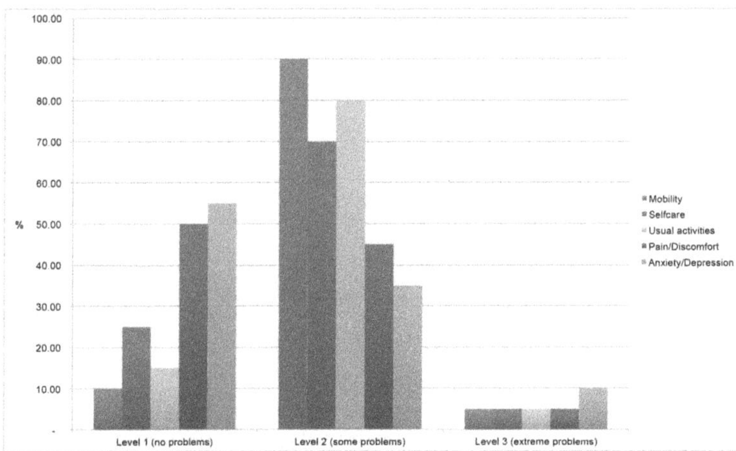

Table 1. Means and standard deviations of EQ-5D VAS scores in three walking aids groups (N=20)

MOBILITY AID	Mean	N	Std. Deviation
Rollator	67.14%	7	9.94%
Crutches	62.50%	4	15.00%
Frame Walker	63.89%	9	25.47%
Total	64.75%	20	18.53%

Table 2. Category frequencies of SF-12 questions

		Count	%
In general, would you say your health is:	Excellent	2	10.0%
	Very Good	5	25.0%
	Good	6	30.0%
	Fair	4	20.0%
	Poor	3	15,0%
Moderate activities, such as moving a table, pushing a vacuum cleaner, bowling, or playing golf	Yes, limited a lot	13	65.0%
	Yes, limited a little	6	30.0%
	No, not limited at all	1	5.0%
Climbing several flights of stairs	Yes, limited a lot	8	40.0%
	Yes, limited a little	9	45.0%
	No, not limited at all	3	15.0%
Accomplished less than you would like	NO	10	50.0%
	YES	10	50.0%
Were limited in the kind of work or other activities	NO	6	30.0%
	YES	14	70.0%
Accomplished less than you would like	NO	10	50.0%
	YES	10	50,0%
Did work or other activities less carefully than usual	NO	13	65.0%
	YES	7	35.0%
During the past four weeks, how much did pain interfere with your regular work (including both work outside the home and housework)	Not at all	11	55.0%
	A little bit	3	15.0%
	Moderately	5	25.0%
	Extremely	1	5.0%

Note (for Table 3 & 4): Values in the same row and subtable not sharing the same subscript are significantly different at $p< 0.05$ in the two-sided test of equality for column proportions. Cells with no subscript are not included in the test (this category is not used in comparisons because its column proportion is equal to zero or one). Tests assume equal variances (tests are adjusted for all pairwise comparisons within a row of each innermost subtable using the Bonferroni correction).

Detailed frequency distribution of the IPA questions is presented in Table 5 & 6.

Note: Values in the same row and sub-table not sharing the same subscript are significantly different at $p<0.1$ in the two-sided test of equality for column proportions. Cells with no subscript are not included in the test (this category is not

Table 3. Category frequencies of SF-12 questions

		Mobility Aid									
		Rollator		Crutches		Frame		Elderly group		Rehab group	
		Count	%	Count	%	Count	%	Count	%	Count	%
SF_12_2b Climbing several flights of stairs	Yes, limited a lot	2_a	28.60	2_a	50.00	4_a	44.40	3_a	27.30	5_a	55.60
	Yes, limited a little	3_a	42.90	2_a	50.00	4_a	44.40	6_a	54.50	3_a	33.30
	No. not limited at all	2_a	28.60	1	0.00	1_a	11.10	2_a	18.20	1_a	11.10
SF_12_3a Accomplished less than you would like	NO	3_a	42.90	2_a	50.00	5_a	55.60	5_a	45.50	5_a	55.60
	YES	4_a	57.10	2_a	50.00	4_a	44.40	6_a	54.50	4_a	44.40
SF_12_3b Were limited in the kind of work or other activities	NO	2_a	28.60	1_a	25.00	3_a	33.30	4_a	36.40	2_a	22.20
	YES	5_a	71.40	3_a	75.00	6_a	66.70	7_a	63.60	7_a	77.80
SF_12_7 During the past four weeks, how much of the time has your physical health or emotional problems interfered with your social activities (like visiting friends, relatives, etc.)?	All of the time	1	0.00	1_a	25.00	1	0.00	1_a	9.10	1	0.00
	Most of the time	1_a	14.30	1_a	25.00	1_a	11.10	3_a	27.30	1	0.00
	Good bit of the time	1	0.00	1	0.00	1	0.00	1	0.00	1	0.00
	Some of the time	1_a	14.30	1	0.00	4_a	44.40	2_a	18.20	3_a	33.30
	Little of the time	1	0.00	1	0.00	1_a	11.10	1_a	9.10	1	0.00
	None of the time	5_a	71.40	2_a	50.00	3_a	33.30	4_a	36.40	6_a	66.70

Table 4. Means and standard deviations of IPA subscales

	Mobility Aid																
	Rollator			Crutches			Frame			Elderly group				Rehab group			
	M	Median	SD	M	Median	SD	M	Median	SD	M	Median	N	SD	M	Median	N	SD
Autonomy indoors	1.27_a	1.43	0.69	0.71_{ab}	0.71	0.58	0.60_b	0.43	0.45	0.69_a	0.57	11	0.51	1.06_a	1	9	0.71
Family role	1.92_a	2.14	1.06	1.75_a	1.57	0.67	1.78_a	1.86	0.4	1.82_a	1.86	11	0.73	1.83_a	1.86	9	0.72
Autonomy outdoors	1.60_a	1.4	0.87	1.85_a	1.8	0.3	1.58_a	1.6	0.95	1.60_a	1.6	11	0.72	1.69_a	1.6	9	0.93
Social life	0.24_a	0.14	0.24	0.14_a	0.14	0.16	0.44_a	0.29	0.44	0.19_a	0.14	11	0.25	0.46_b	0.29	9	0.4
Work education	1.43_a	1.83	0.95	2.04_a	2.08	0.83	2.06_a	2	1.3	1.95_a	2	11	1.29	1.69_a	1.67	9	0.85

Table 5. Frequency distributions of IPA questions (N=20)

	0	1	2	3	4	Total	%
	Count	Count	Count	Count	Count	Count	Score 3-4
@1a	9	6	5	0	0	20	0%
@1b	10	6	4	0	0	20	0%
@1c	1	5	7	6	1	20	35%
@1d	1	2	2	8	7	20	75%
@1e	3	9	7	1	0	20	5%
@2a	6	1	12	1	0	20	5%
@2b	5	4	9	2	0	20	10%
@2c	10	9	1	0	0	20	0%
@2d	10	9	1	0	0	20	0%
@2e	12	6	1	0	1	20	5%
@2f	5	13	2	0	0	20	0%
@3a	2	4	7	5	2	20	35%
@3b	8	3	4	4	1	20	25%
@3c	2	3	4	7	4	20	55%
@3d	4	4	6	4	2	20	30%
@3e	2	0	6	6	6	20	60%
@3f	3	2	8	6	1	20	35%
@3g	2	10	8	0	0	20	0%
@4a	15	3	1	0	1	20	5%
@4b	17	3	0	0	0	20	0%
@5a	8	5	4	3	0	20	15%
@5b	7	7	6	0	0	20	0%
@6a	18	1	1	0	0	20	0%
@6b	19	0	0	0	1	20	5%
@6c	19	0	1	0	0	20	0%
@6d	15	4	1	0	0	20	0%
@6e	17	2	1	0	0	20	0%
@6f	11	7	1	0	1	20	5%
@6g	8	3	6	2	1	20	15%
@6h	7	10	3	0	0	20	0%
@7a	12	5	2	1	0	20	5%
@7b	13	4	3	0	0	20	0%

continues on following page

Table 5. Continued

	0	1	2	3	4	Total	%
	Count	Count	Count	Count	Count	Count	Score 3-4
@8a	1	5	3	5	6	20	55%
@8b	2	3	5	3	2	15	33%
@8c	10	1	2	2	0	15	13%
@8d	8	0	3	4	0	15	27%
@8e	2	2	2	4	5	15	60%
@8f	2	5	8	0	0	15	0%
@9a	10	6	1	1	2	20	15%
@9b	10	9	1	0	0	20	0%
@10	7	9	3	1	0	20	5%

used in comparisons because its column proportion is equal to zero or one). Tests assume equal variances (tests are adjusted for all pairwise comparisons within a row of each innermost subtable using the Bonferroni correction).

The referred comments from the frequency distributions of the IPA open questions were coded and categorized into six main domains (see Figures 2, 3 and 4).

Figure 2. Frequency distributions of IPA open questions (N=20)

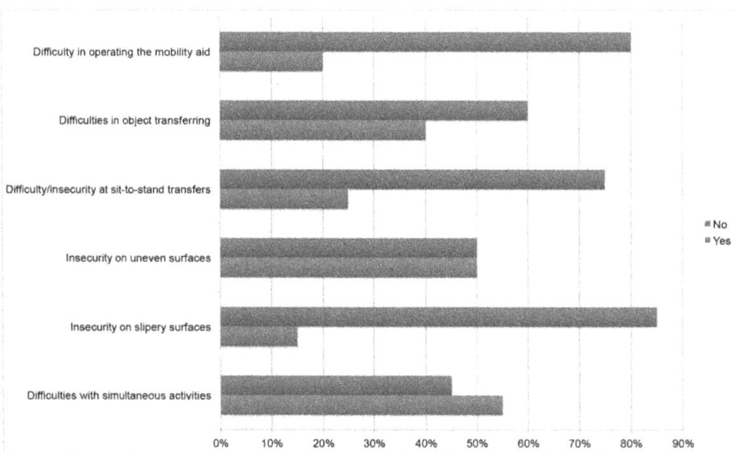

Table 6. Frequency distributions of IPA questions per walking aid group

		Mobility Aid					
		Rollator		Crutches		Frame	
		Count	%	Count	%	Count	%
@1a	0	2_a	28.6%	1_a	25.0%	6_a	66.7%
	1	1_a	14.3%	3_a	75.0%	2_a	22.2%
	2	4_a	57.1%	0[1]	0.0%	1_b	11.1%
@1b	0	3_a	42.9%	1_a	25.0%	6_a	66.7%
	1	1_a	14.3%	3_a	75.0%	2_a	22.2%
	2	3_a	42.9%	0[1]	0.0%	1_a	11.1%
@1c	0	1_a	14.3%	0[1]	0.0%	0[1]	0.0%
	1	2_a	28.6%	0[1]	0.0%	3_a	33.3%
	2	1_a	14.3%	3_a	75.0%	3_a	33.3%
	3	3_a	42.9%	1_a	25.0%	2_a	22.2%
	4	0[1]	0.0%	0[1]	0.0%	1_a	11.1%
@2c	0	2_a	28.6%	2_a	50.0%	6_a	66.7%
	1	5_a	71.4%	2_a	50.0%	2_a	22.2%
	2	0[1]	0.0%	0[1]	0.0%	1_a	11.1%
@2d	0	1_a	14.3%	$2_{a,b}$	50.0%	7_b	77.8%
	1	5_a	71.4%	2_a	50.0%	2_a	22.2%
	2	1_a	14,3%	0[1]	0.0%	0[1]	0.0%
@3a	0	1_a	14.3%	0[1]	0.0%	1_a	11.1%
	1	1_a	14.3%	3_b	75.0%	0[1]	0.0%
	2	3_a	42.9%	0[1]	0.0%	4_a	44.4%
	3	1_a	14.3%	1_a	25.0%	3_a	33.3%
	4	1_a	14.3%	0[1]	0.0%	1_a	11.1%

DISCUSSION

Even though no significant differences in the mean scores of the EQ-5D VAS were found among users of different types of mobility aids [Kruskal Wallis chi-square (df=2, N=20)=0.31, p=0.86], participants that use a rollator as a mobility aid (N=7) characterize their health state with relative higher scores than the ones that use the other two mobility aids (crutches N=4, frame walkers N=9) (see Table 1). An explanation to this could be that those using a rollator may have comprehended their health situation (as a lifetime status), while the others (using crutches or frame

Figure 3. Frequency distributions of IPA open questions per walking aid group

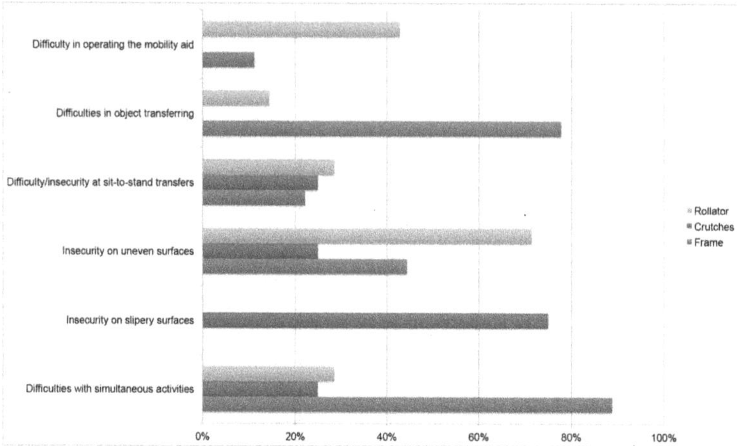

Figure 4. Frequency distributions of IPA open questions for the rehabilitation group and the elderly group

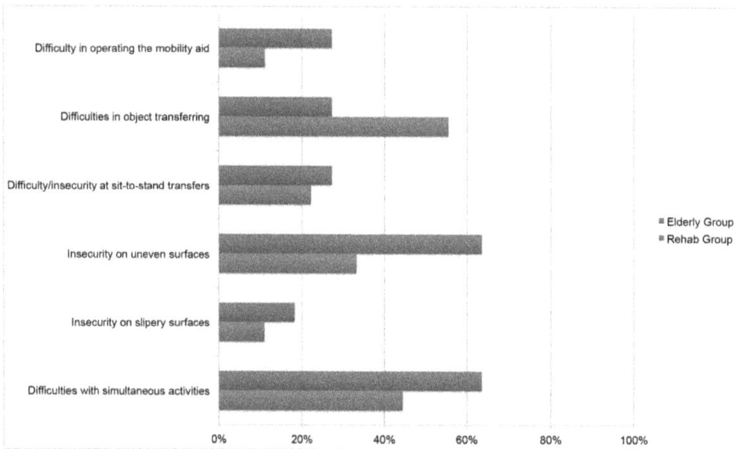

walkers) are in a psychological situation that cannot still accept their health status. Persons belonging in the latter category are on the edge of independent living, and this may be a criterion of continuous thoughts about their health status and agony about not being entirely independent of mobility aids. That is also in line with the fact that 90% of the subjects face depression and anxiety symptoms (Figure 1).

According to the findings of Table 2, the vast majority of mobility aid users (95%) reported limitations in moderate activities (such as moving a table, pushing a vacuum cleaner, etc.), while 65% of them were "limited a lot". Moreover, a high percentage (85%) of the users reported having limitations at climbing several flights of stairs, and 70% were limited in work or other activities as a result of their physical health condition.

According to the data of Table 3, no significant differences were noticed for the selected items. However, as seen at the SF-12, item 7, problems regarding social activities were least frequently mentioned by rollator users (N=5, 71.4%), and more frequently by crutches users (N=2, 50%) and frame users (N=3, 33.3%). Another interesting finding is the 2b item of the SF-12 (limitations when climbing several flights of stairs), where rollator users that answered "not limited at all" are significantly more than frame and crutches users giving the same answer. The results revealed that both groups present a similarly high percentage of limitations when climbing several flights of stairs (elderly group N=9, 81.8% and for the rehabilitation group N=8, 88.9%), as it was anticipated due to their overall health condition. However, the elderly (N=3, 27.3%) reported being "limited a lot" significantly less frequently than the rehabilitation participants (N=5, 55.6%).

Table 4 shows that all participants score high rates (0=very good, 1=good) at "social life" subscale, with the elderly group scoring significantly higher rates (M=0.190) than the ones from the rehabilitation group (M=0.46). At the remaining subscales, group differences are not significant. Both groups score high rates at the "social life" and "autonomy indoors" subscales. On the mobility type based grouping, frame-walker users score significantly higher rates at "autonomy outdoors" subscale (M=0.60) than the rollator ones (M=1.27). No significant differences between the two groups were noticed for the remaining subscales.

According to the findings of Table 5, as it was expected, mobility aid users report severe limitations in activities including outdoor transportation (1d, 3e, 1c), indoor role fulfilment (3a, 3c, 3f) and job-related problems (8a, 8b, 8e). Rollator users reported more significant difficulties in moving around the house. 57.1% of them stated having fair chances of getting around in the house, while all crutches users and 88,9% of frame walker users state to have "very good" or "good" chances of achieving it. The vast majority of the participants (95%) claimed to have "very good" or "good" chances of getting up and going to bed whenever they decide to. Depending on the mobility aid, frame users have significantly better chances of answering "very good" at the IPA_2c question than rollator users. Although 95% of all participants have "very good" or "good" chances of going to the toilet when they wish or need, significant differences appear between rollator users and frame users. As seen at IPA_2d, rollator users have 14.3% chances of answering "very good" at the question, while the respective percentage for frame-walker users reaches 77.8%. For question IPA_3a (my chances of contributing to looking after my house the way I like are), most of the answers for frame-walker users (44.4%) and rollator users (42.9%) were "fair", and no other significant differences for the two groups were found.

More than half of the participants (55%) mentioned difficulties when attempting other activities while using their mobility aid. These difficulties mostly affected frame-walker users (88.9%), while rollator and crutches users were affected at a percentage of 28.6% and 25% respectively. Insecurity while walking on uneven surfaces was mentioned from 50% of the sample. This sense was reported by 71.4% of rollator users, while frame walker users and crutches users reported it as a percentage of 44.4% and 25% respectively. Difficulties in transferring objects were mentioned from 40% of the sample. This restriction mainly concerned frame walker users (77.8%), while for rollator users, it affects only 14.3% of them.

On the other hand, 55.6% of the rehab group reported the same difficulty. Sit-to-stand transfers are reported as a difficult task or as an insecurity-causing task by 25% of the sample. Insignificant differences exist between mobility aid groups and rehabilitation/elderly categorizations. Finally, crutches users (15%) were the only group that mentioned "sense of insecurity while walking on slippery surfaces, independent of the group they were belonging.

No significant differences were found at "autonomy outdoors" subscale scores of the IPA questionnaire between thc three answer categories of the SF_12_2b item, despite the interesting differences observed. These differences describe smaller autonomy level (M=2.00) for those who answered: "Yes, limited a lot" compared to those who answered "No, not limited at all" (M=0.80). Referring to the correlations between 3a and 3b (agreement or disagreement in both questions 3a & 3b of SF-12) and the question 10 of IPA, this was also found insignificant (p=0.08). Mobility aid users that answered "Yes" at both 3a and 3b questions mentioned a lower level (35% scored "2" or "3" at IPA_10 item) compared to those who answered "No" at both 3a and 3b questions (0% scored "2" or "3" at IPA_10 item). That means that those who accomplished less than they would like and were also limited in their work or other activities as a result of their physical health had worse chances of living life the way they want to.

Even though it is significant for a group of older adults with mobility impairments to use the frame walker, it has been observed a difficulty to take the stairs or go up and down on a slope while using the walker. That may occur because of two primary reasons: (i) they are physically too weak to accomplish the previously mentioned functions, and therefore they need assistance from another person, and (ii) the design of walkers themselves is not functional for the previous activities. Our results are in line with another study that recommends an improved walker design for older adults (Cherng-Yee Leung & Po-Chan Yeh, 2008).

Apart from all the above, many other issues are related to the dangers associated with mobility aids. For example, it is possible that the act of lifting the mobility aid (referring to walking frames) can lead to instability in the same way that lifting the foot can cause the Centre of Mass (COM) to fall toward the unsupported side during unassisted gait. By suddenly reducing the Base of Support (BOS), lifting the device could create a state of imbalance in which the COM lies outside the BOS limits. Moreover, the tendency of the walking frame to tip increases with the magnitude of the applied horizontal force and with the height of the walker (Bateni & Maki, 2005). When it comes to gait speed, the use of any walking aid, in particular walkers, results in slower gait speed and requires considerably more energy and cardiovascular fitness than walking unassisted (Martins, Frizera-Neto, Urendes, dos Santos, Ceres & Bastos-Filho, 2012). Also, as mentioned by (Cetin, Muzembo, Pardessus, Puisieux & Thevenon, 2010), with a fixed frame walker, Physiological Cost Index (PCI) was higher in a weakened elderly individual due to heart rate increase and lower walking speed. Several studies have found that use of mobility aid is a prospective predictor of increased risk of falling in older adults or is associated with falls and related injuries.

Furthermore, it appears that frame-walker-related injury can occur as a result of contact and/or "catch" of the mobility aid with environmental objects, such as carpets and doorframes that would not usually be considered obstacles (Bateni & Maki, 2005). Fall-related injuries among older adults are also associated with substantial social and economic costs (Solway, Brooks, Lacasse & Thomas, 2001; Beaupre, Jones, Johnston, Wilson & Majumdar, 2012; Stevens, Thomas, Teh & Greenspan, 2009). There is little evidence to suggest whether the use of a walking aid alone leads to this risk or if it is related to the decreased level of physical function, increased frailty, and poorer general health that users of walking aids may have. However, inappropriate walking aid prescription, inadequate training of the user and un-prescribed use of walking aids are likely to exacerbate the problem (Thomas et al., 2010).

According to the findings of the research, it is crucial to provide new technological solutions to support the needs and overcome most of the problems faced by mobility aid users. Apart from the underlying pathology, mobility aids have been proved crucial for the everyday living of their users. The adoption of some technological innovations could enhance the performance and the acceptance rate of the already existing mobility aids. To this end, several new functionalities could be proved valuable for mobility aid users. More specifically, sit-to-stand support seems to be crucial for most of the users, while a mobility aid that could enhance the safety feeling when moving around slippery and uneven surfaces is also considered critical. Apart from the above, according to open-ended interviews we had with the participants, another critical issue identified was to support them in navigating in unknown spaces. Functionalities that could support them to reach mobility aid when it is at a distance could also provide great support. Finally, providing help when it comes to climbing stairs is valuable, whereas the existence of sitting support while walking is also considered extremely helpful.

The functionalities mentioned above can be implemented using the latest robotics and human-computer interaction techniques. Several robotic intelligent mobility aids have been presented in the literature, divided into two main categories: robotic wheelchairs and robotic walkers (Van der Loos & Reinkensmeyer, 2008). Robotic walkers constitute a mechanized version of the standard walking frame and are further divided into three main groups (Frizera, Ceres, Pons, Abellanas & Raya, 2008): (i) the Zimmer Frame, designed to provide support to a person with a lower limb weakness, (ii) the Rollators which is a standard frame attached with wheels used where balance is the major problem, and (iii) the Reciprocal Frames, similar to the Standard Frames except that the frame is hinged on either side allowing the sides of the frame to be moved alternately. All robotic walkers are a robotized variation of the Rollator frame. They generally present the following functionalities (Martins, Santos, Frizera-Neto & Ceres, 2012):

- physical support;
- cognitive assistance;
- sensorial assistance;
- health monitoring;
- advanced human-machine interface.

Robotic walkers can be divided into passive and active rollators (Ko & Agrawal, 2010). The passive mobility aids can steer or brake, but cannot move forward without a person applying force on them, while the active rollators are equipped with actuators, and their motion can be actively controlled. Several intelligent mobility aids exist nowadays: the iWalker robot (Kulyukin, Kutiyanawala, LoPresti, Matthews & Simpson, 2008), the GUIDO system (Haptica Inc., Dublin, Ireland), the Personal Aids for Mobility and Monitoring “PAMM” SmartWalker (Spenko, Yu & Dubowsky, 2006), a system called SmartWalker (Shin, Rusakov & Meyer, 2016), the JAIST Active Robotic Walker (JARow) (Geunho, Jung, Ohnuma, Chong, & Yi, 2011), the Fraunhofer’s Care-O-bot and Care-O-bot II (Graf, Hans & Schraft, 2004), the LEA robot (Robot Care Systems bv, Den Haag, Zuid-Holland), etc.

In the same direction, an innovative experimental prototype called MOBOT utilized audio-gestural controls, navigation functionality and an actuated robotic rollator (Koumpouros et al., 2017a; Efthimiou et al., 2016; Fotinea et al., 2014). However, further research is required in the above directions in order to conclude in marketable products (lightweight, low cost and highly aesthetics) that can support mobility aid users more efficiently and intuitively. The acceptance and use of innovative assistive technologies among people with cognitive impairment and their caregivers is still challenging (Thordardottir, Malmgren Fänge, Lethin, Rodriguez Gatta & Chiatti, 2019). The performance of daily activities by device-assisted walkers is restrained by several factors, related to the assistive device limitations or/and the limitations emerged from environmental causes. A critical point in the development and further enhancement of mobility aid devices is the successful evaluation of all phases (research, design, development, market entering). As already stated in the Introduction section of the paper, it is difficult to find a single instrument able to capture the subjective satisfaction of the end-users. However, a recent effort in this direction proposes a newly developed tool called PYTHEIA with very encouraging results (Koumpouros, 2016; Koumpouros et al., 2016; Koumpouros, Papageorgiou & Karavasili, 2016). PYTHEIA's capability to capture the satisfaction of the end-users with assistive and robotic technologies, while being able to evaluate any individual features/functionalities implemented is valuable and unique. This is not present in any other scales (QUEST 2.0, ATDPA, etc.). The validation of PYTHEIA scale in population using assistive technology devices (robotic or not) opens new horizons in the subjective assessment of mobility assistive devices, giving the opportunity to researchers and companies to evaluate their products in all stages of design and production.

Although our sample size can be considered adequate for reasoning, it is rather small, thus limiting the statistical power of our study. In order to generalize the findings, a more significant sample is necessary. Moreover, the study was designed in only one center. A multi-center or even multi-country approach would add significant value.

CONCLUSION

The current study attempted to reveal the major limitations, concerns and metrics around mobility aid devices and user needs while presenting an assessment strategy. The user evaluation of assistive devices has been proved to be very challenging (Koumpouros et al., 2017a; Koumpouros et al., 2017b; Efthimiou et al., 2016). A bibliographic survey followed by a real case study on a small size of the population with specific characteristics (mobility aid users, rehabilitation patients or older adults, independent of any associating disease). From the beginning of our searching a necessary assumption was made: the concept of "user needs", being mandatorily unable to be separated from every single dimension that could claim a portion of existence in every individual's needs spectrum will have –as mandatorily- to be described as a multi-dimensional, broad and complex field. Trying to reach conclusions on the relationships between all these complex data (social, psychological, mental, and biological) that will come up whenever entering this field would be a duty that exceeds the capabilities -although not the interests- of this attempt. We attempted, instead, by using three different valid instruments that try to extract from very general to precise information, to cover many aspects of self-perceiving ones' mobility and overall condition. Using multi-dimensional questionnaires helped us consider the full spectrum of user needs and at the same time to correlate data from different dimensions (e.g. mobility limitations and social life). From the EQ5D questionnaire, very general limitations on physical, mental and social functionality can be confirmed and classified. The SF-12 questionnaire includes some targeted questions from which user needs can be specified in more details, exploring in a more detailed level the physical and mental dimensions of QOL. Finally, the more extended IPA questionnaire, has a range of specified questions which cover nine different aspects of participation and autonomy (such as mobility, activities in and around the house, etc.) and also has predicted open-ended comments for each different aspect, allowing user-derived information and ideas on needs and limitations (in general and also in specific for mobility aids, if they exist) to enter the form. Recent studies reveal the lack of appropriate instruments to measure and assess the subjective opinion of users of assistive devices (Koumpouros, 2016) while proposing new tools to this direction (Koumpouros, Papageorgiou & Karavasili, 2016; Koumpouros, Papageorgiou, Karavasili & Koureta, 2016). Unfortunately, the PYTHEIA scale was not present when performing our research and thus we couldn't use it in the assessment strategy. Our next efforts will exploit PYTHEIA's unique characteristics for a more complete and detailed assessment of different mobility aid devices. Concluding, it is evident that there is a great need for better, more intuitive and adaptable mobility aid devices capable of covering the needs of their end users in the modern era.

ACKNOWLEDGMENT

I would like to thank the physical therapists P. Siavelis, D. Alexopoulou, and the physiatrist A. Karavasili, working in the rehabilitation hospital Diaplasis in Kalamata, Greece, that helped in the recruitment process and collection of the data from the participating patients in the study. The work leading to the presented results has received funding from the European Union under grant agreement n°600796.

REFERENCES

Akinbo, S. R., Sokunbi, O., & Ogunbameru, T. (2008). Factors contributing to possession of walking aids among persons with osteoarthritis of the knee. *Nigerian Quarterly Journal of Hospital Medicine*, *18*(2), 64–68. PMID:19068554

Bateni, H., & Maki, B. E. (2005). Assistive Devices for Balance and Mobility: Benefits, Demands, and Adverse Consequences. *Archives of Physical Medicine and Rehabilitation*, *86*(1), 134–145. doi:10.1016/j.apmr.2004.04.023 PMID:15641004

Bateni, H., & Maki, B. E. (2005). Assistive Devices for Balance and Mobility: Benefits, Demands, and Adverse Consequences. *Archives of Physical Medicine and Rehabilitation*, *86*(1), 134–145. doi:10.1016/j.apmr.2004.04.023 PMID:15641004

Beaupre, L., Jones, C., Johnston, D., Wilson, D., & Majumdar, S. (2012). Recovery of function following a hip fracture in geriatric ambulatory persons living in nursing homes: Prospective cohort study. *Journal of the American Geriatrics Society*, *60*(7), 1268–1273. doi:10.1111/j.1532-5415.2012.04033.x PMID:22702238

Brandt, A., Iwarsson, S., & Ståhl, A. (2003). Satisfaction with rollators among community-living users: A follow-up study. *Disability and Rehabilitation*, *25*(7), 343–353. doi:10.1080/0963828021000058495 PMID:12745958

Brooks, R. (1996). EuroQol: The current state of play. *Health Policy (Amsterdam)*, *37*(1), 53–72. doi:10.1016/0168-8510(96)00822-6 PMID:10158943

Cardol, M., de Haan, R., van den Bos, G., de Jong, B., & de Groot, I. (1999). The development of a handicap assessment questionnaire: The Impact on Participation and Autonomy (IPA). *Clinical Rehabilitation*, *13*(5), 411–419. doi:10.1191/026921599668601325 PMID:10498348

Cardol, M., de Haan, R. J., de Jong, B. A., van den Bos, G. A., & de Groot, I. J. (2001). Psychometric properties of the Impact on Participation and Autonomy Questionnaire. *Archives of Physical Medicine and Rehabilitation*, *82*(2), 210–216. doi:10.1053/apmr.2001.18218 PMID:11239312

Cardol, M., de Jong, B., & Ward, C. (2001). *On autonomy and participation in rehabilitation*. Amsterdam: Academic Press.

Cetin, E., Muzembo, J., Pardessus, V., Puisieux, F., & Thevenon, A. (2010). Impact of different types of walking aids on the physiological energy cost during gait for elderly individuals with several pathologies and dependent on a technical aid for walking. *Annals of Physical and Rehabilitation Medicine*, *53*(6-7), 399–405. doi:10.1016/j.rehab.2010.06.003 PMID:20674533

Charron, P., Kirby, R., & MacLeod, D. (1995). Epidemiology of walker-related injuries and deaths in the united states. *American Journal of Physical Medicine & Rehabilitation*, *74*(3), 237–239. doi:10.1097/00002060-199505000-00011 PMID:7779337

De Smedt, D., Clays, E., Doyle, F., Kotseva, K., Prugger, C., Pająk, A., ... De Bacquer, D. (2013). Validity and reliability of three commonly used quality of life measures in a large European population of coronary heart disease patients. *International Journal of Cardiology*, *167*(5), 2294–2299. doi:10.1016/j.ijcard.2012.06.025 PMID:22748284

Demers, L., Monette, M., LaPierre, Y., Arnold, D. L., & Wolfson, C. (2002). Reliability, validity, and applicability of the Quebec User Evaluation of Satisfaction with assistive Technology (QUEST 2.0) for adults with multiple sclerosis. *Disability And Rehabilitation, 24*(1/2/3), 21-30.

Demers, L., Weiss-Lambrou, R., & Bernadette, S. (2002). The Quebec User Evaluation os Satisfaction with Assistive Technology (QUEST 2.0): An overview and recent progress. *Technology and Disability*, *14*(3), 101–105. doi:10.3233/TAD-2002-14304

Demers, L., Weiss-Lambrou, R., & Ska, B. (2000). *Quebec User Evaluation of Satisfaction with Assistive Technology (QUEST Version 2.0). An Outcome Measure for Assistive Technology Devices*. Webster: The Institute for Matching Person & Technology.

Efthimiou, E., Fotinea, S., Goulas, T., Koutsombogera, M., Karioris, P., Vacalopoulou, A., & ... . (2016). The MOBOT rollator human-robot interaction model and user evaluation process. *2016 IEEE Symposium Series On Computational Intelligence (SSCI)*. 10.1109/SSCI.2016.7850061

EuroQol. (1990). EuroQol—A new facility for the measurement of health related quality of life. *Health Policy (Amsterdam)*, *16*(3), 199–208. doi:10.1016/0168-8510(90)90421-9

EuroQol. (2007). *EQ5D Value Sets-inventory, comparative review and user guide. EuroQol group Monographs*. Springer.

Fong, D. Y., Lam, C., Mak, K. K., Lo, S. W., Lai, K. Y., Ho, Y. S., & Lam, T. H. (2010). The Short Form-12 Health Survey was a valid instrument in Chinese adolescents. *Journal of Clinical Epidemiology*, *63*(9), 1020–1029. doi:10.1016/j.jclinepi.2009.11.011 PMID:20189764

Fotinea, S. E., Efthimiou, E., Dimou, A. L., Goulas, T., Karioris, P., Peer, A., ... Stanzyk, B. (2014). Data acquisition towards defining a multimodal interaction model for human - assistive robot communication. In. Lecture Notes in Computer Science: Vol. 8515. *Universal Access in Human-Computer Interaction. Aging and Assistive Environments* (pp. 613–624). Springer International Publishing. doi:10.1007/978-3-319-07446-7_59

Frizera, A., Ceres, R., Pons, J., Abellanas, A., & Raya, R. (2008). The smart walkers as geriatric assistive device. The simbiosis purpose. *Gerontechnology (Valkenswaard), 7*(2). doi:10.4017/gt.2008.07.02.045.00

Gandek, B., Ware, J. E., Aaronson, N. K., Apolone, G., Bjorner, J. B., Brazier, J. E., ... Sullivan, M. (1998). Cross-Validation of Item Selection and Scoring for the SF-12 Health Survey in Nine Countries. *Journal of Clinical Epidemiology, 15*(11), 1171–1178. doi:10.1016/S0895-4356(98)00109-7 PMID:9817135

Geunho, L., Jung, E.-J., Ohnuma, T., Chong, N. Y., & Yi, B.-J. (2011). JAIST Robotic Walker Control Based on a Two-Layered Kalman Filter. *2011 IEEE International Conference on Robotics and Automation*, 3682-3687.

Globe, D., Levin, S., Chang, T., Mackenzie, P., & Azen, S. (2002). Validity of the SF-12 Quality of Life Instrument in Patients with Retinal Diseases. *Ophthalmology, 109*(10), 1793–1798. doi:10.1016/S0161-6420(02)01124-7 PMID:12359596

Graf, B., Hans, M., & Schraft, R. (2004). Care-O-bot II—Development of a Next Generation Robotic Home Assistant. *Autonomous Robots, 16*(2), 193–205. doi:10.1023/B:AURO.0000016865.35796.e9

Hallén, K., Orrenius, U., & Rose, L. (2006). *Ergonomical evaluation of the rollator prototype Walker*. ERAK report 2006-02.

Hill, K., Goldstein, R., Gartner, E. J., & Brooks, D. (2008). Daily Utility and Satisfaction With Rollators Among Persons With Chronic Obstructive Pulmonary Disease. *Archives of Physical Medicine and Rehabilitation, 89*(6), 1108–1113. doi:10.1016/j.apmr.2007.11.032 PMID:18503807

Hoffmann, C., McFarland, B., Kinzie, J., Bresler, L., Rakhlin, D., Wolf, S., & Kovas, A. E. (2005). Psychometric properties of a Russian version of the SF-12 Health Survey in a refugee population. *Comprehensive Psychiatry, 46*(5), 390–397. doi:10.1016/j.comppsych.2004.12.002 PMID:16122541

Hurst, N., Kind, P., Ruta, D., Hunter, M., & Stubbings, A. (1997). Measuring health related quality of life in rheumatoid arthritis: Validity, responsiveness and reliability of EuroQol (EQ-5D). *British Journal of Rheumatology*, *36*(5), 551–559. doi:10.1093/rheumatology/36.5.551 PMID:9189057

Kersten, P., Cardol, M., George, S., Ward, C., Sibley, A., & White, B. (2007). Validity of the impact on participation and autonomy questionnaire: A comparison between two countries. *Disability and Rehabilitation*, *29*(19), 1502–1509. doi:10.1080/09638280601030066 PMID:17852246

Ko, C., & Agrawal, S. (2010). *Walk-Assist Robot: A Novel Approach to Gain Selection of a Braking Controller using Differential Flatness.* In 2010 American Control Conference. Marriott Waterfront, Baltimore, MD.

Kontodimopoulos, N., Pappa, E., Niakas, D., & Tountas, Y. (2007). Validity of SF-12 summary scores in a Greek general population. *Health and Quality of Life Outcomes*, *5*(1), 55. doi:10.1186/1477-7525-5-55 PMID:17900374

Kontodimopoulos, N., Pappa, E., Niakas, D., Yfantopoulos, J., Dimitrakaki, C., & Tountas, Y. (2008). Validity of the EuroQoL (EQ-5D) instrument in a Greek General Population. *Value in Health*, 11. PMID:18489492

Koumpouros, Y. (2016). A Systematic Review on Existing Measures for the Subjective Assessment of Rehabilitation and Assistive Robot Devices. *Journal of Healthcare Engineering*, *2016*, 1–10. doi:10.1155/2016/1048964 PMID:27196802

Koumpouros, Y., Karavasili, A., Efthimiou, E., Fotinea, S., Goulas, T., & Vacalopoulou, A. (2017a). User Evaluation of the MOBOT Rollator Type Robotic Mobility Assistive Device. *Technologies*, *5*(4), 73. doi:10.3390/technologies5040073

Koumpouros, Y., Karavasili, A., Efthimiou, E., Fotinea, S., Goulas, T., & Vacalopoulou, A. (2017b). User Evaluation of the MOBOT rollator type robotic mobility assistive device. *Proceedings Of The 10Th International Conference On Pervasive Technologies Related To Assistive Environments - PETRA '17*. 10.1145/3056540.3076183

Koumpouros, Y., Karavasili, A., Papageorgiou, E., & Siavelis, P. (2016). Validation of the Greek version of the device subscale of the Quebec User Evaluation of Satisfaction with Assistive Technology 2.0 (QUEST 2.0). *Assistive Technology*, *28*(3), 152–158. doi:10.1080/10400435.2015.1131758 PMID:26854178

Koumpouros, Y., Papageorgiou, E., & Karavasili, A. (2016). Development of a new psychometric scale (PYTHEIA) to assess the satisfaction of users with any assistive technology. *7th International Conference on Applied Human Factors and Ergonomics, AHFE 2016. Florida, USA: IEEE Proceedings.*

Koumpouros, Y., Papageorgiou, E., Karavasili, A., & Koureta, F. (2016). PYTHEIA: A Scale for Assessing Rehabilitation and Assistive Robotics. *International Journal of Medical, Health, Biomedical, Bioengineering and Pharmaceutical Engineering, 10*(11), 522–526.

Kulyukin, V. A., Kutiyanawala, A., LoPresti, E., Matthews, J. T., & Simpson, R. (2008). iWalker: Toward a Rollator-Mounted Wayfinding System for the Elderly. *2008 IEEE International Conference on RFID*, 303-311.

Lezzoni, L. I., Rao, S. R., & Kinkel, R. P. (2009). Patterns of mobility aid use among working-age persons with multiple sclerosis living in the community in the United States. *Disability and Health Journal, 2*(2), 67–76. doi:10.1016/j.dhjo.2008.12.001 PMID:21122745

Lim, L., & Fisher, J. (1999). Use of the 12-item short-form (SF-12) health survey in an Australian heart and stroke population. *Quality of Life Research: An International Journal of Quality of Life Aspects of Treatment, Care and Rehabilitation, 8*(1-2), 1–8. doi:10.1023/A:1026409226544 PMID:10457733

Martins, M., Frizera-Neto, A., Urendes, E., dos Santos, C., Ceres, R., & Bastos-Filho, T. (2012). A novel human-machine interface for guiding: The neoasas smart walker. *Biosignals and Biorobotics Conference (BRC)*. 10.1109/BRC.2012.6222195

Martins, M., Santos, C., Frizera-Neto, A., & Ceres, R. (2012). Assistive mobility devices focusing on Smart Walkers: Classification and review. *Robotics and Autonomous Systems, 60*(4), 548–562. doi:10.1016/j.robot.2011.11.015

Minor, M., & Minor, S. (2013). *Patient care skills* (7th ed.). Pearson.

Nilsson, E., Wenemark, M., Bendtsen, P., & Kristenson, M. (2007). Respondent satisfaction regarding SF-36 and EQ-5D, and patients' perspectives concerning health outcome assessment within routine health care. *Quality of Life Research: An International Journal of Quality of Life Aspects of Treatment, Care and Rehabilitation, 16*(10), 1647–1654. doi:10.100711136-007-9263-8 PMID:17922304

Papadopoulos, A., Ikonomakis, E., Kontodimopoulos, N., Frydas, A., & Niakas, D. (2007). Assessment of health-related quality of life for diabetic patients type 2. *Archives of Hellenic Medicine, 24*(1), 66–74.

Pezzilli, R., Morselli-Labate, A., Frulloni, L., Cavestro, G., Ferri, B., Comparato, G., & … . (2006). The quality of life in patients with chronic pancreatitis evaluated using the SF-12 questionnaire: A comparative study with the SF-36 questionnaire. *Digestive and Liver Disease, 38*, 109–111. PMID:16243011

Resnik, L., Allen, S., Isenstadt, D., Wasserman, M., & Iezzoni, L. (2009). Perspectives on use of mobility aids in a diverse population of seniors: Implications for intervention. *Disability and Health Journal, 2*(2), 77–85. doi:10.1016/j.dhjo.2008.12.002 PMID:20160951

Roman de Mettelinge, T., & Cambier, D. (2015). Understanding the Relationship Between Walking Aids and Falls in Older Adults. *Journal of Geriatric Physical Therapy, 38*(3), 127–132. doi:10.1519/JPT.0000000000000031 PMID:25594520

Rubenach, S., Shadbolt, B., McCallum, J., & Nakamura, T. (2002). Assessing health-related quality of life following myocardial infarction: Is the SF-12 useful? *Journal of Clinical Epidemiology, 55*(3), 306–309. doi:10.1016/S0895-4356(01)00426-7 PMID:11864802

Shin, J., Rusakov, A., & Meyer, B. (2016). SmartWalker: Towards an Intelligent Robotic Walker for the Elderly. *Journal of Ambient Intelligence and Smart Environments, 1*, 1–5.

Sibley, A., Kersten, P., Ward, C., White, B., Mehta, R., & George, S. (2006). Measuring autonomy in disabled people: Validation of a new scale in a UK population. *Clinical Rehabilitation, 20*(9), 793–803. doi:10.1177/0269215506070808 PMID:17005503

Siu, S., Wong, M., Shah, A., Li, H., Soong, A., & Cao, R. (2008). Redesign of the Rollator's (Walker's) Parking Brake System. In *Proceedings of the IASTED International Conference on Telehealth* (pp. 129-132). ACTA Press.

Soer, R., Reneman, M. F., Speijer, B. L., Coppes, M. H., & Vroomen, P. C. (2012). Clinimetric properties of the EuroQol-5D in patients with chronic low back pain. *The Spine Journal, 12*(11), 1035–1039. doi:10.1016/j.spinee.2012.10.030 PMID:23199409

Solway, S., Brooks, D., Lacasse, Y., & Thomas, S. (2001). A Qualitative Systematic Overview of the Measurement Properties of Functional Walk Tests Used in the Cardiorespiratory Domain. *Chest, 119*(1), 256–270. doi:10.1378/chest.119.1.256 PMID:11157613

Stahl, E., Jansson, S., Jonsson, A., Svensson, K., Lundback, B., & Andersson, F. (2003). Health-related quality of life, utility, and productivity outcomes instruments: Ease of completion by subjects with COPD. *Health and Quality of Life Outcomes, 1*(1), 18–24. doi:10.1186/1477-7525-1-18 PMID:12809558

Stevens, J., Thomas, K., Teh, L., & Greenspan, A. (2009). Unintentional Fall Injuries Associated with Walkers and Canes in Older Adults Treated in U.S. Emergency Departments. *Journal of the American Geriatrics Society*, *57*(8), 1464–1469. doi:10.1111/j.1532-5415.2009.02365.x PMID:19555423

Thomas, S., Halbert, J., Mackintosh, S., Cameron, I. D., Kurrle, S., Whitehead, C., ... Crotty, M. (2010). Walking aid use after discharge following hip fracture is rarely reviewed and often inappropriate: An observational study. *Journal of Physiotherapy*, *56*(4), 267–272. doi:10.1016/S1836-9553(10)70010-2 PMID:21091417

Thordardottir, B., Malmgren Fänge, A., Lethin, C., Rodriguez Gatta, D., & Chiatti, C. (2019). Acceptance and Use of Innovative Assistive Technologies among People with Cognitive Impairment and Their Caregivers: A Systematic Review. *BioMed Research International*, *2019*, 1–18. doi:10.1155/2019/9196729 PMID:30956989

United Nations, Department of Economic and Social Affairs, Population Division. (2015). *World Population Ageing 2015* (ST/ESA/SER.A/390). Author.

United States Census Bureau. (2019). *Mobility is Most Common Disability Among Older Americans*. Retrieved 11 September 2019, from https://www.census.gov/newsroom/press-releases/2014/cb14-218.html

University of Oxford. (n.d.). *Patient Reported Outcomes Measurement Group*. Retrieved May 24, 2014, from http://phi.uhce.ox.ac.uk/inst_types.php

Utah Department of Health. (2001). *Interpreting the SF-12*. Utah Health Status Survey, Utah Department of Health.

Van der Loos, H. M., & Reinkensmeyer, D. J. (2008). Rehabilitation and Health Care Robotics. In B. Siciliano & O. Khatib (Eds.), *Springer Handbook of Robotics*. Berlin: Springer. doi:10.1007/978-3-540-30301-5_54

Vazirinejad, R., Lilley, J., & Ward, C. (2003). The 'Impact on Participation and Autonomy': Acceptability of the English version in a multiple sclerosis outpatient setting. *Multiple Sclerosis Journal*, *9*(6), 612–615. doi:10.1191/1352458503ms936oa PMID:14664475

Vilagut, G., Forero, C., Pinto-Meza, A., Haro, J., de Graaf, R., & Bruffaerts, R. (2013). The Mental Component of the Short-Form 12 Health Survey (SF-12) as a FP7 - MOBOT – 600796 74 Measure of Depressive Disorders in the General Population: Results with Three Alternative Scoring Methods. *Value in Health*, *16*, 564–573. doi:10.1016/j.jval.2013.01.006 PMID:23796290

Walsh, T., Caraceni, A., Fainsinger, R., Foley, K., Glare, P., & Goh, C. (2009). *Palliative Medicine* (1st ed.). Elsevier.

Ware, J. Jr, Kosinski, M., & Keller, S. (1996). A 12-Item Short-Form Health Survey: Construction of scales and preliminary tests of reliability and validity. *Medical Care, 34*(3), 220–233. doi:10.1097/00005650-199603000-00003 PMID:8628042

Ware, J., Snow, K., Kosinski, M., Gandek, B., & Institute, N. E. (1993). *SF-36 health survey: manual and interpretation guide*. The Health Institute, New England Medical Center.

WHO. (1980). International classification of impairments, disabilities and handicaps: a manual of classification relating to the consequences of disease (ICIDH). Geneva: World Health Organization (WHO).

WHO. (2001). The international classification of functioning, disability and health - ICF. Geneva: World Health Organization (WHO).

WHO. (2019). *Ageing and health*. Retrieved 11 September 2019, from https://www.who.int/news-room/fact-sheets/detail/ageing-and-health

Whynes, D., McCahon, R., Ravenscroft, A., Hodgkinson, V., Evley, R., & Hardman, J. (2013). Responsiveness of the EQ-5D Health-Related Quality-of-Life Instrument in Assessing Low Back Pain. *Value in Health, 16*(1), 124–132. doi:10.1016/j.jval.2012.09.003 PMID:23337223

Yfantopoulos, J. (2001). The Greek version of the EuroQol (EQ-5D) instrument. *Archives of Hellenic Medicine, 18*(2), 180-191.

KEY TERMS AND DEFINITIONS

Activities of Daily Living (ADLs): ADLs are the basic activities people should be able to do in order to rake care themselves. Self-care activities include toileting, mobility (ambulation), eating, bathing, dressing, grooming, and personal device care. Assistive technology can ameliorate the effects of disabilities that limit the ability to perform ADLs.

Human-Computer Interaction (HCI): It is the study of how people interact with computers and to what extent computers are or are not developed for successful interaction with human beings. HCI consists of three parts: the user, the computer, and the ways they work together. HCI helps to produce usable, functional and safe systems. According to HCI, people should be at the center of any design process in order for the developed solution to meet their needs, capabilities and preferences for conducting various tasks. To this end, the system should be designed to match their requirements. Usability is one of the main concepts in HCI.

Human-Robot Interaction (HRI): HRI is related to the study of people's behavior and attitudes towards robots in relationship to the physical, technological and interactive features of the robots. The main goal of HRI is to develop efficient and acceptable robots. Societal and emotional needs of their end-users should also be taken into account in the design process, according to HRI.

Mobility Aids: Mobility aids are devices designed to assist walking and improve the mobility of people with mobility impairment. There are various walking aids nowadays: wheelchairs, mobility scooters, canes, crutches, rollators, robotic rollators, and many others. The term refers to those devices whose use enables a freedom of movement similar to that of unassisted walking or standing up from a chair. Latest technological advances are being exploited in order to increase the scope of these devices considerably—for example, the use of sensors and audio or tactile feedback.

Usability: Is defined as the ease of use and learnability of a human-made object such as a tool or device. It comprises effectiveness, efficiency, learnability, flexibility, robustness, and utility. A usable system should be easy to learn, easy to remember how to use, effective to use, efficient to use, safe to use and enjoyable to use. In software engineering, is related to the degree to which a software can be used by the end-users to achieve quantified objectives with effectiveness, efficiency, and satisfaction in a quantified context of use. Needs analysis and the study of the principles behind an object's perceived efficiency or elegance are in the frames of usability. In human-computer interaction and computer science, usability studies the elegance and clarity with which the interaction with a computer program or a web site is designed. User satisfaction and utility are quality components of usability.

Chapter 8
The Clinical Laboratory and the Commitment to Quality:
Update on Best Practices and Regulatory Requirements

Marilena Stamouli
Naval and Veterans Hospital of Athens (NNA), Greece

Antonia Mourtzikou
University General Hospital "ATTIKON", Greece

ABSTRACT

The main role that clinical laboratories play in the detection, diagnosis, and treatment of diseases is clearly evident. Clinical laboratories need to sustain a commitment to quality and demonstrate a certifiable level of compliance. Many strategies are used to reduce laboratory errors, including internal QC procedures, external quality assessment programs, implementation of QIs and six-sigma methodology. All strategies should be consistent with the requirements of the international standard for medical laboratory accreditation and suitable for promoting corrective/preventive actions. They must promote total quality and patient safety and be consistent with the definition of a laboratory error. Harmonization process is in progress; however, further efforts must be made. Total quality management must be evaluated periodically. For a patient-centered approach, there is the need to assure that each and every step of the total testing process is correctly performed, that weaknesses are recognized, and that corrective and preventive actions are designed and implemented.

DOI: 10.4018/978-1-7998-2390-2.ch008

INTRODUCTION

Clinical laboratories play an important essential role in the detection, diagnosis and treatment of diseases. Patient management, treatment, detection of complications, hospital admission and discharge, are based on laboratory test results, (Mourtzikou et al.,2013; Mourtzikou & Stamouli, 2017).

It is estimated that about 251,000 patients die every year in the U.S. due to medical errors, making medical errors the third most common cause of death in the U.S. Mistakes in medication and treatment, diagnostic errors and erroneous laboratory results are contributing mainly to these estimations (Makary & Daniel, 2016). In the United States between 7 and 10 billion laboratory tests are reported annually, while a15% of patients receive either incorrect or delayed reports (Noble, 2009), (Stamouli et al., 2019).Thus, the laboratory has an ethical obligation to produce reliable, unambiguous and reproducible analytic measurements and to provide clinicians with relevant information for the prevention, diagnosis, treatment and management of the disease (Plebani et al., 2019).

Clinical laboratory work is highly complex and with an absolute need for accuracy, confidentiality, time effectiveness and cost-effectiveness. It includes both technical and management activities; coordination between them is essential for the production of high-quality and error-free test results. Concerns about the quality of the test results have led to increased regulation and guideline establishment, and the development of quality improvement programs. The guidelines for quality can be found in government regulations, accreditation standards, and national practice standards such as CLIA (Clinical Laboratory Improvement Amendments), JCAHO (Joint Commission on the Accreditation of Healthcare Organizations), NCCLS (National Committee for Clinical Laboratory Standards), ISO 15189:2012, ISO/IEC 17025 (International Organization for Standardization), as well as in the detailed guidelines from CAP (College of American Pathologists) and COLA (Commission of Office Laboratory Accreditation). Laboratories need to follow constantly the changes of these regulatory requirements and the addition of new ones.

Moreover, since clinical laboratories must ensure the quality, integrity, and reliability of a wide range of patient results, they need to sustain a commitment to quality and demonstrate a certifiable level of compliance. The purpose of our study is to provide the latest update on best practices and regulatory requirements, for the improvement of clinical laboratory services through quality. The data and the examples presented in this study are based on our work and experience at biochemistry laboratories in NHS hospitals.

BACKGROUND

Laboratory Testing Process

The Pre-Analytical Phase

The laboratory testing process is divided into three phases; the pre-analytical, the analytical and the post-analytical phase. In order to provide reliable test results, the laboratory must follow best practices for the prevention and detection of errors at all steps (Stamouli et al., 2019; Lippi et al., 2017; Lippi et al., 2011; Lippi et al., 2019; Hammerling, 2012; Lao et al., 2017).

The pre-analytical phase includes test request, patient preparation, patient and specimen identification, specimen collection, specimen transportation, specimen centrifugation and handling (Flegar-Mestric, et al., 2017; Gimenez-Marin, et al., 2014; Lippi, et al., 2017; Simundic, et al., 2015; Simundic, et al., 2014). Although errors can arise at any of the threephases, many studies have shown that the pre-analytical phase accounts for 46% to 68.2% of errors observed during the total testing process (Barak & Jaschek, 2013; Hawkins, 2012).This phase is most prone to errors as the steps involved are directly dependent on humans and are out of direct control of the laboratory (Neoggi, et al., 2016; Lippi et al., 2019; Plebani, 2019).

Evidence presented in the literature shows that pre-analytical error rates are lower when the laboratory staff performs the collection, identification, labeling, handling and transportation of patient samples, and this, in turn, represents a key issue in defining strategies for reducing the risk of errors in the pre-analytical steps (Jegede et al., 2015; Kemp et al.2012;Lippiet al., 2015; Plebani et al., 2015). Pre-analytical errors can be reduced with the right training, close coordination among all the members of staff involved (clinician, phlebotomist and laboratory staff) and implementation of good laboratory practices such as using appropriate technology for patient and sample identification (wristbands, barcodes, RFID identification), automated detection of serum interference indices (such as the hemolysis, lipemic and icterus indices), and link to the Laboratory Information System. The use of appropriate blood collection systems, sample tubes and anticoagulants may contribute significantly to quality (Hawkins, 2012; Söderberg et al., 2009; Lippi et al., 2019).

All laboratories must have written procedures about patient preparation, patient identification, specimen collection, specimen identification, specimen transportation and preparation for analysis (Lippi et al., 2019).They should also establish rejection criteria for specimens and should follow them carefully, as well as corrective actions that should take place in such a case.

The use of Quality Indicators (QIs) is of utmost importance for detecting errors made in the different steps of the pre-analytical phase (Plebani et al., 2015).The Institute of Medicine (IOM 2005) defines the QI as an objective measure that potentially evaluates all critical care domains, such as patient safety, effectiveness, equity, patient-centeredness, timeliness and efficiency. It is based on information and evidence associated with the critical care domains and can be implementedconsistently and comparably across settings and over time (Shahangian & Snyder, 2009). Moreover, according to the International Standard for medical laboratories accreditation ISO 15189:2012, the laboratory shall establish Quality Indicators (QIs) to monitor and evaluate the performance throughout critical aspects of the entire testing process, and the process of monitoring QIs shall be planned, which includes establishing the objectives, methodology, interpretation, limits, action plan and duration of measurement (ISO 15189:2012).Thus, the clinical laboratory must establish QIs covering pre-analytical, analytical and post-analytical phases, in order to comply with the requirements of the International Standard and achieve accreditation.

In order to develop new QIs, appropriate methods and criteria for identification, selection, implementation and evaluation must be applied. Defining a QI needs a lot of effort and work, including thesetting of achievable goals and a detailed review of the literature. During the last decade, laboratories have used various methods to develop QIs, in order to comply with the requirements of accreditation standards and to monitor and improve quality and patient safety. The QIs must be measurable, objective, designed to identify those events that reflect the actual situations in question, user-friendly, understandable, robust, they must provide reliable and valid information for continuous improvement and encourage prompt and suitable corrective or preventive actions. QIs should have clear and unambiguous definition and interpretation, whereas the ability to measure the indicator is a prerequisite for its successful implementation, reproducible application, and monitoring.

Moreover, a QI must have a clinical or empirical rationale for its use, should measure an essential aspect of clinical laboratory quality, and it should be related to other indicators intended to measure the same or related aspects of quality. Sometimes looking at groups of indicators together provides a complete picture of laboratory quality performance (Gimenez-Marin et al., 2014; Njoroge & Nichols, 2014).QIs can either be measures of processes, outcomes or contribution of the laboratory to the patient care, but can also indicate the quality of many processes, such as organization and management, supplies, equipment maintenance, laboratory staff education, environmental safety and health worker safety, communication, resolving of complaints and nonconformities (David & Dobreanu, 2015;Njoroge & Nichols, 2014).Since all these are activities that have a substantial effect on the overall quality of laboratory work, it is imperative to monitor some indicators of those strategic and support processes.

The number of QIs to be monitored varies depending on the size of the laboratory, the quality goals, and the workload. The number of QIs can change with time, and new QIs can be defined to replace the previous ones, as a step of the PDCA (Plan-Do-Check-Act) quality cycle for the continuous improvement. Many organizations, such as the College of American Pathologists, the Centers for Disease Control and Prevention, the Institute for Quality in Laboratory Medicine, the Joint Commission on Accreditation of Healthcare Organizations and the Centers for Medicare and Medicaid Services have developed QIs for clinical laboratory performance. Moreover, the IFCC Working Group "Laboratory Errors and Patient Safety" has developed a model of QIs and has collected data from several laboratories at an international level.Other programs on QIs have been organized and implemented in several countries (Barth, 2012; Shcolnik et al., 2012).The extended use of QIs emerged the need for their harmonization, based on sound criteria.QIs should be consistent with the requirements of the International Standard for medical laboratories accreditation ISO 15189: 2012, suitable for promoting corrective and preventive actions, promote total quality and patient safety and consistent with the definition of laboratory error, as it is specified in the ISO/TS 22367 (Plebani et al., 2014; Plebani et al., 2015). In addition to the list of harmonized QIs, the system for data collection and reporting should also be harmonized, in order to allow the comparison of data between different laboratories. Although the harmonization process is in progress, further efforts must be made to raise the awareness of all health personnel involved in the total testing process and to highlight the importance of QIs implementation for improving the quality of laboratory services and patient safety (Plebani et al., 2017). The most widely applied QIs for the evaluation of the pre-analytical phase at the biochemistry laboratory isas follows (Lippi et al., 2018):

- number of misidentified samples/ total number of samples
- number of requests with erroneous data/ total number of requests
- number of samples collected in wrong specimen tube/ total number of samples
- number of hemolysis samples/total number of samples
- number of samples not received/ total number of samples
- number of samples with insufficient volume/total number of samples

Examples of QIs for the evaluation of support processes are (Cadamuro et al., 2018):

- Number of training events organized for all staff per year (employee competence)
- Number of employees that obtained all credits of continuous medical education required in a year/total number of employees (employee competence)

- Number of laboratory information system unplanned downtime episodes, per year (LIS efficiency)
- Number of incident/adverse events occurred in the laboratory concerning the health and safety of laboratory staff (staff safety).

The Analytical Phase

The analytical phase is described as the sum of activities occurring from the time the sample arrives at the laboratory for verification (Smith et al., 2013). Due to automation and information technology, the analytical phase shows the lowest rate of errors in the whole total testing process; approximately 7-13% of laboratory errors. However, errors occurring in the analytical phase can have a detrimental effect on patient care because they can lead to incorrect diagnosis and improper treatment decisions. There are multiple areas of concern regarding the analytical phase, including interfering substances, reagent stability, calibration, performance and monitoring of quality control, instrumentation malfunction, as well as failure to follow standard procedures for both patient testing and equipment maintenance. Thus, it is critical that clinical laboratory staff adhere to accreditation and regulatory requirements such as the use of standard operating procedures, the performance of quality control measurements, instrument calibration schedules, instrument preventative maintenance schedules and participation in external quality control schemes. The most frequently reported errors during the analytical phase are attributed to insufficient sample volume, hemolysis samples giving poor results, internal quality control (IQC) failures, failures of analyzers during the analytical process and contradicting results upon re-testing.

Internal Quality Control

Internal quality control is a set of procedures undertaken by laboratory staff for the continuous monitoring of operations and the results of measurements, in order to decide whether results are reliable enough to be released (Thompson & Wood, 1995). Internal quality control is based on the use of control samples and statistical methods. Control samples are biological samples (serum, whole blood, urine, etc.), usually lyophilized, that contain analytes in concentrations close to the medical decision limits.The choice of appropriate IQC material is very important. For most routine analyses commercial material is readily available, usually provided from the reagent kit manufacturers. However, extra quality control material prepared from an independent source to the kit manufacturer should also be employed. The composition of IQC material should be close to patient samples, and they should be stored, handled and prepared according to the manufacturer's instructions. The manufacturer should provide sufficient amounts of the same lots of control samples, for at least one year, because this will provide long-term quality assurance for the laboratory and will make the process as efficient as possible (Ceriotti et al.,2015; Lippi et al., 2016; Lund et al., 2015). The requirements for the control samples are set by the In Vitro Diagnostic Directive (IVDD) 98/79/EC, ISO 17511:2003 and ISO 18153:2003. Laboratories use two or three different control samples which contain analytes in different concentrations/levels, such as low, borderline, medium, high, in order to check the performance of laboratory methods across the whole range of measurement (García-Lario J.V.,& Boned Juliani, B., 2012). Control materials are lyophilized and need reconstitution. However, the act of reconstitution can introduce an error to the control material, such as instability in specific analytes or contamination from the diluent. Each laboratory should perform stability testing for control material after reconstitution or thawing and control material in long term storage.

The most widely used tool for internal quality control is the Shewhart or Levey-Jennings chart. In order to prepare the Shewhart chart for an analyte, the laboratory assays the control samples for at least 20 consecutive days. Then the mean (m) and the standard deviation (SD) are calculated from the observed data. Further results are then plotted on the graph daily and, if normally distributed, 95% of these should fall between the mean±3SD limits (García-Lario J.V.,& Boned Juliani B., 2012). James Westgard proposed a series of rules and criteria which allow interpretation of the data shown in the Shewhart charts. These criteria are in use in many laboratories worldwide, and if the internal quality control fails to meet them, the laboratory must take corrective actions. Westgard rules use a combination of decision criteria in order to decide whether an analytical run is in or out-of-control. They are generally used with 2 or 4 control measurements per run, which means they are appropriate when two different control materials are measured 1 or 2 times per material, which is the case in many clinical chemistry applications. Some alternative control rules are more suitable when three control materials are analyzed, which is typical for applications in haematology, coagulation, and immunoassays.The Westgard rules are simple to use routinely. They improve capacity for detecting real analytical errors, give a low level of false assay rejections, indicate the type of error, and help with problem-solving (Westgard et al., 2002). The Westgard rules applied routinely at the clinical laboratories are:

1. one point outside ±2 SD of the target value
2. two successive points outside ±2 SD of the target value
3. one point outside ±3 SD of the target value
4. four successive points outside ±1 SD of the target value on one side of the target value

5. there is a difference of 4 SD between successive points
6. ten successive points on one side of the target value.

Westgard rules 3 and 5 identify random errors, which are represented by an increased scatter around the baseline value [Figure 1]. Rules 2, 4, and 6 are designed to identify systematic failures; they will identify either a gradual trend of the data away from the baseline value or a step change in baseline.

The Shewhart chart analyzes only the information included in the last point signaled on the chart and evaluates if this point signals a special cause of variation. It ignores any information given by the entire series of points. This fact makes Shewhart chart insensitive to slight changes in the process, on the order of 1.5 standard deviations or less. CUSUM (Cumulative Sum) and EWMA (Exponentially Weighted Moving Average) charts are used to monitor processes that are subjected to small shifts, by incorporating both current and previous data values from the process. The CUSUM chart plots the cumulative sums of the deviations of the sample values from a target value (T). For a process that remains in control and centered at the target value, the cumulative sum will vary randomly around a mean of zero. However, if the mean shifts upwards or downwards to some value μ, (μ> T; μ<T), then an upward or downward trend respectively, will quickly develop in the cumulative sum. Whenever the CUSUM chart indicates an out of control process, we suspect an assignable cause of variation, which can be very quickly detected [Figure 2]. The EWMA

Figure 1. Shewhart chart glucose, based on internal quality control results, created with Minitab 17 statistical package (control material was provided by Medicon Hellas SA; measurements were performed at the Department of Biochemistry, Naval and Veterans Hospital, Athens, Greece).

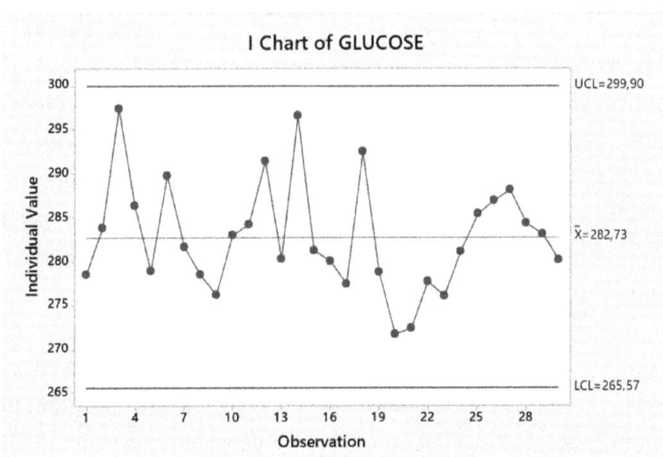

Figure 2. CUSUM chart for glucose, based on internal quality control results, created with Minitab 17 statistical package (control material was provided by Medicon Hellas SA; measurements were performed at the Department of Biochemistry, Naval and Veterans Hospital, Athens, Greece). From measurement 1 until measurement 35 process remains in control and the cumulative sum varies randomly around a mean of zero. From measurement 36 and on the mean shifts downwards, and a downward trend is detected. Thus, the CUSUM chart indicates an out of control process.

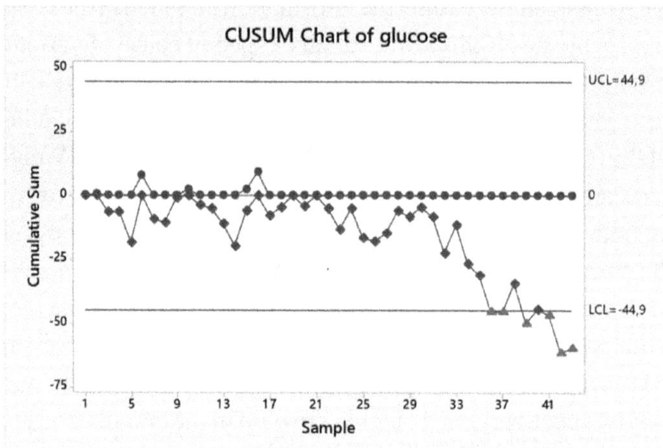

chart has similar properties to the CUSUM chart and is also useful for detecting smaller shifts in the process mean. Each EWMA value is a weighted average of the current preprocessed result and previous results, with the weights decreasing exponentially with the age of the reading. EWMA weights samples in geometrically decreasing order so that the most recent samples are weighted most highly while the most distant samples contribute very little.Thus, this type of chart incorporates the process history into the current evaluation of the process [Figure 3].

It should be noted that runs, trends, or zone rules that have been developed for Shewhart control charts do not apply to the CUSUM and EWMA charts, due to data autocorrelation. We conclude that the process is out of control only when a point exceeds the control limits. CUSUM and EWMA charts have been widely applied in infection control and hospital epidemiology, public health surveillance, cardiac surgery performance, for the detection of abnormal patient arrivals at hospital emergency department and recently for the monitoring of blood glucose in type-II diabetes patients (Neuburger et al.,2017; Aslam et al., 2019).

Internal quality control checks the accuracy and precision of the analytical method applied. Accuracy is defined as the closeness of agreement between a measured quantity value and a true quantity value of a measurand (VIM). Precision

Figure 3. EWMA chart for urea, based on internal quality control results, created with Minitab 17 statistical package (control material was provided by Medicon Hellas SA; measurements were performed at the Department of Biochemistry, Naval and Veterans Hospital, Athens, Greece). The EWMA chart indicates a process in control. The chart limits vary with time, approaching asymptotic limits as time increases.

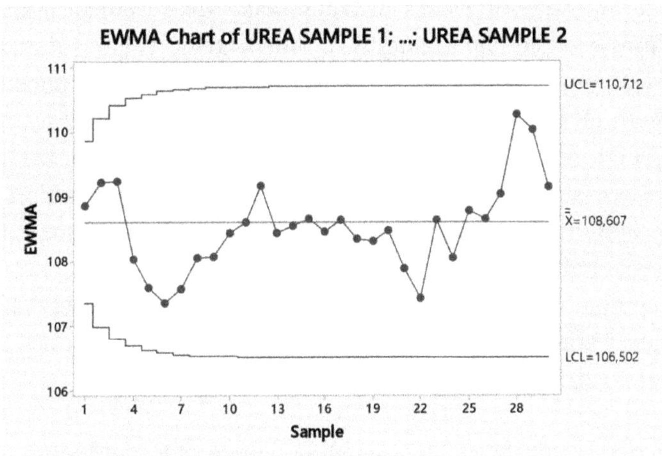

is defined as the closeness of agreement between indications or measured quantity values obtained by replicate measurements on the same or similar objects under specified conditions (VIM). Any change in accuracy, such as a systematic shift or drift, would result in a change in the mean value of the control, which would be shown by a shift in the chart (Ceriotti F et al., 2015; Lund et al., 2015). The precision can be expressed by the coefficient of variation CV=(SD/XX)*100, where SD is the standard deviation for a statistically significant number of measurements. The precision of an assay can be described in terms of intrabatch and interbatch CVs. Intrabatch CV is obtained by determining the mean (XX) and SD for an analyte, measured on the same sample a given number of times (usually 10 or more) within the same batch. The inter-batch CV is obtained by determining the mean and SD for an analyte, measured on the same sample a given number (usually 10 or more) of times between batches. In all assays, the inter-batch CVs for a given analyte should be greater than the intrabatch CVs and laboratories should regularly check the precision of assays to evaluate their performance.

ISO 15189: 2012 requires that laboratories shall determine measurement uncertainty for each measurement procedure in the analytical phase. Measurement uncertainty is defined as the interval around the measured value, where the true value lies with some probability. The measurement uncertainty is the half-width of that interval and is always non-negative. There are two sources of variation that contribute to measurement uncertainty in the clinical laboratory: there is variation associated with the calibrators used in the medical laboratory methods, and there is also random variation associated with repetitive testing of the same sample in the test system. Since several contributors influence its value, the collection of data for its estimation should include testing with different operators at different times with different analyzers or pieces of equipment. Measurement uncertainty must be reported as expanded uncertainty (U). This statistic value is derived from two statistical precursors, standard uncertainty (u) and combined uncertainty (UC). Standard uncertainty (u) is expressed as a standard deviation for a set of n replicates in a sample. Combined uncertainty (UC) accounts for multiple sources of variability within a process, such as methods of measurement, contamination of reagents, interferences, volume and mass measurements, variable instrument backgrounds (Panteghini M., et al., 2017; Padoan et al., 2017).

Another approach to monitoring the analytical quality of analytical runs is based on patient data. Patient data can be used in several different ways (Karkalousos & Evangelopoulos, 2011):

- AON (Average Of Normals), which is a method based on the principle that the mean value of all normal results fluctuates between well-defined limits
- Bull's algorithm used for hematology analyzers
- Delta check, which is the difference between the current value of one person and the previous one
- Patient duplicate results
- Discordance checks between different analytes (such as urea and creatinine, total and direct bilirubin, total serum protein and serum albumin etc.)
- Anion gaps.

As a conclusion we can comment that IQC offers confidence and validity of the test results, helps in monitoring the performance and output of a laboratory process, shows problems or deficiencies that might exist, helps decision making about the results and provides a statistical basis from which the results can be judged.

External Quality Control

The term EQA is used to describe a method that allows the comparison of a laboratory's performance to a source outside the laboratory, such as a peer group of laboratories or a reference laboratory. The term is sometimes used interchangeably with proficiency testing, where an external provider sends unknown samples for testing to a set of laboratories. These samples are analyzed, and the results of all laboratories are sent to the provider. The provider evaluates the results and reports the evaluation to the laboratories. However, EQA can also be carried out using other processes, such as participation in schemes organized by national and international professional, scientific societies, by professionals on behalf of governments or by commercial companies (IFCC). Participation in any of these schemes demonstrates a commitment to improving performance and to deliver unbiased, reliable and accurate results.

Moreover, it provides testing laboratories with the necessary evidence that their practices meet quality standards. Performance specifications in EQA programs are very different due to a range of factors, such as the rationale for setting the criteria, the clinical setting and the available economic resources in different countries. The need for harmonized EQA quality performance specifications is of great importance, but harmonization can only be achieved with hard work, significant collaborative effort, sharing data, clearly defined goals and agreed approaches.

Moreover, the need for harmonization of test results between different laboratories is also very importantin order to avoid misinterpretation of results, wrong treatments and adverse patient outcomes (Jones G.R.,&Koetsia S., 2014; Jones G.R., 2016). In Europe, there is an initiative to promote harmonization activities of the Total Testing Process among the 40 European Federation of Clinical Chemistry and Laboratory Medicine (EFLM) member societies. The responsible experts consist of the Working Group on the Harmonization, which is chaired by F. Ceriotti (Ceriotti, 2016; Plebani, 2016). Some activities that are already being promoted are:

- Pre-analytical phase: test requesting, demand management, reflex testing, harmonized test profiles, guidelines and position papers, best practices for patient preparation, sample collection, sample handling, and transport, quality indicators.
- Analytical phase: use of traceable assays, development of commutable secondary reference materials, harmonization of mass spectrometry methodology.
- Post-analytical phase: standardization of reporting units and terminology, harmonization of calculated parameters, common reference intervals, decision limits for immunoassay analytes where there is method bias standardization of report formatting, harmonized processes for management and communication of critical results, list of critical tests, harmonization of commenting for EQA, harmonized approach to validation of quality of biological variation data for use with reference change values interpretation, quality indicators.

For laboratory tests where there is reference measurement procedure available, the metrological concepts of standardization, calibration traceability to reference materials and measurements, and measurement uncertainty are described in the International Organization for Standardization (ISO) standards ISO 17511 and 18153. Calibration material with accurately defined concentrations is usually available for all analytes. The concentration of analytes in serum-based calibration material is determined by a reference method, such as inductively coupled plasma mass spectrometry (ICP-MS). Therefore, a very accurate result can be ascribed to that material, and the routine method used by the laboratory can be calibrated against this result. Reference methods are available for most commonly measured analytes.

Moreover, the manufacturers of the reagents should be able to show the traceability of results back to these or similar materials. However, harmonization is required to achieve uniform results among different measurement procedures for the same laboratory test where there is no reference measurement procedure available. For this purpose, an international consortium for harmonization of clinical laboratory results (ICHCLR- International Consortium for Harmonization of Clinical Laboratory Results) has been formed, focused on organizing and coordinating these global harmonization efforts made by different organizations (Myers, G.L.,& Miller, W.G., 2016).

The Post-Analytical Phase

According to the ISO15189:2012 standard for a medical laboratory, the post-analytical phase is a process following the analytical phase, which includes a review of the results, retention, and storage of clinical material, handling and disposal of the samples and laboratory waste. Moreover, the post-analytical phase includes the formatting, releasing, reporting and retention of the examination results for future access (ISO 15189:2012; Sikaris, 2015). The majority of laboratory results are quantitative; they provide information on the amount of analytes in the sample. Quantitative results are reported numerically and are compared against a reference interval for interpretation. However, some test results are qualitative; they identify the presence or absence of the analyte (pathogen, toxin, antigen, antibody etc) and they are reported converted either to an ordinal scale (such asAnti-Nuclear-Antibodies negative, equivocal or positive) or not (such as blood group determination and the results of haemoglobin electrophoresis, where a particular pattern is observed and interpreted).The quality of quantitative tests can be measured as imprecision, bias, total error and measurement uncertainty (VIM). Since the quality of qualitative tests cannot be expressed by the same parameters, the International Standard for Proficiency Testing ISO/IEC 17043defines these tests as a separate class and recognizes that the quality of their interpretation depends on more on a participant's competence in identifying a certain pattern rather than the technical assessment of the laboratory, in general (ISO/IEC 17043;Nordin, 2015; Sikaris, 2015). Interpretive comments are applied mainly to histopathology, immunophenotyping, flow cytometry, microbiology, molecular biology, autoimmunity, and genetics, and there is some evidence that they lead to improved outcomes (Claustres, 2014; Sikaris, 2015). Quantitative test results are usually interpreted against reference intervals or clinical decision intervals. Reference intervals are statistical confidence limits for the results of a healthy reference population, and they are designed to confirm health with high specificity. Reference intervals can vary depending on the patient's gender and age. Since children are not small adults, adult reference intervals are not appropriate for pediatric patients. Pediatric patients require a unique medical approach, as significant differences exist in disease frequencies, specimen collection, test performance and test interpretation. Gender, diet, life-style habits, ethnicity and socio-economic conditions may also affect the physiology of a population so that measures of normal physiological functions differ between different population groups. Special forms of reference limits also exist, regarding substances that are not typically found in healthy individuals (such as detection limits for toxins or drugs of abuse, therapeutic ranges for drug levels and legal limits for alcohol) (Gerostamoulos, 2013; Ye, 2013). Defining reference intervals is a major challenge because of the difficulty in recruiting volunteers to participate and testing samples from a large number of healthy reference individuals (Koerbin, 2014; Miri-Dashe, 2014). Clinical decision limits are clinically focused, are determined by medical evidence and aim to confirm the presence of a particular disease or clinical risk with high sensitivity (Devgun, 2015; SolingerandRothman, 2013; Tate,2014). As a conclusion, we can say that the quality of the laboratory report lies in its ability to support clinical decision-making and to ensure improved outcomes for patients.

Four of the post-analytical indicators that are widely applied are transcription errors, turnaround time (TAT), incorrect reports and delay in critical result notification. However, defining performance criteria for these post-analytical indicators is very difficult. Since manual transcription of numerical data is prone to error, transcription errors can be eliminated by the implementation of a laboratory information system (LIS). Many post-analytical errors such as dilution errors, calculations, improper validation, incorrect units and incorrect reports could also be reduced by the implementation of LIS (Sadiq,2014). Reports with missing tests can cause a delay in patient management and are usually attributed to input errors of the requested tests. TAT is a post-analytical quality indicator; however, the analytical TAT is usually only a fraction of the complete diagnostic TAT, which includes pre-analytical sample collection, sample transportation and the time to review and validate laboratory results before report release. Excessively prolonged TAT can be attributed to unforeseen and unavoidable problems. Reduction of TAT improves the quality of service because timeliness is very important to the clinician. Apart from delays in the analytical phase, delayed and lost test requisitions and delayed reports are major contributing factors prolonging result TAT (Rodríguez-Borja, 2014; Sadiq,2014).

TAT can be evaluated by the use of Pareto chart, a basic quality tool that helps us identify the most frequent defects, complaints, or factors which contribute to a problem. It is based on the "80/20 rule," which postulates that 80% of the problems come from 20% of the causes. The lengths of the bars at the Pareto chart represent frequency and are arranged with the longest bars on the left and the shortest to the right. In this way, the chart visually depicts which situations are more significant. For example, TAT of laboratory tests is a key contributor to the Emergency Department workflow. Appropriate triage and discharge of patients are being impacted by the timely return of laboratory test results. By applying the Pareto chart, we can confirm if the 60-minute goal for the processing of stat specimens are being met.

Moreover, we can estimate during which shift is recorded the prolonged TAT. Data can be collected from the HIS database. TAT start time is defined as the time of specimen arrival at the laboratory; end time is defined as the time of completion of the last test ordered, including the 20-minute clotting step. Outliers are defined as more than 60 minutes for biochemistry measurements. The time taken to transport blood samples to the laboratoryis excluded. Full day work cycle can be divided into2-hour intervals, and TAT can be evaluated during each interval [Figure 4].

Critical test results (also called panic or alert results) are those test results that fall significantly outside the reference interval, may represent life-threatening conditions and require rapid communication to the responsible physician. A delay in taking action to respond to the critical result may lead to serious adverse outcomes for the patient. Rapid and accurate communication of critical laboratory test results is required by the Clinical Laboratory Improvement Amendments (CLIA) regulations, by laboratory accreditation standards and by the World Health Organization's World Alliance for Patient Safety (Campbell & Horvatrh, 2014; Zeng, 2013).Various national surveys have demonstrated that critical test lists and critical limit lists vary significantly. These variations can be attributed to different patient populations, different settings, and different laboratory methods. Laboratory staff must be appropriately trained to identify, verify and handle critical results. Laboratories may have different levels of alarms and procedures in place to check the validity of critical results (Kopcinovic,2015;Rashid, 2015; Zeng, 2013). It is a common practice in clinical laboratories that critical results are automatically repeated, in order to exclude errors related to pre-analytical problems, common interferences, interferences by certain medications and analytical problems. According to study results, no errors are detected in routine repeat testing. Therefore automated repeats do not offer any advantage over a single run (Deetz, 2012).

Figure 4. Pareto chart for the evaluation of biochemistry result TAT at the Emergency Department, created with Minitab 17 statistical package. The 60-minute goal for the processing of ED specimens was not being met for 10.5% of the samples. A percentage of 60.3% of the prolonged TAT was recorded from 06:00 to 10:00 every day, which coincides with healthcare personnel shift changes at 07:00, as well as high volume of testing, work load and internal quality control process during this time interval.

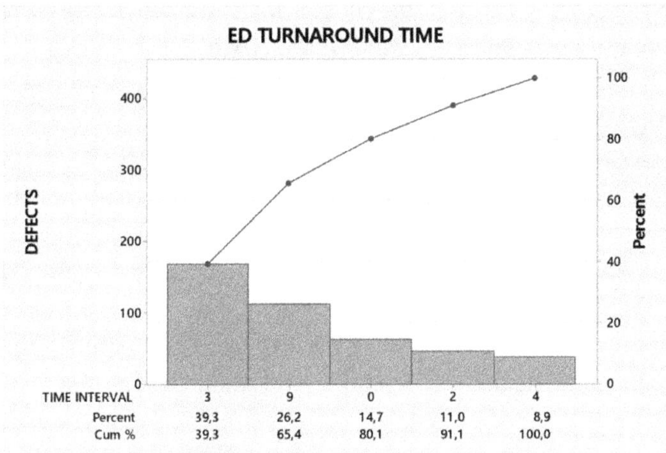

Moreover, with this practice, reporting of critical results is further delayed. Laboratories implement different alarm systems for critical result notification. For example, the LIS systems identify critical results in zones with red color, which indicates danger or significant morbidity (Rashid et al., 2015; White et al., 2014). Some laboratories implement automated notification systems, which are automated alerting systems or computerized reminders using mobile phones, email or other personal electronic devices to alert the responsible healthcare provider. Others use call centers, which are centralized units for the communication of critical laboratory test results via telephone. Conclusions from many surveys demonstrate that phone calling directly by lab staff is still the most utilized method of communication of critical results to the physicians. With the advancement of information technology, it is expected that automated alerts become more widespread and efficient (Campbell and Horvatrh, 2014; Liebow, 2012; Rashid, 2015). Harmonization is necessary for the timely notification of laboratory results that represent potential patient safety hazards. Laboratories need to define critical tests and critical limits based on work published by experts in order to harmonize the critical lists. The procedures for reporting critical results should be discussed and agreed between the laboratory and the physicians.

Moreover, laboratories and physicians must audit, update and continuously improve their critical result management practices in order to provide safe and reliable care to patients (Campbell and Horvatrh, 2014; Zeng, 2013). Laboratories need to design procedures for identifying critical results, rules for confirming the validity of those results, algorithms for the communication of those results and alternative procedures for cases that these results cannot be communicated to the primary physician. Laboratories must keep records of critical results, which must include patient identification, laboratory staff and physician identification, the time of the communication, the critical result and the receipt of result communication (Lam, 2016).

The Six Sigma Approach

Six-sigma methodology is a strategy of quality measurement and improvement, which is widely implemented in business and industry. It was adopted by Motorola in the early 1990s and won the Malcolm Baldridge Quality Award. The core of the Six Sigma Methodology is the DMAIC cycle, which stands for define, measure, analyze, improve, and control. The DMAIC cycle is summarized as follows (Fursule,2012;Hekmatpanah, 2013;Ying-Jiun Hsieh, 2012):

- *Define*: identify a potential project, evaluate the project, select project, prepare problem and mission statement for the project, select and launch project team, set goals striving for customer satisfaction and aligning business objectives.
- *Measure:* plan for data collection, validate the measurement system, measure the process by collecting relevant data to realize issues and for future comparison, measure the process capability.
- *Analyze:* to verify the connection between different factors, causes of variation and causes of problems and defects, analyze collected data and check for sources of variation, check for cause and effect relationships.
- *Improve:* the process by reducing variation based upon the analysis, optimize process capability, evaluate alternative solutions and deal with resistance to change.
- *Control:* the process and maintain the reduction of variation, document the improved process, determine new process capability, ensure that the new process is indeed capable and in control.

Six-sigma methodology aims to reduce the processes variation, suggesting the existence of a direct correlation between the number of products with defects, percentage of revenues wasted with these defects and the level of customer satisfaction with the offered product or service. A Six Sigma process produces no more than 3.4 defects per million opportunities, where the defect is defined as any feature of the product or service outside the specifications desired by the customer. The adequate implementation of the Six Sigma methodology in an organization can result in a competitive advantage because it provides control, continuous and robust improvement in processes performance and adds value to the product or service offered to customers. The effective incorporation of this methodology in the quality culture of the organizations is not simple and should be implemented gradually (Cloete,2012;Nanda &Rey, 2013). The most utilized six sigma tools during each phase of the DMAIC cycle are (Hekmatpanah, 2013;Bubshait&Al-Dosary, 2014):

- Define phase: project charter, value stream mapping, process flowchart, SIPOC (Suppliers, Inputs, Process, Outputs, and Customers) diagram, FMEA, understanding CTQs (Critical To Quality), stakeholder analysis, cause and effect matrix, DMAIC (Define, Measure, Analyze, Improve and Control) work breakdown structure, voice of the customer
- Measure phase: process flowchart, cause and effect matrix, FMEA, data collection plan/example, benchmarking, measurement system analysis, Gage R & R (Gage repeatability and reproducibility), voice of the customer, process sigma metrics calculation
- Analyze phase: histogram, Pareto chart, time series/run chart, scatter plot, regression analysis, cause and effect/fishbone diagram, 5 whys, process map review and analysis, statistical analysis, hypothesis testing, non-normal data analysis
- Improve phase: brainstorming, mistake proofing, design of experiments, house of quality, FMEA, simulation software
- Control phase: process sigma metrics calculation, control charts (variable and attribute), cost savings calculations, control plan.

Sigma metric has been widely introduced as a metric for measuring defects and improving quality. Any process can be evaluated in terms of a sigma metric that describes how many sigmas fit within the tolerance limits. Measurement of process outcome is done by calculating defects per million (DPM) and converting it into sigma metric. Quality is assessed on the sigma scale with a criterion of 3 σ as the minimum allowable sigma for regular performance and a sigma of 6 σ being the goal for world-class quality. Sigma metrics can be used effectively for clinical laboratory services (Lippi &Plebani, 2018).

It helps to assess analytical methodologies, augment laboratory performance and acts as a guide for planning quality control strategy (Afrifa,2015;Lakshman, 2015).

Sigma value for a laboratory analyte can be calculated using the formula sigma value = (TEa- bias) / CV%. TEa (total allowable error) is the total allowable difference from the accepted reference value seen in the deviation of single measurement from the target value. TEa values of various laboratory analytes can be estimated from CLIA guidelines. Bias is the systematic difference between the expected results obtained by the laboratory's test method and the results that would be obtained from an accepted reference method. It is calculated from the external quality control results for each laboratory analyte. CV% (coefficient of variance) is the analytical coefficient of variation of the test method. It is calculated from the internal quality control results for each laboratory analyte. Tests with sigma values ≥ 6 are considered excellent and can be evaluated using one quality control per day, alternating control levels between days and one rule. Tests with sigma values between 4 and 6 are suited for the purpose and are evaluated with two levels of quality control per day and one rule. Tests with sigma values between 3 and 4 are poor performers, and their evaluation needs the use of a combination of rules with two levels of quality control per day. Tests with sigma values of less than 3 show significant problems. Their evaluation is based on the maximum quality control (3 levels threetimes a day) and testing of specimens in duplicate (Stoiljkovic, 2014; Usha,2015).

The Process Capability Analysis is performed in order to ensure that the process outcomes are capable of meeting certain requirements or specifications [Figure 5]. A process capability index is a metric used to indicate the performance of the process relative to requirements, as indicated by the following equations: $C_p=(USL-LSL)/6\sigma$ and $C_{pk}=\min\{(USL-\mu)/3\sigma, (\mu-LSL)/3\sigma\}$, where USL and LSL are the upper specification limit and lower specification limit, respectively, σ is standard deviation, and μ is the mean of the process.Assuming the process distribution is normal, and the process average is exactly centered between the engineering requirements, a Cp index of 1 or less would give an inadequate process. A Cp index between 1.00 and 1.33 would give a marginally capable process, while a Cp index between 1.33 and 1.67 a satisfactory process. If the Cp index is 1,67 or more, the process is considered as excellent. In general, the larger the Cp is, the better. For a Six Sigma process, the value of Cp would be 2. The Cp index cannot be used unless there are both upper and lower specifications, and it does not account for process centering. If the process average is not exactly centered relative to the engineering requirements, the Cp index will give misleading results. The value of Cpk tells us if the process is truly capable of meeting requirements (Chen, 2014; El-Hashmi &Gnieber, 2014).

ISO 15189:2012 incorporates the approach to risk reduction and risk management, according to which clinical laboratory staff must identify unwanted events and incidents and adopt improvements systematically, in order to reduce or eliminate risks and minimize consequences to patient care (International Organization for Standardization, 2012 ; Mourtzikou&Stamouli, 2017;Mourtzikou, Stamouli, &Athanasiadi, 2013; Mourtzikou, Stamouli, Athanasiadi, &Marasidi, 2015;Pouliakis, Athanasiadi, et al., 2014; Pouliakis, Margari, et al., 2014; Vavoulidis et al., 2016a, 2016b,2016c, 2016d).

Figure 5. Process Capability Report for Amylase created with Minitab 17 statistical package (based on internal quality control results for amylase; control material was provided by Medicon Hellas SA; measurements were performed at the Department of Biochemistry, Naval and Veterans Hospital, Athens, Greece). This figure is an example of Process Capability Analysis. Details about the sample used for this analysis are observed in the upper left frame of the figure. Capability indices are observed at the right frame of the figure, C_{pl} measures how close the process mean is running to the lower specification limit, C_{pu} measures how close the process mean is running to the upper specification limit and C_{pk} equals the lesser of C_{pu} and C_{pl}. The frame at the lower part of the figure shows results of the process performance. PPM<LSL indicates the number of nonconforming parts less than the lower specification limit. PPM>USL indicates the number of nonconforming parts greater than the upper specification limit. PPM Total indicates the total number of nonconforming parts outside both specification limits. By comparing PPM values before and after a process improvement, you can get a concrete sense of how much a process improvement has actually reduced the number nonconforming parts on both ends of the process curve.

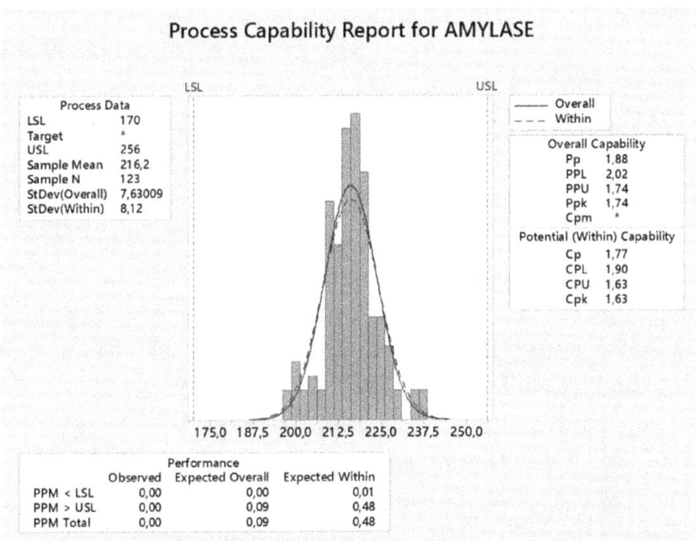

FMEAis a systematic approach to identifying and preventing product and process problems and adverse events before they occur. Since in healthcare services there are many different ways that a process or sub-process can fail to provide the anticipated result, it is frequently employed to avoid possible errors in healthcare (Stamouli, 2019; Dehnavieh, 2014;Hung, 2015; Mendes,2013). The following steps are included in an FMEA:

- define clearly the process to be studied (e.g. the pre-analytical phase)
- assemble a multidisciplinary team including experts on the subject
- develop and verify the flow chart of the process
- number each step identified in the process flow chart. If the process is complex, such as the pre-analytical phase, identify the area of the process to focus on (e.g. blood specimen collection, specimen transportation, specimen centrifugation)
- use various six sigma tools (such as including triggering questions, brainstorming, cause and effect chart) to identify all possible/potential failure modes for the process steps identified in the previous step. Failure modes include anything that could go wrong that would prevent the process step from being carried out (e.g. wrong sample identification, insufficient sample, wrong collection tube, haemolysis)
- number each failure mode and transfer it to the FMEA form
- list all possible/potential effects of the failure mode. Effects include anything that could happen if the failure occurs
- determine the severity (S) of each effect by using the Severity Rating table and document it on the FMEA form
- determine the potential causes of each failure mode. Each failure mode may have multiple failure mode causes (e. g. haemolysis causes might be prolonged tourniquet, variability in the training, skills, and frequency of phlebotomy practice of the nonlaboratory staff, puncturing small and fragile veins, the needle can transfer wet alcohol from the skin into the blood specimen, needle size, improper syringe draws, biological causes such as haemolyticanaemiaetc)
- document the causes on the FMEA form
- determine the probability of occurrence (O) for each of the potential causes by using the Probability Rating table and record it on the FMEA form
- determine the probability of detection (D) for each of the potential causes by using the Probability Rating table and record it on the FMEA form
- determine the Risk Priority Number (RPN) by multiplying (S) by (O) and (D)
- if the RPN is high, strong consideration should be given to developing an action plan
- record a corrective action for each failure mode on the FMEA form. Multiple actions can be implemented in the process to control a single hazard. An action can be used more than once in the process
- identify process and/or outcome measures that will be used to analyze and test the redesigned process
- identify a single, responsible individual to complete the corrective action
- record the corrective action, responsibility and target date on the FMEA form

- when the corrective actions have been implemented, the RPN should be lower
- calculate new RPN and documentit on the FMEA form.

A cause and effect chart, also known as an Ishikawa or "fishbone" chart, is a graphic tool used to explore and display the possible causes of a certain effect. In the classic fishbone diagram, different causes group naturally under the categories of Materials, Methods, Equipment, Environment, and People [Figure 6]. A cause and effect chart helps the user understand that there are many causes that contribute to an effect, it displays graphically the relationship of the causes to the effect and helps to identify areas for improvement (Ilie,2010).

Fault Tree Analysis (FTA) is a logical and diagrammatic tool that helps to estimate the probability of an event to occur based on the occurrence or non-occurrence of other events. In order to carry out an FTA, a leadingor top event has to be determined; this top event is a critical situation that can cause the system's failure. The tree formation starts with the definition of the top event, then the events that may lead to the top event are identified and connected to the top event with a logic gate. Further, the events leading to each next event are identified and connected with logic gates [Figure 7]. This process continues until all the basic causes of the top event are

Figure 6. A fishbone chart used to explore and display all the possible causes of a clinical laboratory specimen haemolysis, based on our experience. Haemolysis causes are divided in six main causes-branches (specimen collection. Specimen handling, specimen centrifugation, specimen transportation, in vivo haemolysis, and specimen storage). Each cause is analyzed in deeper and more detailed levels of causes.

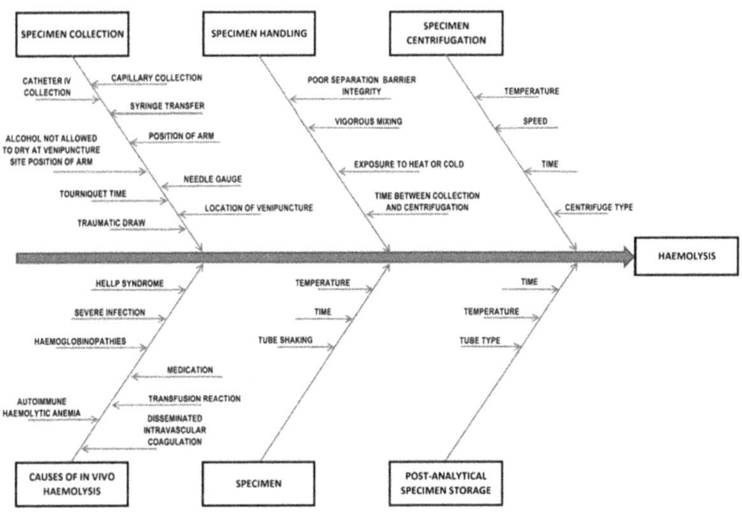

Figure 7. Fault Tree Analysis (FTA) used to explore and display all the possible causes of "no result reported from the biochemistry analyzer", based on our experience. Causes are divided in two categories: barcode label failure and samples failure.

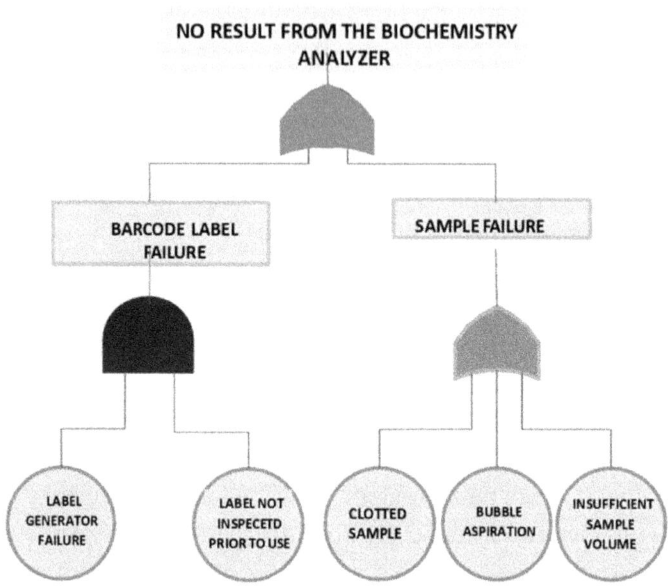

identified, FTA is a binary analysis, meaning that all events can either hap pen or not; there are no other options. Moreover, FTA may be qualitative, quantitative or both depending on the information available and the goals of the analysis.

Laboratory Waste Management

During the last decade, there is a significant increase in public concern about medical waste disposal, in order to reduce the transmission of infections, prevent environmental contamination and avoid public health risks. Waste management considerations derive from state laws and regulations, European directives, local regulations and non-regulatory requirements, such as the safety and environmental standards from the Joint Commission on Accreditation of Healthcare Organizations (JCAHO) and the College ofAmerican Pathologists (CAP), (El-Gilany et al., 2017; Awasthi et al., 2018; Ho&Chen,2018; Ho, 2019;National Research Council (US) Committee on Prudent Practices in the Laboratory.Washington (DC): National Academies Press (US); 2011.Prudent Practices in the Laboratory: Handling and Management of Chemical Hazards: UpdatedVersion).The total volume of waste generated per laboratory is estimated to more than 30,000 tons per year. Laboratory waste may be divided into the following categories:

- chemical waste (reagents, disinfectants, hypochlorite, ethanol, extraction solvents)
- solid and liquid infectious waste (blood samples, biological specimens, contaminated cotton pads, slides covered with cell substrates, blood cultures)
- sharps (needles, razors, blades, laboratory slides and cover slips, broken glass)
- low-level radioactive waste, such as specimens from patients receiving radioactive substances for diagnostic purposes
- wastes with multiple hazards (fluids generated form laboratory analyzers, laboratory stains)
- different kinds of solid waste for recycling, such as packaging waste, paper, plastic material
- used batteries
- printer ink and toner cartridges
- e-waste.

Managing waste generated in the clinical laboratory is a core element of the laboratory risk management program, (www.medical laboratory observer- Online.com), (https://www.mun.ca/sgs/current/chem_waste.pdf; www.medical laboratory observer- Online.com), (http://www.elinyae.gr/el/category_details.jsp?cat_id=2864;http://www.nomotelia.gr/photos/File/99738-19.pdf;

https://epoptes.wordpress.com/2018/02/22/;Laboratory Waste Management: A Guidebook (ACS Professional Reference Book) by ACS Task Force on Laboratory and Chemical Waste Management (2012-09-13) by ACS Task Force on Laboratory and Chemical Waste Management I Jan 1, 1744). All laboratory generated waste is considered the responsibility of the laboratory until its final disposition. Each laboratory should have a waste management program which includes waste determination according to its hazards and characteristics, separation and segregation of generated waste, recycling process for paper, bottles and aluminium cans, storage, transportation, and disposal operations.The procedure of removal from the laboratory must minimize the risk of spills, accidents and staff exposure.

Moreover, there must be a written contingency plan for emergencies such as leaks, spills, hood failures, and employee exposures to infectious and hazardous substances. Staff training in proper waste segregation, storage, labelling, and movement of waste in and out of the laboratory must be continuously subject to internal audits in order to correct any nonconformities discovered. It is also very important to have a commitment for sustainability and apply “green” practices, such as recycling of different disinfected waste streams, substitution of hazardous chemicals for less hazardous ones when possible, reduction of energy and water consumption (such as the turn off of biosafety cabinets and equipment when not in use and the use of reverse osmosis or ion exchange methods).

CONCLUSION

Clinical laboratories must ensure the quality, integrity, and reliability of a wide range of patient results. Moreover, they need to sustain a commitment to quality and demonstrate a certifiable level of compliance. Many strategies are used to reduce laboratory errors, including internal QC procedures, external quality assessment programs, implementation of QIs and six-sigma methodology. All strategies should be consistent with the requirements of the International Standard for medical laboratories accreditation [ISO 15189: 2012] and suitable for promoting corrective/preventive actions. They must promote total quality and patient safety and be consistent with the definition of a laboratory error; as it is specified in the ISO/TS 22367: 2008. Harmonization process is in progress. However, further efforts must be made to raise the awareness of all health personnel involved in the total testing process. Total quality management, which encompasses all the steps involved in sample processing, beginning from test order to the final interpretation of results by the clinicians, must be evaluated periodically to reduce or eliminate the errors that may arise during the various steps. For a patient-centered approach, there is the need to assure that every step of the total testing process is correctly performed, that weaknesses are recognized and that corrective and preventive actions are designed and implemented.

REFERENCES

Adeli, K., Raizman, J. E., Chen, Y., Higgins, V., Nieuwesteeg, M., Abdelhaleem, M., ... Blais, D. (2015). Complex biological profile of hematological markers across pediatric, adult, and geriatric ages: Establishment of robust pediatric and adult reference intervals based on the Canadian Health Measures Survey. *Clinical Chemistry*, *61*(8), 1075–1086. doi:10.1373/clinchem.2015.240531 PMID:26044509

Afrifa, J., Gyekye, S. A., Owiredu, W. K., Ephraim, R. K., Essien-Baidoo, S., Amoah, S., ... Arthur, A. R. (2015). Application of sigma metrics for the assessment of quality control in clinical chemistry laboratory in Ghana: A pilot study. *Nigerian Medical Journal*, *56*(1), 54–58. doi:10.4103/0300-1652.149172 PMID:25657495

Aslam, M., & Srinivasa Rao, G. (2019). Control Charts for Monitoring Process Capability Index Using Median Absolute Deviation for Some Popular Distributions. *Processes, 7*(5), 287. Doi.org/10.3390/pr7050287. doi:10.3390/pr7050287

Awasthi, A. K., Wang, M., Wang, Z., Awasthi, M. K., & Li, J. (2018). E-waste management in India: A mini-review. *Waste Management & Research, 36*(5), 408–414. doi:10.1177/0734242X18767038 PMID:29732961

Barak, M., & Jaschek, R. (2013). A new and effective way for preventing preanalytical laboratory errors. *Clinical Chemistry and Laboratory Medicine, 50*(4), 1–4. doi:10.1515/cclm-2013-0597

Barth, J. H. (2012). Clinical quality indicators in laboratory medicine. *Annals of Clinical Biochemistry, 49*(1), 9–16. doi:10.1258/acb.2011.011126 PMID:22042979

Berte, L. M. (2007). Improvement of Clinical Laboratory Services through Quality. *Clinics in Laboratory Medicine, 27*(4), 771–790. doi:10.1016/j.cll.2007.07.008 PMID:17950897

Bubshait, A., & Al-Dosary, A. (2014).Application of Lean Six-Sigma Methodology to Reduce the Failure Rate of Valves at Oil Field. *Proceedings of the World Congress on Engineering and Computer Science WCECS, 2*.

Campbell, C. A., & Horvath, A. R. (2014). Harmonization of critical result management in laboratory medicine. *Clinica Chimica Acta, 432*, 135–147. doi:10.1016/j.cca.2013.11.004

Cantalejo, R. F. (2010). Evaluación de métodos y validez de pruebasdiagnósticas. Estudio de las característicasmetrológicas de un test. In *CursoIVCongresoNacionaldel LaboratorioClinico*. CAPCollege of American Pathologists. Retrieved from http://www.cap.org/

CDC Center of Disease Control and Prevention. (n.d.). Retrieved from http://www.cdc.gov/

Ceriotti, F. (2016). Harmonization initiatives in Europe. *EJIFCC, 27*, 5–14. PMID:27683503

Ceriotti, F., Brugnoni, D., & Mattioli, S. (2015). How to define a significant deviation from the expected internal quality control result. *Clinical Chemistry and Laboratory Medicine, 53*(6), 913–918. doi:10.1515/cclm-2014-1149 PMID:25870962

Chen, M. S., Wu, M. H., & Lin, M. C. (2014). Application of Indices Cp and Cpk to Improve Quality Control Capability in Clinical Biochemistry Laboratories. *The Chinese Journal of Physiology*, *57*(2), 63–68. doi:10.4077/CJP.2014.BAB170 PMID:24694196

Claustres, M., Kožich, V., Dequeker, E., Fowler, B., Hehir-Kwa, J. Y., Miller, K., ... Barton, D. E. (2014). Recommendations for reporting results of diagnostic genetic testing (biochemical, cytogenetic and molecular genetic). *European Journal of Human Genetics*, *22*(2), 160–170. doi:10.1038/ejhg.2013.125 PMID:23942201

CLIA Clinical Laboratory Improvement Amendments. (n.d.). Retrieved from https://www.cms.gov/Regulations-and uidance/Legislation/CLIA/index.html?redirect

Cloete, B. C., & Bester, A. (2012). A Lean Six Sigma approach to the improvement of the selenium analysis method. *The Onderstepoort Journal of Veterinary Research*, *79*(1), E1–E13. doi:10.4102/ojvr.v79i1.407 PMID:23327320

COLA Commission on Office Laboratory Accreditation. (n.d.). Retrieved from http://www.ama-assn.org/ama/pub/physician-resources/clinical-practice-improvement/clinical-quality/accreditation-collaboration/cola.page

Dallas Jones, G. R. (2015). Analytical performance specifications for EQA schemes –need for harmonization. *Clinical Chemistry and Laboratory Medicine*, *53*(6), 919–924. doi:10.1515/cclm-2014-1268

David, R. E., & Dobreanu, M. (2015). Risk Management in Clinical Laboratory: From Theory to Practice. *Acta Medica Marisiensis*, *61*(4), 372–377. doi:10.1515/amma-2015-0086

Deetz, C. O., Nolan, D. K., & Scott, M. G. (2012). An examination of the usefulness of repeat testing practices in a large hospital clinical chemistry laboratory. *American Journal of Clinical Pathology*, *137*(1), 20–25. doi:10.1309/AJCPWPBF62YGEFOR PMID:22180474

Dehnavieh, R., Ebrahimipour, H., Molavi-Taleghani, Y., Vafaee-Najar, A., Noori Hekmat, S., & Esmailzdeh, H. (2014). Proactive risk assessment of blood transfusion process, in pediatric emergency, using the Health Care Failure Mode and Effects Analysis (HFMEA). *Global Journal of Health Science*, *7*(1), 322–331. doi:10.5539/gjhs.v7n1p322 PMID:25560332

Devgun, M. S., Chan, M. K., El-Nujumi, A. M., Abara, R., Armbruster, D., & Adeli, K. (2015). Clinical decision limits for interpretation of direct bilirubin—A CALIPER study of healthy multiethnic children and case report reviews. *Clinical Biochemistry*, *48*(1-2), 93–96. doi:10.1016/j.clinbiochem.2014.10.011 PMID:25445233

El-Gilany, A. H., El-Shaer, S., Khashaba, E., El-Dakroory, S. A., & Omar, N. (2017). Knowledge, attitude, and practice (KAP) of 'teaching laboratory' technicianstowards laboratory safety and waste management: A pilot interventional study. *The Journal of Hospital Infection, 96*(2), 192–194. doi:10.1016/j.jhin.2017.02.007 PMID:28268025

El-Hashmi, K., & Gnieber, O. K. (2014). Applying Process Capability Analysis in Measuring Clinical Laboratory Quality - A Six Sigma Project. *Proceedings of the 2014 International Conference on Industrial Engineering and Operations Management Bali, Indonesia. Abstract Book*, 1780-1789.

Flegar-Meštrić, Z., Perkov, S., Radeljak, A., Kardum Paro, M. M., Prkačin, I., & Devčić-Jeras, A. (2017). Risk analysis of the preanalytical process based on quality indicators data. *Clinical Chemistry and Laboratory Medicine, 55*(3), 368–377. doi:10.1515/cclm-2016-0235 PMID:27580180

Fursule, N.V., Bansod, S.V., & Fursule, N.S. (2012). Understanding the benefits and limitations of Six Sigma Methodology. *International Journal of Scientific and Research Publications, 2*(1), 1-9.

García-Lario, J. V., & Boned Juliani, B. (2012). Control de la CalidadInterno: Una PrácticaMuyActual. *EdCont Lab Clín, 15*, 97–111.

Gerostamoulos, D. (2013). Urinary drug screening. *Australian Prescriber, 36*(2), 62–64. doi:10.18773/austprescr.2013.025

Gimenez-Marin, A., Rivas-Ruiz, F., Perez-Hidalgo, M. M., & Molina-Mendoza, P. (2014). Preanalytical errors management in the clinical laboratory: A five-year study. *Biochemical Medicine, 24*(2), 248–257. doi:10.11613/BM.2014.027 PMID:24969918

Hammerling, J. A. (2012). A Review of MedicalErrors in Laboratory Diagnostics and WhereWe Are Today. *Laboratory Medicine, 43*(2), 41–44. Doi.org/10.1309/LM6ER9WJR1IHQAUY. doi:10.1309/LM6ER9WJR1IHQAUY

Hawkins, R. (2012). Managing the pre- and post-analytical phases of the total testing process. *Annals of Laboratory Medicine, 32*(1), 5–16. doi:10.3343/alm.2012.32.1.5 PMID:22259773

Hekmatpanah, M., Ravichandran, N., Shahin, A., & Ahmadi, H. (2013). Investigating the Application of Six Sigma Methodology and Quality Control Tools and Techniques in Sepanhan Oil Company. *The Global eLearning Journal, 2*(3), 1-24.

Hsieh, Y. J., Huang, L. Y., & Wang, C. T. (2012). A framework for the selection of Six Sigma projects in services: Case studies of banking and health care services in Taiwan. *Service Business, 6*(2), 243–264. doi:10.100711628-012-0134-1

Hung, S. H., Wang, P. C., Lin, H. C., Chen, H. Y., & Su, C. T. (2015). Integration of Value Stream Map and Healthcare Failure Mode and Effect Analysis into Six Sigma Methodology to Improve Process of Surgical Specimen Handling. *Journal of Healthcare Engineering*, *6*(3), 377–398. doi:10.1260/2040-2295.6.3.377 PMID:26753440

IFCC. (n.d.). Retrieved from http://www.ifcc.org/ifccfiles/docs/fundamentals-for-eqa.pdf

Ilie, G., & Ciocoiu, C. N. (2010). Application of Fishbone Diagram to Determine the Risk of an Event with Multiple Causes. *Management Research and Practice*, *2*(1), 1–20.

In vitro diagnostic medical devices 98/79 EC.

Institute of Medicine (IOM). (2005). *Performance Measurement: Accelerating Improvement*. Washington, DC: NationalAcademy Press.

ISO 15189:2012. (2012). *Medical laboratories – requirements for quality and competence*. Geneva, Switzerland: International Organization for Standardization.

ISO 17511:2003. (2003). *In vitro diagnostic medical devices -Measurement of quantities in biological samples - Metrological traceability of values assigned to calibrators and control materials*. ISO.

ISO 18153: 2003. (2003). *In vitro diagnostic medical devices – Measurement of quantities in biological samples – metrological traceability of values for catalytic concentration of enzymes assigned to calibrators and control materials*. ISO.

ISO/IEC 17025:2005. (2005). *General requirements for the competence of testing and calibration laboratories*. ISO.

ISO/IEC 17043 (2010). *Conformity assessment — General requirements for proficiency testing*. ISO.

ISO/TS 22367: 2008. (2008). *Medical laboratories —Reduction of error through risk management and continual improvement*. ISO.

JCAHO Joint Commission. (n.d.). *Accreditation, Health care, certification*. Retrieved from www.jointcommission.org

Jegede, F. E., Mbah, H. A., Aminu, M., Yakubu, T. N., & Torpey, K. (2015). Evaluation of Laboratory Performance withQualityIndicators in Infectious DiseaseHospital, Kano, Nigeria. *Open Journal of Clinical Diagnostics*, *5*(01), 1–9. doi:10.4236/ojcd.2015.51001

Jones, G. R. (2016). Average of delta: A new quality control tool for clinicallaboratories. *Annals of Clinical Biochemistry, 53*(1), 133–140. doi:10.1177/0004563215581400 PMID:25800407

Jones, G. R., & Koetsia, S. D. (2014). Combinedreferenceintervals and analytical EQA. *The Clinical Biochemist. Reviews / Australian Association of Clinical Biochemists, 35*(4), 243–250.

Karkalousos, P., & Evangelopoulos, A. (2011). *Quality Control in Clinical Laboratories, Applications and Experiences of Quality Control*. In Tech. Retrieved from http://www.intechopen.com/books/applications-and-experiences-of-quality-control/quality-control-in clinical-laboratories.

Kemp, G. M., Bird, C. E., & Barth, J. H. (2012). Short-term interventions on wards fail to Reducepreanalytical errors: Results of two prospective controlled trials. *Annals of Clinical Biochemistry, 49*(2), 166–169. doi:10.1258/acb.2011.011133 PMID:22169099

Koerbin, G., Sikaris, K. A., Jones, G. R., Ryan, J., Reed, M., & Tate, J. (2014). Evidence-based approach to harmonized reference intervals. *Clinica Chimica Acta, 432*, 99–107. doi:10.1016/j.cca.2013.10.021 PMID:24183842

Kopcinovic, L. M., Trifunović, J., Pavosevic, T., & Nikolac, N. (2015). Croatian survey on critical results reporting. *Biochemia Medica, 25*(2), 193–202. doi:10.11613/BM.2015.019 PMID:26110031

Kumar, N. S., & Ray, L. (2013). Application of Sigma Metrics in Medical Biochemistry. *Journal of Clinical and Diagnostic Research: JCDR, 7*(12), 2689–2691. doi:10.7860/JCDR/2013/7292.3700 PMID:24551613

Lakshman, M., Ravindra Reddy, B., & Bhulaxmi, P. (2015). Evaluation of sigma metrics in a Medical Biochemistry lab. *International Journal of Biomedical Research, 6*(03), 164–171. doi:10.7439/ijbr.v6i3.1709

Lam, Q., Ajzner, E., Campbell, C. A., & Young, A. (2016). Critical risk results – an update on international initiatives. *EJIFCC, 27*(1), 66–76. PMID:27683507

Lao, E.G., García, A.S., Figuerola, M.B., Ester Moreno, E., & Paraire, A.H. (2017). Errors of Clinical Laboratory and Its Impact on Patient Safety. *Open Journal of Social Sciences, 5*, 243-253.

Liebow, E. B., Derzon, J. H., Fontanesi, J., Favoretto, A. M., Baetz, R. A., Shaw, C., ... Epner, P. (2012). Effectiveness of Automated Notification and CustomerServiceCallCenters for Timely and Accurate Reporting of Critical Values: A Laboratory Medicine Best Practices Systematic Review and Meta-Analysis. *Clinical Biochemistry*, *45*(13-14), 979–987. doi:10.1016/j.clinbiochem.2012.06.023 PMID:22750773

Lippi, G., Baird, G. S., Banfi, G., Bölenius, K., Cadamuro, J., Church, S., ... Simundic, A.-M. (2017). Improving quality in the preanalytical phase through innovation, on behalf of the European Federation for Clinical Chemistry and Laboratory Medicine (EFLM) Working Group for Preanalytical Phase (WG-PRE). *Clinical Chemistry and Laboratory Medicine*, *55*(4), 489–500. doi:10.1515/cclm-2017-0107 PMID:28231060

Lippi, G., Becan-McBride, K., Behúlová, D., Bowen, R. A., Church, S., Delanghe, J., ... Simundic, A.-M. (2013). Preanalytical quality improvement: In quality we trust. *Clinical Chemistry and Laboratory Medicine*, *51*(1), 229–241. doi:10.1515/cclm-2012-0597 PMID:23072858

Lippi, G., Betsou, F., Cadamuro, J., Cornes, M., Fleischhacker, M., Neumaier, M., & ... . (2019). Working Group for Preanalytical Phase (WG-PRE), European Federation of Clinical Chemistry and Laboratory Medicine (EFLM).Preanalytical challenges - time for solutions. *Clinical Chemistry and Laboratory Medicine*, *57*(7), 974–981. doi:10.1515/cclm-2018-1334 PMID:30710481

Lippi, G., & Cadamuro, J. (2017). Novel opportunities for improving the quality of preanalytical phase. A glimpse to the future? *Journal of Medical Biochemistry*, *36*(4), 1–6. doi:10.1515/jomb-2017-0029 PMID:30581325

Lippi, G., Chance, J. J., Church, S., Dazzi, P., Fontana, R., Giavarina, D., ... Simundic, A.-M. (2011). Preanalytical quality improvement: From dream to reality. *Clinical Chemistry and Laboratory Medicine*, *49*(7), 1113–1126. doi:10.1515/CCLM.2011.600 PMID:21517699

Lippi, G., Mattiuzzi, C., & Favaloro, E. J. (2015). Pre-analytical variability and quality of diagnostic testing. Looking at the moon and gazing beyond the finger. *N Z J Med Lab Sci*, *69*, 4–8.

Lippi, G., & Plebani, M. (2018). A Six-Sigma approach for comparing diagnostic errors in healthcare-where does laboratory medicine stand? *Annals of Translational Medicine*, *6*(10), 180. doi:10.21037/atm.2018.04.02 PMID:29951502

Lippi, G., Plebani, M., & Graber, M. L. (2016). Building a bridge to safe diagnosis in health care. The role of the clinical laboratory. *Clinical Chemistry and Laboratory Medicine*, *54*(1), 1–3. doi:10.1515/cclm-2015-1135 PMID:26630697

Lippi, G., von Meyer, A., Cadamuro, J., & Simundic, A. M. (2019). Blood sample quality. *Diagnosis (Berl)*, *6*(1), 25–31. doi:10.1515/dx-2018-0018 PMID:29794250

Lund, F., Petersen, P. H., Fraser, C. G., & Sölétormos, G. (2015). Calculation of limits for significant bidirectional changes in two or more serial results of a biomarker based on a computer simulation model. *Annals of Clinical Biochemistry*, *52*(4), 434–440. doi:10.1177/0004563214555163 PMID:25249664

Mendes, M. E., Ebner, P. R., Romano, P., Neto, M. P., Sant'anna, A., & Sumita, N. M. (2013). Practical aspects of the use of FMEA tool in clinical laboratory risk management. *Jornal Brasileiro de Patologia e Medicina Laboratorial*, *49*(3), 174–181. doi:10.1590/S1676-24442013000300004

Miri-Dashe, T., Osawe, S., Tokdung, M., Daniel, N., Choji, R. P., Mamman, I., ... Abimiku, A. (2014). ComprehensiveReferenceRanges for Hematology and Clinical Chemistry Laboratory Parameters Derived from Normal Nigerian Adults. *PLoS One*, *9*(5), e93919. doi:10.1371/journal.pone.0093919 PMID:24832127

Mourtzikou, A., & Stamouli, M. (2017). An Update On Best Practices and Regulatory Requirements for the Improvement of Clinical Laboratory Services through Quality. *International Journal of Reliable and Quality E-Healthcare*, *6*(1), 1–17. doi:10.4018/IJRQEH.2017010101

Mourtzikou, A., Stamouli, M., & Athanasiadi, E. (2013). Article. *International Journal of Reliable and Quality E-Healthcare*, *2*(2), 38-46. Doi: 104018/ijrqeh.2013040103

Myers, G. L., & Miller, W. G. (2016). The International Consortium for Harmonization of Clinical Laboratory Results (ICHCLR) – A pathway for harmonization. *EJIFCC*, *27*(1), 30–36. PMID:27683504

Nanda, S. K., & Ray, L. (2013). Quantitative Application of Sigma Metrics in Medical Biochemistry. *Journal of Clinical and Diagnostic Research*, *7*(12), 2689–2691. doi:10.7860/JCDR/2013/7292.3700 PMID:24551613

Neuburger, J., Walker, K., Sherlaw-Johnson, C., van der Meulen, J., & Cromwell, D. A. (2017). Comparison of control charts for monitoring clinical performance using binary data. *BMJ Quality & Safety*, *26*(11), 919–928. doi:10.1136/bmjqs-2016-005526 PMID:28947635

Njoroge, W. S., & Nichols, H. J. (2014). Risk Management in the Clinical Laboratory. *Annals of Laboratory Medicine*, *34*(4), 274–278. doi:10.3343/alm.2014.34.4.274 PMID:24982831

Noble, M. (2009). *Quality Management for the Medical Laboratory*. Retrieved from www.polqm.ca/.../qmformedlab2008

Nordin, G. (2015). Before defining performance criteria we must agree on what a "qualitative test procedure" is. *Clinical Chemistry and Laboratory Medicine*, *53*(6), 939–941. doi:10.1515/cclm-2015-0005 PMID:25879322

Padoan, A., Antonelli, G., Aita, A., Sciacovelli, L., & Plebani, M. (2017). Issues and challenges in applicability of measurement uncertainty estimation in medical laboratories. *Journal of Laboratory and Precision Medicine*, *2*, 69–72. doi:10.21037/jlpm.2017.08.10

Panteghini, M., Ceriotti, F., Jones, G., Oosterhuis, W., Plebani, M., & Sandberg, S. (2017). Strategies to define performance specifications in laboratory medicine: 3 years on from the Milan Strategic Conference. *Clinical Chemistry and Laboratory Medicine*, *55*(12), 1849–1856. doi:10.1515/cclm-2017-0772 PMID:29031018

Plebani, M. (2016). Harmonization of clinical laboratory information – current and future strategies. *EJIFCC*, *27*(1), 15–22. PMID:27683502

Plebani, M., Astion, M. L., Barth, J. H., Chen, W., de Oliveira Galoro, C. A., Escuer, M. I., ... Sumarac, Z. (2014). Harmonization of quality indicators in laboratory medicine. A preliminary consensus. *Clinical Chemistry and Laboratory Medicine*, *52*(7), 951–958. doi:10.1515/cclm-2014-0142 PMID:24622792

Plebani, M., Laposata, M., & Lippi, G. (2019). Driving the route of laboratory medicine: A manifesto for the future. *Internal and Emergency Medicine*, *14*(3), 337–340. doi:10.100711739-019-02053-z PMID:30783946

Plebani, M., Sciacovelli, L., & Aita, A. (2017). Quality Indicators for the Total Testing Process. *Clinics in Laboratory Medicine*, *37*(1), 187–205. doi:10.1016/j.cll.2016.09.015 PMID:28153366

Plebani, M., Sciacovelli, L., Aita, A., Pelloso, M., & Chiozza, M. L. (2015). Performance criteria and quality indicators for the pre-analytical phase. *Clinical Chemistry and Laboratory Medicine*, *53*(6), 943–948. doi:10.1515/cclm-2014-1124 PMID:25719322

Rashid, G., Goldman, J., Weinstein, D., Tohami, T., Neumark, E., & Weiss, E. (2015). Reporting Critical Lab Results, a Challenge for the lab and the Physician - A Summary of Four Years of Experience in MeirMedicalCenter Laboratories. *Harefuah, 154*(8), 494–498, 541. PMID:26480612

Rodríguez-Borja, E., Villalba-Martinez, C., & Carratalá–Calvo, A. (2014). Enquiry time as part of turnaround time: When do our clinicians really consult our results? *Journal of Clinical Pathology, 67*(7), 642–644. doi:10.1136/jclinpath-2013-202102 PMID:24706264

Ryu, J. H., & Hong Wan, H. (2010). Optimal Design of a CUSUM Chart for a Mean Shift of Unknown Size. *Journal of Quality Technology, 42*(3), 311–326. doi:10.1080/00224065.2010.11917826

Sadiq, F., Yasmeen, F., Mumtaz, A., Hussain, W., Butt, A. T., Qureshi, S. A., & Ibrahim, M. (2014). Frequency of Errors in Clinical Laboratory Practice. *Iranian Journal of Pathology, 9*(1), 45–49.

Shahangian, S., & Snyder, S. R. (2009). Laboratory medicine quality indicators: A review of the literature. *American Journal of Clinical Pathology, 131*(3), 418–431. doi:10.1309/AJCPJF8JI4ZLDQUE PMID:19228647

Shcolnik, W., de Oliveira, C. A., de São José, A. S., de Oliveira Galoro, C. A., Plebani, M., & Burnett, D. (2012). Brazilian laboratory indicators program. *Clinical Chemistry and Laboratory Medicine, 50*(11), 1923–1934. doi:10.1515/cclm-2012-0357 PMID:23096110

Sikaris, K. (2015). Performance criteria of the post-analytical phase. *Clinical Chemistry and Laboratory Medicine, 53*(6), 949–958. doi:10.1515/cclm-2015-0016 PMID:25894643

Simundic, A.M., Cornes, M., Grankvist, K., Lippi, G.,andNybo, M. (2014).

Simundic, A. M., Kackov, S., Miler, M., Fraser, C. G., & Petersen, P. H. (2015). Terms and symbols used in studies on biological variation: The need for harmonization. *Clinical Chemistry, 61*(2), 438–439. doi:10.1373/clinchem.2014.233791 PMID:25403815

Söderberg, J., Brulin, C., Grankvist, K., & Wallin, O. (2009). Preanalytical errors in primary healthcare: A questionnaire study of information search procedures, test request management and test tube labelling. *Clinical Chemistry and Laboratory Medicine, 47*(2), 195–201. doi:10.1515/CCLM.2009.048 PMID:19191726

Solinger, A. B., & Rothman, S. I. (2013). Risks of mortality associated with common laboratory tests: A novel, simple and meaningful way to set decision limits from data available in the Electronic Medical Record. *Clinical Chemistry and Laboratory Medicine*, *51*(9), 1803–1813. doi:10.1515/cclm-2013-0167 PMID:23729574

Stamouli, M., Mourtzikou, A., Karkalousos, P. L., Athanasiadou, Z., Marasidi, E., & Skliris, A. (2019). Application of Failure Modes and Effects Analysis (FMEA) During the Pre-analytical Phase in a Greek Biochemistry Laboratory. *International Journal of Reliable and Quality E-Healthcare*, *4*(3), 22–35. doi:10.4018/IJRQEH.2019070102

Standardization of collection requirements for fasting samples: for the Working Group on Preanalytical Phase (WG-PA) of the European Federation of Clinical Chemistry and Laboratory Medicine (EFLM). (n.d.). *ClinChimActa, 15*(432), 33-7. Doi:10.1016/j.cca.2013.11.008

Stoiljkovic, V., Milosavljevic, P., Mladenovic, S., Pavlovic, D., & Todorovic, M. (2014). Improving the Efficiency of the Center for Medical Biochemistry clinical Center, by Applying Lean Six Sigma Methodology. *Journal of Medical Biochemistry*, *33*(3), 299–307. doi:10.2478/jomb-2014-0012

Tate, J. R., Sikaris, K. A., Jones, G. R., Yen, T., Koerbin, G., Ryan, J., ... Graham, P. (2014). Harmonising Adult and Paediatric Reference Intervals in Australia and New Zealand: An Evidence-Based Approach for Establishing a First Panel of Chemistry Analytes. *The Clinical Biochemist. Reviews / Australian Association of Clinical Biochemists*, *35*(4), 213–235. PMID:25678727

Thompson, M., & Wood, R. (1995). Harmonized guidelines for internal quality control in analytical chemistry laboratories. *Pure and Applied Chemistry*, *67*(4), 649–666. doi:10.1351/pac199567040649

Usha, S., Adiga, U. S., Preethika, A., & Swathi, K. (2015).Sigma metrics in clinical chemistry laboratory – A guide to quality control. *Al Ameen J Med Sci, 8*(4), 281-287.

Westgard, J. O., Barry, P. L., Quam, E. F., Shermeyer, S. S., Plaut, D., & Statland, B. E. (2002). *Chapter6 in Basic QC Practices, Training in StatisticalQuality Control for Healthcare Laboratories* (2nd ed.). Madison, WI: Westgard QC, Inc.

White, G. H., Campbell, C. A., & Horvath, A. R. (2014). Is this a critical, panic, alarm, urgent or markedly abnormal result? *Clinical Chemistry*, *60*(12), 1589–70. doi:10.1373/clinchem.2014.227645 PMID:25189694

Ye, Z. K., Tang, H. L., & Zhai, S. D. (2013). Benefits of therapeutic drug monitoring of vancomycin: A systematic review and meta-analysis. *PLoS One*, *8*(10), e77169. doi:10.1371/journal.pone.0077169 PMID:24204764

Yuh-Shan, H. (2019). Comment on Chen, J.; Su, Y.; Si, H.; Chen, J. Managerial Areas of Construction and Demolition Waste: A Scientometric Review. *Int. J. Environ. Res. Public Health* 2018, *15*, 2350. *International Journal of Environmental Research and Public Health, 16*(10), 1837. doi:10.3390/ijerph16101837

Zeng, R., Wang, W., & Wang, Z. (2013). National survey on critical values notification of 599 institutions in China. *Clinical Chemistry and Laboratory Medicine, 51*(11), 2099–2107. doi:10.1515/cclm-2013-0183 PMID:23839815

KEY TERMS AND DEFINITIONS

Coefficient of Variance: It is the analytical coefficient of variation of the test method, expressed in CV%.

External Quality Control: It describes a method that allows the comparison of a laboratory's performance to a source outside the laboratory, such as a peer group of laboratories or a reference laboratory.

Inductively Coupled Plasma Mass Spectrometry: It is a reference method that determines the concentration of analytes in serum-based calibration material.

Internal Quality Control: It is the use of control samples and statistical methods, where control samples are biological samples (serum, whole blood, urine, etc.), usually lyophilized, that contain analytes in concentrations close to the medical decision limits.

Quality Indicator: It is an objective measure that potentially evaluates all critical care domains.

Standard Deviation: A quantity expressing by how much the members of a group differ from the mean value for the group.

Turn Around Time: It is the amount of time taken to complete a process or fulfill a request.

Chapter 9
A Model for Determining Process-Wise CTQs for Testing Laboratories

Pranil Vijay Sawalakhe
Debre Tabor University, Ethiopia

ABSTRACT

Ensuring the quality of testing laboratory services plays an important role in the field of service sector. Acknowledging the revolution of Six Sigma (SS) in the corporate world and service sector, testing laboratories can also be benefited by the application of the same. SS focuses on process improvement that is a major determinant of customer satisfaction. CTQ (critical to quality) is a quality characteristic of a product or a service that is required to be improved from a customer's point of view. CTQs are the key measurable indicators of a product or process whose performance standards or specification limits must be met in order to satisfy the customer. The aim of this research is to develop a model for establishing CTQ for testing laboratory. The focus is on establishing process-wise CTQ characteristics from the voice of customer taken from direct and indirect customers associated with testing laboratories. The list of established CTQs will be a useful guide for both practitioners and academics willing to evaluate performance of testing laboratories.

INTRODUCTION

With the development of product certification, more and more attention has been given to testing laboratories in order to serve the health care and industry sector more efficiently and effectively.

DOI: 10.4018/978-1-7998-2390-2.ch009

Various types of testing laboratories that incorporate advanced testing have been introduced and also are in the process of being expanded. As a result, the testing process is becoming increasingly complex, and the number of tests to be processed is increasing. Many research studies have been conducted to develop and deliver high-quality services in laboratories. However, in order for a more substantial and successful management program, it is necessary to translate broad customer needs into specific, actionable, measurable performance requirements.

Quality of service is a critical determinant of testing laboratory performance. Also, it can be a critical factor in determining the long-term viability of a testing laboratory. Therefore, assessing the laboratory user's needs are critical factors to the success of modern testing laboratory. This study aims to develop a model for establishing CTQ and identify the critical attributes affecting the quality of testing laboratory.

BACKGROUND

What is CTQ

The Six Sigma methodology uses facts and data to search for the root cause of problems that dissatisfy customers. An important issue that we must come to grips with is how to take customer requirements and turn them into characteristics that we can measure to see how well we are meeting the requirements. We need to define what is known as Critical to Quality Characteristics (CTQ's) based on the Voice of the Customer. Customers know what they want in general terms, but are often not capable of expressing those needs concretely and objectively.

Critical To Quality (CTQ) characteristics are features by which customers evaluate the product or, and that can be used as measures for a project. CTQ stands for Critical to Quality. CTQs are translated from VOC. VOC is often vague, emotional or merely generalizations about products or services. CTQ's are the quantifiable, measurable and meaningful translation of VOC.

Method for Determining CTQs

A critical to quality (CTQ) is the flowchart process of finding out quality features or characteristics of the customer with the perspective to identify the problems. However, critical to quality determines the inputs and outputs of processes in order to find out the path that influences the standard or quality of process outputs. CTQs are the central unit to measure features of a process whose presentation values or

Table 1: Definition of CTQ by various researchers

Researchers	Definition of CTQ
Kenworthy (2004)	Key measurable characteristics of a product or process that must be met to satisfy customer and shareholder needs
Al Juboury (2012)	Measurable characteristics and requirements that are identified by the customer to ensure the improvements in order to guarantee his/her satisfaction
	Tools to apply scales and improve the goals which are considered the primary basis to understand the current process requirements and that allow fulfilling the future process requirements
Knop (2016)	CTQ tree is a tool proposed within the Six Sigma concept, which decodes customer language (needs, expectations, requirements) into product/services specifications
	CTQs are the internal critical quality parameters that relate to the wants and needs of the customer

specification limits must be qualified in order to meet the customers' requirements. They bring into design efforts or line improvement with the requirements of the customers.

CTQs correspond to the service characteristics that are comprehensively defined by both the internal as well as the external customers. They may include the lower and upper specification limits or factors that are related to the service or product. According to the opinion of valued customers, a complete CTQ analysis is an actionable and qualitative business specification methodology.

The CTQ method helps to bring a clear structure to what these requirements are. The method also helps to set priorities to manage quality. The method of determining CTQs are followed by three steps, as shown below.

Step 1: Identify Critical Needs

Firstly, there is a need to identify the critical needs that our service has to meet. During this first need, the criticality of service is a significant concern. Therefore, it is best to define these needs in broad terms; this will help ensure that not a single important thing is missed in the next steps.

If it is not possible to ask customers directly about their needs then one should go brainstorming their needs with people who deal with customers directly – salespeople and customer service representatives – as well as with your team. These can be done smoothly by using the Voice of Customer (VOC) tools like customer interviews, surveys, focus groups, customer surveys, market research, observations and test customers.

Step 2: Identify Quality Drivers

Secondly, there is a need to identify the specific quality drivers that have to be in place to meet the needs that are identified in the previous step. These are those characteristics, attributes, factors or process features that play a critical or critical role in influencing the fulfilment of that need. Tools like Kano Analysis and Five product level play an essential role in identifying process features that will delight the customers.

Step 3: Identify Performance Requirements

After determination of quality drives, the aim is to set up a range of results that will be acceptable in order for the customer to be satisfied. Finally, the minimum performance requirements are to be identified to satisfy each quality driver in order to provide a quality service. It is crucial to evaluate the ability to deliver the requirements like sufficient equipment and machines, human resources, materials, methodologies in place etc. After completion of a CTQ Tree for each critical need, there will be a list of measurable requirements that must be met to deliver a high-quality service.

Studies Related to Establishing CTQs

Many studies based on establishing CTQ for service sector were studied. These studies are mainly focused on the application of Six Sigma in the service industry for enhancing quality standards concerning customer satisfaction. That was done by identifying CTQs through the VOC. The study provides in-depth information about the usage of CTQs and their impact in multiple disciplines of the service sector.

Table 2 containing Researcher, number of identified CTQs and List of identified CTQs was developed.

Limitations of the Studies Related to CTQs

From the above mentioned CTQs by various researchers, It is observed that CTQs are normally used in the service sector like hospitals, education bodies, laboratories etc. These studies are carried out by conducting surveys and interviews with internal and external customers. From these studies, it is evident that some issues related to establishing CTQs are not covered in a detailed way. These issues are as follows:

a) A detailed structure, i.e. Process map for which CTQs are developed.
b) Detailed layout of the method in establishing CTQs

Figure 1. Conversion of customer requirements into CTQs

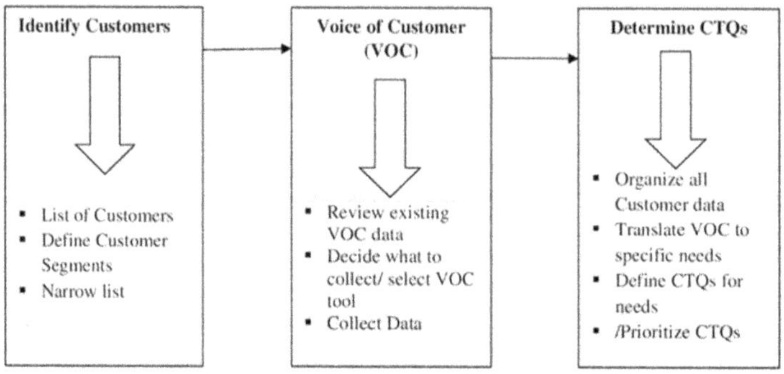

Figure 1. Conversion of Customer requirements into CTQs

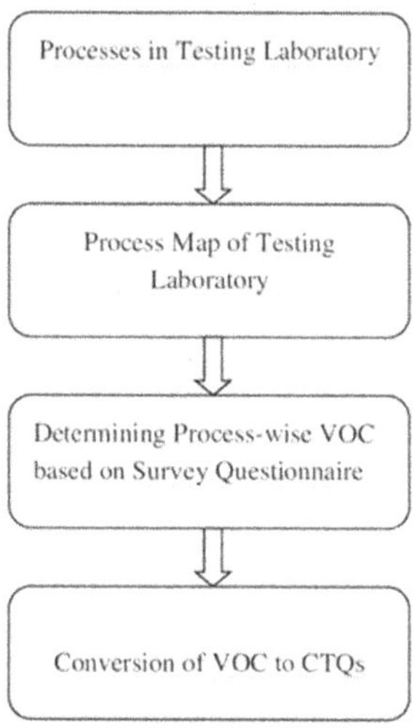

c) Model for establishing process-wise CTQs
d) Coverage of all the CTQs for the mentioned process.

The above are some limitations of the studies which are carried out by various researchers. These limitations are in-depth studied and are resolved by implicating these issues in establishing CTQs.

Need for Establishment of CTQS

The Six Sigma methodology uses facts and data to search for the root cause of problems that dissatisfy customers. An important issue that we must come to grips

Table 2. Identification of CTQs in the service sector by various researchers

Sr. No.	Researchers	Number of CTQs	Identified CTQs
01	Stahl (2003)	12	▪ Accuracy of diagnosis. ▪ Appropriateness of treatment. ▪ Timeliness of service ▪ Wait times. ▪ Exam and treatment. ▪ Testing and report turnaround. ▪ Staff availability. ▪ Bed availability in the emergency department and hospital. ▪ Responsiveness to squads. ▪ Satisfaction of patient and referring doctor. ▪ Cost of operations. ▪ Productivity and workflow.
02	Chakrabarty, A., & Tan, K. C. (2008)	11	▪ Representative responsiveness ▪ Patient preparation time ▪ Timely and accurate claims reimbursement ▪ Accuracy in the allocation of cash ▪ Accurate information to customers ▪ Time-waiting time, Treatment time cycle time, service time, turnaround time ▪ Employee behaviour ▪ Time to respond and restore ▪ Customer complaints ▪ Timely and accurate information to the customer ▪ Service cost
03	Yun, E. K., & Chun, K. M (2008)	09	▪ Accuracy of input patient demographic ▪ Medical data - Adequate patient data ▪ Properly documented records ▪ Competence of medical professionals ▪ Quality of recommendation- Trustworthiness of information provided to the customer ▪ Cost ▪ Time- Preparation time (data input), Processing time (transmission), Delayed time ▪ Follow up procedure ▪ Number of unsolved cases
04	Chakraborty, A., & Tan, K. C. (2012)	14	▪ Waiting time, service time, cycle time ▪ Response time to customer complaints ▪ Service Cost ▪ Billing error ▪ Occupancy rate ▪ Inventory reduction ▪ Wastage/pilferage ▪ Ease of use(documents) ▪ Assessment consistency(documents) ▪ Timely information to the customer ▪ Clinical outcome time (service time, waiting time, cycle time) ▪ Accurate information to the customer ▪ Time to restore customer complaints ▪ Time to respond to customer complaints
05	Indrawati (2012)	07	▪ Wrong dimension ▪ Failure in the whole process ▪ Cracked part ▪ Scratch /tool mark ▪ Non- conforming parts for the next process ▪ Layer defect did not match with part process sheet ▪ Wrong and wrong application of chemical addition

continues on following page

Table 2. Continued

Sr. No.	Researchers	Number of CTQs	Identified CTQs
06	Aminudin, O., & Zainol, M. (2014)	04	▪ Time- service time, waiting time, and cycle time ▪ Cost ▪ Employee behaviour ▪ Information- accurate and timely information
07	Taner et al. (2014)	05	• Patient's eye anatomy • Experience of ophthalmic surgeon • Quality of surgical equipment • Quality and type of suture • Experience of staff
08	Knop (2016)	36	▪ Construction of the walls and pillars of the load box ▪ System of tilting ▪ Tilting angle of the load box to the sides ▪ Shape of the load box platform ▪ Opening and closing system of the walls of the load box ▪ Number of levers to open the walls of load platforms ▪ Height of load box platform from the ground (land) ▪ Manufacturer of profiles trailers ▪ Way of walls stabilizing ▪ Sheet thickness of walls/floor ▪ Number of cargo handles on the floor ▪ Shape of the frame ▪ Type of profiles on the frame ▪ Grade of steel used on the frame ▪ Type of steel used on the floor ▪ Quality of the paint coating ▪ Construction of the walls and pillars of the load box ▪ Loading surface ▪ Load capacity ▪ Height of walls of the load box ▪ Length of the load box inside ▪ Width of the load box inside ▪ Overall dimensions ▪ Opening and closing system of the walls load box ▪ Type of equipment of the rear wall of the load box ▪ Tipping angle of the load box to back ▪ Maximum design speed ▪ Type of additional equipment ▪ Construction of the walls and pillars of the load box ▪ Type of protection against load box falling ▪ Type of document regarding approval to the public road traffic ▪ Way of stopping the trailer ▪ Type of additional equipment ▪ Number of items of standard equipment ▪ Overall weight ▪ Price

with is how to take customer requirements and turn them into characteristics that we can measure to see how well we are meeting the requirements. We need to define what is known as Critical to Quality Characteristics (CTQ's) based on the Voice of the Customer. Customers know what they want in general terms, but are often not capable of expressing those needs concretely and objectively. Critical to Quality (CTQ) focuses on the key metrics of customer satisfaction. A CTQ tree will translate the initial customer requirements to numerical or quantified requirements for testing laboratory.

These are the detailed critical requirements for the organization to satisfy. These can be regarded as critical results of the process. The development of a CTQ tree would go from the general requirement to the specific, or from "hard to measure" to "easy to measure". It helps identify Critical to Quality (CTQ) characteristics, features by which customers evaluate the product or service, and that can be used as measures for the project. CTQ stands for Critical to Quality. CTQs are translated from VOC. VOC is often vague, emotional or merely generalizations about products or services. CTQ's are the quantifiable, measurable and meaningful translation of VOC.

Model for Establishing CTQs for Testing Laboratory

Many studies and articles based on CTQs in the service sector were studied. It is but evident that CTQs are obtained from the VOC taken from various internal and external customers. In many of the articles, CTQs are directly identified without showing the VOC of a particular process. The sequences of the process or sub-process for which the CTQs are to be developed are not adequately explained with flowcharts, process map. Etc. These studies lack a model for establishing CTQs for testing laboratory.

A testing laboratory has its full application in the service sector. The processes in the laboratory are to be explained in a detailed manner. In order to get a clear understanding of input, output and process flow. The process map for each process in the laboratory will be analysed. Then the process map for each process is then critically reviewed for determining sub-processes related to direct and indirect customers.

For establishing CTQ, a questionnaire-based survey of direct and indirect customers related to the testing laboratory is carried out, and voice of the customer (VOC) is derived from laboratory employees (Indirect Customer) and daily customers (Direct Customer). This VOC is then converted into measuring indicators, i.e. CTQ. The step by step process for the establishment of CTQs can be demonstrated by the use of the following model.

The above model helps in identifying process-wise CTQs for testing laboratory. It gives in-depth information on the processes involved in the testing laboratory, Process map of those processes, determination of process-wise VOC using different methods and finally conversion of VOC to CTQs.

Process Map for a Testing Laboratory

To gain a clear understanding of processes and identification of internal and external customers in a testing laboratory, a process map ishas to be developed. Work in the laboratory can be described as a series of individual tasks or steps. The point of mapping these steps is to make them visual, making the connections and feedback loop visible, to improve the overall process. Laboratories often use it to gain an understanding of their existing functional processes and a clear sense of their needs. That enhances their ability to develop a deliberate course of action to improve the timeliness and quality of services.

It establishes a clear and comprehensive picture of how the testing laboratory currently works or plans to work. It visually displays starting and ending points for functional activities, standards, and quality of input sequences throughout the process. The process could belong to a department, equipment or an employee. It also documents relationships of each function to understand existing processes and purpose for the outcome.

There are many different processes involved in testing laboratories, such as Laboratory Personnel, Employee Training, Purchasing & Inventory, Documents and Record, Inter-Lab Comparison; Uncertainty Measurement; Management Review; Internal Audit, Equipment: Equipment Maintenance; Calibration, Customer Requirement, Sample Collection, Testing of Sample, Results & Report Preparation, Housekeeping, Quality Control, Corrective & Preventive Action.

Let us consider a process of sample collection from the processes mentioned above in a testing laboratory. In this process, the sample is collected and stored to the rack. The travel of sample from the collection re-centre/laboratory section till storage consists of many activities like labelling, checking for environmental and storage conditions etc. These activities are to be connected by arrows, rectangle and diagonal in such a way that the process starts with the input and ends by giving specific output. Detailed process map for the sample collection process is shown in the figure below.

Likewise, process maps for the above mentioned eighteen (18) processes have been made by carrying out the same procedure.

Determining the VOC for a Testing Laboratory

VOC is standing for the voice of the customer; it is a term used to discover what the laboratory customers (Internal or External) want the testing laboratory to provide. These are used to describe the customers' needs, and their perceptions regarding the tests carried out in a laboratory. The laboratory people identify and respond to the expectations, wants, and needs of customers, to improve customer satisfaction, loyalty and driving business change. The VOC is different with regards to the type of customer being associated, i.e. internal customer may have needs concerning equipment calibration, equipment maintenance etc. while the external customer may deal with processes like customer requirements, report preparation etc. Testing laboratories which are aligned to VOC continually improve their overall competitive value proposition, increase market share and improve profitability.

The voice of the customer can be obtained in many different ways, including surveys, focus groups, interviews, listening posts, and mystery shopping. For determining the VOC for a testing laboratory, a questionnaire-based survey is carried out.

Surveys are a designed set of questionnaire which is sent out to potential or existing customers. These are tried and have been used in many laboratories and the service sector, like a snail mail tool, and now, e-mail surveys or questionnaires which are the norms. This VOC tool can be successful as long as questions are kept short, offer yes or no answers, or a way to mark a block on a scale of like or dislike. This technique includes a list of questionnaires formed by highlighting critical areas associated with internal and external customers of the laboratory. The VOC determined for sample collection in the testing laboratory is as shown in the table below. Table 3 gives an idea of the process for which the VOC is derived and the data resource from where the customer requirements are taken.

Likewise, VOC for 18 different processes of testing laboratory is determined using the same procedure.

Table 3: Developing VOC for sample collection in testing laboratory

Process	VOC	Method Adopted	Data Resources
SAMPLE COLLECTION	Sufficient storage space is available for the labeled sample.	Questionnaire based Survey	Questionnaire for Lab Employees
	The lab is following Standardized procedure for collecting the sample.		Questionnaire for Lab Employees, Lab test Manual
	Lab instruments are neat and clean		Questionnaire for Lab Employees
	Staffs are technically competent at collection centers.		Questionnaire for Lab Employees
	Collected Sample is stored ensuring proper environmental conditions.		Questionnaire for Lab Employees
	Bar Coding and labelling are accurate and precise.		Questionnaire for Lab Employees
	Test Samples are retained for stipulated time for further reference		Questionnaire for Lab Employees
	Transportation of samples to the laboratory within a time frame		Questionnaire for Lab Employees
	Development of criteria for acceptance or rejection of sample		Questionnaire for Lab Employees

Converting VOC to CTQs

VOCs collected might be very naïve, vague, emotional or merely generalizations about products or services and raw. It needs careful business insight to be converted into requirements. A group of experts should thoroughly go through the VOCs and identify the requirements of the customers as parameters. These parameters are to be short, numerical or quantified requirements.

Not all the customer requirements are Critical or hold equal importance in the eyes of customers. There are some “Must Have” features and some “Pleased to have” features. The project team should be able to identify the different features and where they stand in the eyes of the customer. Tools such as KANO model will be beneficial for this. For example, in sample collection, according to the VOC; “the laboratory should follow a standardized procedure for collecting the sample”. Then accordingly, the CTQ is “SOP for sample collection”

Table 4. Conversion of VOC to CTQ in sample collection of a testing laboratory

Process	VOC	CTQ	Measuring Criteria for CTQ
SAMPLE COLLECTION	Sufficient storage space is available for the labelled sample.	Sufficient storage space	Measurement of sample Storage area
	The lab is following a standardized procedure for collecting the sample.	SOP for sample collection	Authorized guidelines for the test by the medical council
	Lab instruments are neat and clean	Sterilized instrument	The physical appearance of the instrument
	Staffs are technically competent at collection centers.	Skilled lab technician	Qualification and experience of the employee
	Collected sample is stored ensuring proper environmental conditions.	Proper storage & environmental conditions.	Physical appearance temperature check & humidity check
	Barcoding and labelling are accurate and precise.	Accuracy in barcode & labeling	Physical appearance/ Verifying record from the data register
	Test samples are retained for stipulated time for further reference	Retention of test samples	Physical checking of storage of Sample
	Transportation of samples to the laboratory within a time frame	Sample transportation time	Measuring the time for transport
	Development of criteria for acceptance or rejection of sample	Sample acceptance/ rejection criteria	Physical checking of SOP

Likewise, the VOC for the eighteen (18) processes of the testing laboratory is converted into CTQs. Table 5 below shows the process-wise CTQ, which are established using the same procedure as above.

Impact of CTQ On the Performance of a Testing Laboratory

Likewise the manufacturing sector, it is not easy to convert a customer requirement for a product into a measurable form in the service sector. A Customer requirement plays a vital role in the uplifting performance of the testing laboratory. Therefore, Critical to Quality (CTQ) plays a role in measuring customer demands regarding the service sector.

CTQ is that continuous improvement tool which involves understanding different facets of the organization, for instance, how it adds value to customers. Also, using the information obtained from the customers on what they consider to be of value and what they have indicated can be improved. It is essential to get the best return on investment for both customers as well as for the organization.

They are the product or service characteristics required to be met in order to satisfy a customer need. (Ayon, (2008)

CTQs are what customers expect of a product or service. They are the key measurable indicators of a product or service whose performance standards or specification limits must be met in order to satisfy the customer. (Omar, (2014) CTQs align improvement or design efforts with customer requirements.

It is a systematic approach for assessing needs of laboratory customers, called critical-to-quality (CTQ) in Six Sigma, with a purpose of continuous quality improvement. (Kyoung, 2008)

CTQ is defined in different ways in the literature. However, mostly, it is agreed that CTQ is a quality characteristic of a product or a service which is required to be improved on from a customer's point of view.

CONCLUSION

The primary aim of this study was to develop a model for establishing process-wise CTQ and to explore critical to quality (CTQs) in the testing laboratory which led to the Six Sigma initiative, the process of Six Sigma implementation through proper

Table 5. Process wise CTQ for a testing laboratory

Customer Requirement	Sample Collection	Testing of Sample	Employee Training	Inventory Control
▪ Lab Accreditation/ Recognition ▪ Expertise in Test ▪ Staff availability ▪ Availability of instrument and equipment ▪ Standard operating procedure (SOP) for each process and equipment ▪ Physical hygiene of staff ▪ Safety regulations ▪ Timely reports ▪ Accurate reports ▪ Adequate emergency Facility ▪ Adequate emergency staff ▪ emergency Cost ▪ Sufficient lab space	▪ Sufficient storage space ▪ SOP for sample collection ▪ Sterilized instrument ▪ Skilled lab technician ▪ Proper storage & environmental conditions ▪ Accuracy in barcode & labelling ▪ Retention of test samples ▪ Sample transportation time ▪ Sample acceptance/rejection criteria	▪ Proper handling of the sample ▪ Proper composition of reagents ▪ Calibration of instruments & equipment ▪ Maintenance of instruments & equipment ▪ Training of staff ▪ Record keeping of test procedure ▪ Service time ▪ Test processing time	▪ Employee list for training ▪ Well organized training plan ▪ Competent training institutes ▪ Properly organized schedule plan ▪ Evaluation of the effectiveness of Training	▪ Check stock for expiry, damage & obsolete ▪ Stock as per requirement ▪ Quantity & quality check of inventory ▪ Record keeping of inward & outward stock ▪ Proper storage and environmental conditions ▪ Check for deviation of stock
Equipment Maintenance	**Calibration**	**Housekeeping**	**Inter-Lab Comparison**	**Uncertainty Measurement**
▪ Preventive maintenance equipment list ▪ Annual maintenance equipment list ▪ Well organized schedule plan ▪ Maintenance by a competent agency ▪ Regularity ▪ Calibration check after maintenance ▪ Record keeping of maintenance	▪ Calibration by NABL lab ▪ Calibration as per schedule. ▪ Calibration certificate ▪ Calibration detail label ▪ Regularity in calibration ▪ Calibrated reference material ▪ Record keeping of Calibration	▪ Neat and clean lab area ▪ Well organized Housekeeping plan ▪ Sufficient lighting at workplace ▪ Record of housekeeping ▪ Display of lab details ▪ Availability of safety devices ▪ Housekeeping checks ▪ First aid facility ▪ Regularity ▪ Neatness and cleanliness ▪ Location of equipment and material	▪ Interlaboratory comparison plan ▪ Proficiency testing by NABL accredited reference labs ▪ The sample is checked for proper storage & environmental conditions ▪ Results approved from NABL	▪ Calibration of instruments & equipment ▪ The minimum value of UOM ▪ Proper environmental condition ▪ Trained employee ▪ Homogenous sample ▪ Number of tests having UOM value

continues on following page

Table 5. Continued

Equipment Purchase	Quality Control	Internal Audit	Corrective & Preventive Action (CAPA)	Management Review
■ Purchase as per specification ■ Trial run of purchased stock ■ Technical assistance regarding purchased stock ■ Training of staff on Purchased equipment	■ Certified reference material ■ Proficiency Testing ■ Replication of test ■ Retesting of retained items ■ Statistical techniques ■ Records of corrective action of QC tolerance limits ■ QC system design	■ Internal audit system design ■ Regular internal audit ■ Compliance of audit report ■ Fulfilment of nonconformity ■ Distribution of audit report to management ■ Tracking of the current status of deviations in the previous audit ■ Internal audit recordkeeping	■ Non conformity CAPA ■ CAPA for deviations ■ CAPA records ■ CAPA for QC & Inter lab comparison ■ Effectiveness check of CAPA	■ Yearly management review ■ Half-yearly management representative meeting ■ Management review of the compliance of internal audit report ■ Management review of trend analysis of results of QC ■ Management review of staff and training needs ■ Management review for setting objectives and quality policy ■ Management review of trend analysis of results of PT ■ Management review of trend analysis of customer feedback and complaints ■ Management review of estimates of new work, staff and equipment
Record-Keeping Control	**Documentation**	**Results & Report Preparation**		
■ Master List of records ■ Authorized access of records ■ Storage and retrieve of retained records ■ Backup of records ■ Retention period of records	■ Identification of documents ■ Documentation format ■ Master list of documents ■ Easy Retrieval of retained documents ■ Storage of documents	■ Retention of test reports ■ Authorized signatory on test results ■ Paper & printing quality of test reports ■ Readable & understandable test reports ■ Test results delivery ■ record-keeping for interpretation of test results ■ content of Test Report ■ storage and retrieval of test results		

identification of CTQs which display the improvements due to Six Sigma. The Model for establishing CTQs was developed.

Meeting customer expectations and maintaining a high level of quality throughout the laboratory processes are regulatory requirements. These are to be fulfilled in order to provide robust services that will perform at near perfection. The Voice of the Customer (VOC) is a vital tool used in six sigma to capture customer needs and requirements. Accurate translation of these needs and requirements into measurable form takes place using Critical to Quality (CTQs).

CTQs are the key measurable indicators of a product or process whose performance standards or specification limits must be met in order to satisfy the customer. (Ayon, 2012)

Six Sigma focuses on process improvement, and improving the service process is a significant determinant of customer satisfaction.

Our findings have many implications for researchers and practitioners. The findings include 126 CTQs in the testing laboratory that acted as a guide for practitioners in Six Sigma implementation for evaluation of the performance of testing laboratories. Quality of service is a critical determinant of the testing laboratory performance. Additionally, al, it can also be a critical factor in determining the long-term viability of a laboratory service provider. Therefore, assessing the laboratory user's needs are critical factors to the success of modern testing laboratories.

An investigation of relevant publications, references and citations were carried out using multiple databases. These studies provide evidence of the utility of CTQs in the service sector and their impact in enhancing performance in the service industry (the detailed process map of the involved processes and model for establishing CTQs are not evident in these studies). Therefore, these limitations are rectified by providing a detailed process map and model for the same.

The study aimed to provide a service quality framework and to identify the critical attributes affecting quality in testing laboratories. That would be useful for testing laboratories seeking to control and improve.

REFERENCES

Al Juboury, M. I. A., & Al Debag, Z. G. T. (2012). *The Effect Of Critical To Quality Factors In Identification Excellence Strategic Dimensions.* Paper presented at the International Conference on Business Intelligence and Knowledge Economy.

Aminudin, O., & Zainol, M. (2014). Implementation of Six Sigma in Service Industry. *Journal of Quality Measurement and Analysis*, *10*(2), 77–86.

Chakrabarty, A., & Tan, K. C. (2008). *Case study analysis of Six Sigma in Singapore service organizations*. Paper presented at the 2008 International Conference on Service Systems and Service Management.

Chakraborty, A., & Tan, K. C. (2012). Case study analysis of Six Sigma implementation inservice organisations. *Business Process Management Journal*, *18*(6), 992–1019. doi:10.1108/14637151211283384

Indrawati, S., Firmansyah, A., & Sunaryo. (n.d.). *Manufacturing Performance Improvement through Integrated Six Sigma: An Aircraft Industry Case Application*. Retrieved from http://iieng.org/images/proceedings_pdf/7171E0114558.pdf

Kenwothy, H. W. (2004). *Critical to quality-Aligning Improvement/Design efforts with customer requirements*. Retrieved 11 Sep., 2019, from https://www.slideshare.net/Vijay_Bijaj/critical-to-quality-aligning-improvement-design-efforts-with-customer-requirements

Knop, K. (2016). Using a QFD method and CTQ Tree to identify the areas needing Improvement in the Product-Farm Truck Trailer. Academic Press.

Stahl, R. (2003). Customers rarely feel the average performance of a system–instead, they tend to experience the variability. *Six Sigma Forum Magazine*, 17-26. Retrieved from http://asq.org/healthcaresixsigma/pdf/healthcares_horizon.pdf

Taner, M. T. K., Gamze, C. S., Erbas, E. K., & Kemal, M. (2013). Formation of Six Sigma Infrastructure for the Coronary Stenting Process. *International Review of Management and Marketing*, *3*(4), 232–242.

Yun, E. K., & Chun, K. M. (2008). Critical to quality in telemedicine service management: Application of DFSS (Design for Six Sigma) and SERVQUAL). *Nursing Economics*, *26*(6), 384–388. PMID:19330973

KEY TERMS AND DEFINITIONS

Critical to Quality (CTQ): The internal critical quality parameters that relate to the wants and needs of the customer.

Customer: A person who buys goods or services from a shop or business.

Process Map: A process map provides insight into a process, helps teams brainstorm ideas for process improvement, and increases communication and provide process documentation.

Service Sector: The service sector is the third of the three traditional economic sectors.

Six Sigma: A disciplined, statistical-based, data-driven approach and continuous improvement methodology for eliminating defects in a product, process, or service.

Standard: Something used as a measure, norm, or model in comparative evaluations.

Voice of Customer (VOC): A term that describes the customer's feedback about his experiences with and expectations for the products or services.

Chapter 10
Security Improvements for Safer Cross-Border E-Health Services in Europe

Dimitrios G. Katehakis
https://orcid.org/0000-0002-3763-191X
Foundation for Research and Technology – Hellas, Greece

George Pangalos
Aristotle University of Thessaloniki, Greece

Andriana Prentza
University of Piraeus, Greece

ABSTRACT

Preserving patient safety, patient rights, and safeguarding trust are crucial components for the provision of high-quality medical treatments across borders. This chapter focuses on required technological improvements to address quality challenges through the adoption of generic building blocks (BBs) towards enabling seamless care between European healthcare systems. The authors present important considerations that are relevant to incremental, cross-sectorial advancements for the enhancement of the technology used for the implementation of the directive on the application of patients' rights in cross-border healthcare. These include cross-domain technical BBs to support non-repudiation, capability lookup, dynamic service location, and electronic identification. The authors use cross-border electronic prescription and patient summary, as a case to discuss the use of related international interoperability standards, together with recommendations for future work relevant to the introduction of better quality, trustworthy, cross-border, electronic health services in Europe.

DOI: 10.4018/978-1-7998-2390-2.ch010

INTRODUCTION

The use of electronic prescription and patient summary services (eP/ PS) has been recognized as an important strategic policy to improve health care across Europe and to support access to safe and high-quality, cross-border healthcare (Tinholt et al., 2013). Electronic prescribing has already proved that can help patients by providing easier prescription and medication pick-up procedures, fewer difficulties over prescription insurance coverage and an increase in patient safety (e.g. by checking legible prescriptions for harmful interactions) (Hollingworth et al., 2007; Wang et al., 2009). Key benefits of electronic prescription (eP) have been identified as improving the quality of health care services, increasing the efficiency and effectiveness of prescribing and dispensing medications, reducing medication errors, and health care cost savings (Pangalos et al., 2013). Failure to implement properly eP systems can result in new types of errors that can reduce workflow efficiency, increase medication cost, and threaten patient safety (Zadeh & Tremblay, 2016).

The Directive on cross-border healthcare (European Parliament, 2011) regulates patients' rights to cross-border care and makes provision for the continuity of their care through a shared patient summary (PS) and the deployment of eP. It also creates the initial legal framework for cross-border care in the EU. It also establishes the need of a digital infrastructure for the cross-border exchange of health data. The deployment of electronic health (eHealth) solutions for eP/ PS is expected to increase safety and quality of care throughout the European Union and associated countries (EU) by ensuring continuity of care across borders and by providing immediate clinical information needed for unplanned care. What is envisioned is fewer concerns about possible adverse interactions with current treatment and health conditions (allergies, drug interaction, etc.) and the provision of safer healthcare, in cases of emergency or on occasional basis abroad. Other benefits foreseen include lower cost and improved efficiency, through the mutual exploitation of some technological assets with other domains, in order to enable sustainability of eHealth cross-border services through maintenance cost reduction.

Despite favorable attitudes towards both cross-border eP/ PS, multiple perceived barriers impede their incorporation and integration in clinical practice. Until very recently, infrastructures were not in place in all EU countries to support the system and stakeholders in some jurisdictions were reluctant to embrace eHealth due to the high cost and the lack of security of the systems (Kierkegaard, 2013). Patient identification and consent processes were laborious and somewhat time consuming, and member states have varying degrees of health care policy, privacy enforcement and laws concerning data protection (Milieu Ltd & time.lex, 2014). In most of the cases integration with national, health information technology (IT) systems was, and still in some cases is, missing. A lot of progress has been made during the past few years (Staffa et al., 2018; Nalin et al. 2019) and digital exchange of eP & PS is already supported and some health records of patients are already exchanged in the EU.

The chapter presents how epSOS (https://ec.europa.eu/digital-single-market/en/news/cross-border-health-project-epsos-what-has-it-achieved) use cases for eP and PS cross-border exchange have been enhanced with cross-domain BBs to support a safer environment for citizens traveling within the EU to safeguard the continuing applicability and legitimacy of clinical data processing. Work described was conducted within the context of the e-SENS (http://www.esens.eu/) Large Scale Pilot (LSP) project (2013-2017), and is built on top of assets developed in previous LSP projects to provide common solutions for seamless public service delivery across borders (Katehakis et al., 2015; Wisniewski et al., 2016; Mondorf, 2016; Katehakis et al., 2017b). The author focus on the introduction and enhancements of BBs to support non-repudiation, capability lookup, dynamic service location, and electronic identification (eID). Non-repudiation supports evidence emission when backend systems exchange documents, data and/ or messages through access points, registers any attempted access to a patient's protected health information and provides evidence for disputes resolution. Service location and capability lookup provide trusted, secure and efficient mutual configuration for national contact points for eHealth. EID provides the proper authentication strength for patients when seeking health care in a cooperating EU member state, safeguarding their fundamental access rights.

The objective of the presented work is to facilitate cross-border access to health services within the EU and to enhance the technology used with cross-domain technical BBs in order to improve efficiency, cost-effectiveness, safety, and confidentiality in a cross-border use case scenario of high priority for EU member states. The authors present specific work, conducted for the provision of operational cross-border eP and PS services in Europe and discuss on prospective issues. They also make recommendations for future work.

BACKGROUND

The efficient cross-border exchange of electronic health record (EHR) data among countries is a major priority in the EU. According to (European Court of Auditors, 2019) approximately two hundred thousands patients a year take advantage of the systems put in place under Directive 2011/24/EU to receive healthcare treatments abroad. Both the use cases for eP and PS aim towards allowing a patient who is abroad (e.g. visitor to the country of care, or one that lives in one country but works in another) to receive medical treatment, equivalent to the one that he would receive in his home country.

In the case of eP the patient visits a pharmacy in another EU country to obtain medication prescribed in his/ her home country. Initially the pharmacist must request the validation of the identity of the patient. The request is conveyed to the patient's country of affiliation. Once the identity of the patient is electronically validated and the patient consent is verified, the pharmacist selects the requested eP and dispenses the medicinal product, generating an electronic Dispensation document (eD). The eD is transmitted through the national contact point implementation for eHealth (NCPeH) to the country of affiliation, to allow the update of the corresponding eP. If a prescribed medicinal product is not available abroad, the attending pharmacist may, depending on the circumstances, dispense a different brand or package size of a comparable product to the patient.

In the case of PS, the use case begins when a health professional (HP) abroad receives a request for healthcare assistance from a patient from an affiliated country. The HP requests the validation of the identity of the patient. The request is conveyed to the patient's country of affiliation, which in return provides the patient's identity and consent confirmation to the HP. Once the identity of the patient is validated, the patient consent is verified and the HP at the country of care can request for the PS. If the PS exists, country of affiliation provides the PS to the HP. The PS of the patient seeking for healthcare treatment abroad is displayed to the HP.

If the identity of the patient cannot be properly validated in country of affiliation or the eP and/ or the PS of the patient does not exist or cannot be retrieved, then country of treatment, and subsequently the end user, is informed of the failure.

The provision of the current cross-border services and the future extensions are expected to take place within the framework of existing European legislation, such as those for eID and trust services (eIDAS) (Melin et al., 2016), the network and information systems directive (NIS Directive) (Michels & Walden, 2018), as well as the general data protection regulation (GDPR) (Lovell & Foy, 2018). Other relevant policy tools include the Connecting Europe Facility (CEF) (Pernice, 2016), and the eHealth Network (European Commission, 2015).

Regulation (EU) No 910/2014, commonly known as eIDAS (European Parliament, 2014), aims at providing a common, pan-European authentication scheme for notifiable eID, enabling national eID being properly consumed by service providers across the EU, regardless of where it was issued or is operated. EIDAS provides with legal grounds for the mutual recognition of eIDs across borders (Iglezakis, 2015). The idea is to create technical gateways that broker trust across Europe by issuing, authenticating, translating, certifying, and maintaining eID and their relevant attributes.

The eHealth Network, a European eHealth governance structure, has been established at the political level to bring together national authorities, responsible for eHealth, on a voluntary basis, to work on common orientations in this area and to promote an interoperable and sustainable eHealth implementation across Europe. At the strategic level, the European eHealth Governance Initiative eHGI (http://www.ehgi.eu/) has developed strategies, priorities, recommendations, and guidelines designed to deliver eHealth in Europe in a coordinated way (Stroetmann, 2011). At the operational level, projects like epSOS, EXPAND (https://ec.europa.eu/digital-single-market/en/news/expand-deploying-sustainable-cross-border-ehealth-services-eu), e-SENS, eStandards (http://www.estandards-project.eu/), and VALUeHEALTH (http://www.valuehealth.eu/) have worked in trying to resolve European level compatibility and sustainability of the underlying national infrastructures required to support the reliable and secure exchange of medical data, as well as the readiness to address continuously evolving interoperability, legal and security requirements in a cross-border setting.

PS guidelines on data that can be exchanged electronically across borders (eHealth Network, 2013) provided the first draft of the guidelines. Their purpose was not only to describe what data is to be included in the PS, but also to assess the implications of adopting such a PS in practice, especially in terms of organizational, technical and semantic requirements. The second release of the document (eHealth Network, 2016b) provided updated content and guidelines, while (DG SANTE, & CEF eHealth DSI, 2018d) describes the use cases to be found on the eHealth digital services infrastructure (DSI) PS services, identifying the needed requirements, the dataset of information to be exchanged and possible issues from the users' point of view. It is up to the willingness of each member state to adopt the guidelines and hence ensure that its national PS becomes suitable for both cross-border and national use.

The eP guidelines adopted in 2014 (eHealth Network, 2014) indicate areas where further work is required in order to ensure that clinical need and patient safety requirements are taken into account. The second release of the document (eHealth Network, 2016a) provided updated content and guidelines, while (DG SANTE, & CEF eHealth DSI, 2018c) describes the uses cases to be found on the eHealth DSI, identifying the needed requirements, information to be exchanged and possible issues from the users' point of view.

As of January 2016, the OpenNCP (Fonseca et al., 2015) governance model shifted under the direct responsibility of the European Commission, Directorate General for Health and Food Safety (DG SANTE). The goal set was to move the epSOS eHealth pilot OpenNCP into the global European CEF framework project (https://ec.europa.eu/inea/en/connecting-europe-facility) under the umbrella of a CEF digital service infrastructure, the eHealth DSI (https://ec.europa.eu/cefdigital/wiki/display/EHOPERATIONS/eHDSI+Mission). Priorities set regarding cross-border eP/ PS relate to the improvement of existing cross-sectorial BB solutions to become operational ready so that member states can adopt them. In this context, all related integration is conducted within the OpenNCP framework, which is the selected NCPeH reference implementation (eHealth Network, 2015), to support cross-border eP/ PS.

Figure 1 presents a schematic diagram of the eHealth DSI services system. Central services are linked to configuration and consist of a single EU wide instance. Terminology services are out of the scope in this chapter. There is one run-time instance of NCPeH per country.

Currently, the EU, in order to secure the citizen's access to and sharing of health data, is moving towards the development of specifications for a European EHR exchange format, based on open standards, taking into consideration the potential use of data for research and other purposes. The recommendation on a European EHR exchange format (European Commission, 2019) sets out a framework to achieve secure, interoperable, cross-border access to, and exchange of, eHealth data in the EU. The framework includes:

Figure 1. Schematic diagram of the eHealth DSI services system (simplified view)

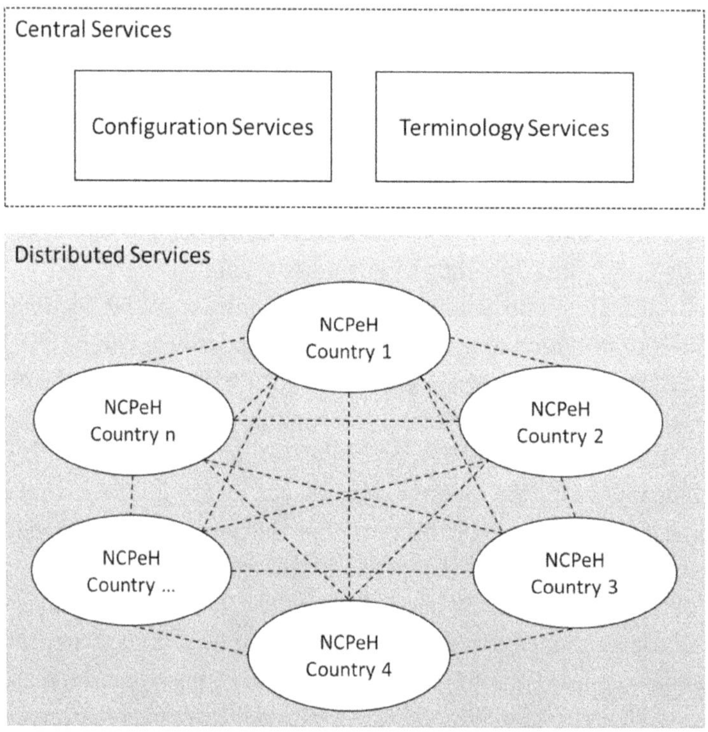

- a set of principles that should govern access to and exchange of electronic health records (EHRs) across borders in the EU;
- a set of common technical specifications for the cross-border exchange of data in certain health information domains;
- a process to take forward the further elaboration of a European EHR exchange format.

The aim is to deliver the right data, at the right time, for citizens and healthcare providers, and allow for the secure access, sharing and exchange of EHRs. The baseline moves beyond patient summaries (PSs) and eP/ eD to include laboratory reports, medical images and reports, and hospital discharge reports, in alignment with established priorities at a European level.

Security Improvements

Priorities set by member states are dictated by common needs for proper identification of the subject of care, end user authentication, as well as guaranteeing confidentiality, integrity, availability of the communicated information in a cross-border environment. The enhancements considered for non-repudiation, capability lookup, dynamic service location, and eID are built on top OpenNCP, by means of developed BBs on already available technologies, upon an architectural framework based on TOGAF (Haren, 2011). The first enhancement is the integration of the evidence emitter BB to effectively support non-repudiation by electronic means. The second enhancement is related to the realignment of the openNCP central services (for configuration management) with more generic standards for capability lookup and dynamic service location. Finally, the third enhancement is strongest patient identification and a better capture of the patient consent by means of a multi-stage approach to support different levels of member state readiness.

All three enhancements included BB integration in the OpenNCP reference implementation framework for an NCPeH. The facilitation of the secure exchange of eP/ PS, with the incorporation of each non-domain specific BB supporting technology for non-repudiation, capability lookup, serviced location, and eID are presented in the following subsections including the rationale behind each BB's adoption, development made for their incorporation in OpenNCP, issues resolved, status, and outlook.

Non-Repudiation

The need of having non-repudiation services emerged since the beginning of the epSOS project, but then left unimplemented due to piloting relaxations. As described in (Katehakis et al., 2017a), the epSOS solution aimed at having audit trail and node authentication (ATNA) (IHE, 2018) achieved, by means of mutual transport layer security (TLS).

Non-repudiation services are necessary in order to generate, collect, maintain, make available and validate evidences concerning a claimed event or action to resolve disputes about the occurrence or non-occurrence of an event or action. Managing non-repudiation aspects in a real-life setting, where backend systems do not exchange documents, data and/ or messages directly but through gateways deployed in each member state (i.e. the NCPeH), under the responsibility of a service provider (public or private sector), is not a trivial task. The International Standards Organization and International Electrotechnical Commission (ISO/ IEC) 13888-3 standard (ISO/ IEC, 2009) defines four types of non-repudiation tokens, namely non-repudiation of origin, of receipt, of delivery, and of submission. EpSOS transactions were defined for communications between national contact points only, in a synchronous fashion, thus requiring mandatory non-repudiation of receipt tokens (namely, the audit trails) and optional non-repudiation of origin (digital signatures).

The e-SENS solution for non-repudiation (evidence emitter) provides a flexible and horizontal model to generate and emit electronic evidence used for non-repudiation purposes, based on respective regulations and technological needs. The non-repudiation architecture for the BB enables different domains to implement their own non-repudiation protocol with the properties needed to achieve their business needs.

The e-SENS Evidence Emitter BB (http://wiki.ds.unipi.gr/display/ESENS/ABB+-+Non-Repudiation), originating from the eJustice domain (project eCODEX, http://www.e-codex.eu/), enables all four corners of the technical architecture model (see Figure 2) to generate and emit electronic evidence and has already been implemented and incorporated in the NCPeH reference implementation software to ensure electronic evidence of the transmission and reception of information.

The delivered solution aimed at enhancing the epSOS approach with a more formal account of evidence, thus enabling the NCPeH to have European Telecommunications Standards Institute (ETSI) Registered Electronic Mail (REM) (Ruggieri, 2010) evidences. The OpenNCP community released a stable release (2.2.0), following the full integration of the e-SENS evidence emitter BB (https://ec.europa.eu/cefdigital/wiki/pages/viewpage.action?pageId=35201410) and the solution was first presented and tested during the 15th European IHE Connectathon event (Luxembourg, April 2015, http://www.ihe-europe.net/connectathon/connectathon-2015), and later in the Expandathon event (Lisbon, December 2015, https://gazelle.ihe.net/content/expandathon-lisbon-december-2015). Additional releases with further improvements have followed since then.

Figure 2. Four-corner architecture model

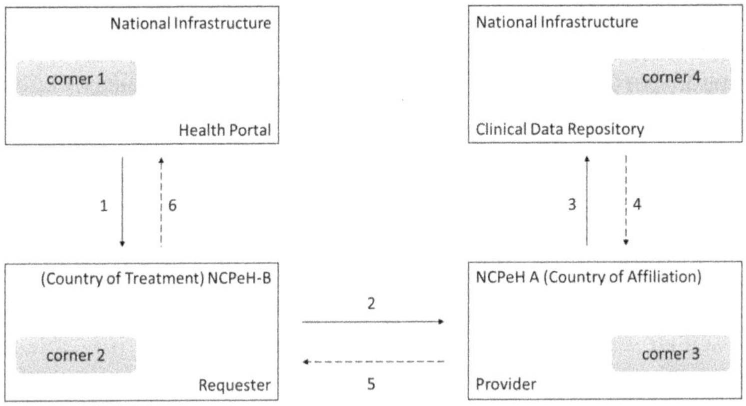

As of June 2019, only the Evidence Recording Service (Evidence Emitter) was agreed (DG SANTE & CEF eHealth, 2018a) and implemented by the current eHealth DSI solution. Future extensions are expected to include a dispute resolution algorithm and evidence exchange among the NCPeH. The orchestration of these services enables full compliance with the ISO 13888 and ETSI REM.

Capability Lookup and Dynamic Service Location

In order to send a message, a sender needs to discover where the information about the receiver is stored. EpSOS used central services for discovering the needed information about a receiver and OpenNCP relied on a set of static configuration entries mapping the remote capabilities. A capability lookup can provide metadata about the communication partner's interoperability capabilities on all levels defined in the European Interoperability Framework (EIF) for legal, organizational, semantic and technical interoperability levels (European Commission, 2017). A service location can be used to retrieve metadata about the receiver. The metadata can be used to dynamically set interoperability parameters and ambitions between the sender and receiver. The epSOS Central Services rationale (architecture and services) evolved by adopting the e-SENS Capability Lookup BB (http://wiki.ds.unipi.gr/display/ESENS/ABB+-+Capability+Lookup+-+1.6.0) and e-SENS Service Location BB (http://wiki.ds.unipi.gr/display/ESENS/ABB+-+Service+Location+-+1.1.0). This step had significant impact at the NCPeH level where refactoring was required to be made in order to allow the improved articulation model between NCPeH.

The service location BB enables the dynamic discovery of the location of other NCPeH-declared interoperability capabilities. The capability lookup BB enables the publishing and fetching of the latter. Together they automate the peer's dynamic discovery and fetch of NCPeH self-declared capabilities (metadata). End point detection uses a distributed mechanism to store and locate public configuration information using the OASIS (https://www.oasis-open.org/) standards service metadata publisher (SMP) and business document metadata service location (BDXL) (OASIS, 2017a) and service metadata publishing (BDX-SMP) (OASIS, 2017b). The service metadata locator (SML) guides the sender towards the location where the information about the receiver is stored, which is called SMP. SMP allows for the publishing of definitions of the provider services as well for the discovery of the definition of those services. SMP exposes the services metadata interface which enables senders to discover service metadata about specific target participants. Once the sender discovers the address of the receiver's SMP it is able to retrieve the needed information (i.e. metadata) about the receiver. With such information the message can be sent. The SML is used to add/ update/ delete information about the participants' SMP location on a Domain Name System (DNS). To retrieve a remote configuration, the NCPeH performs DNS-based queries to SML to obtain a reference to the SMP server (see Figure 3). With SMP, the XML metadata following the data model defined by BDX-SMP is exposed in a RESTful way under the DNS-served URLs.

The initial incorporation of the BBs under consideration, originating from the eProcurement domain (project PEPPOL, http://www.peppol.eu/), was first presented and tested during the Expandathon event in Lisbon, Dec 9-11 2015 (the NCPeH providing its public configuration in an SMP record and pushing it to an SMP server). The new approach leaves the original ad-hoc model, which is based on trust-service status lists behind in favor of a more standardized and robust architecture.

The eHealth DSI Configuration Services is currently composed by the Service Metadata Publisher and Service Metadata Locator (SMP/SML) implemented under CEF eDelivery (https://ec.europa.eu/cefdigital/wiki/display/CEFDIGITAL/eDelivery). This technology adds dynamic capability look-up through the BDXL specification.

Figure 3. Discovery of a peer's metadata (left) and fetch and usage of the metadata (right) (Katehakis et al., 2017a)

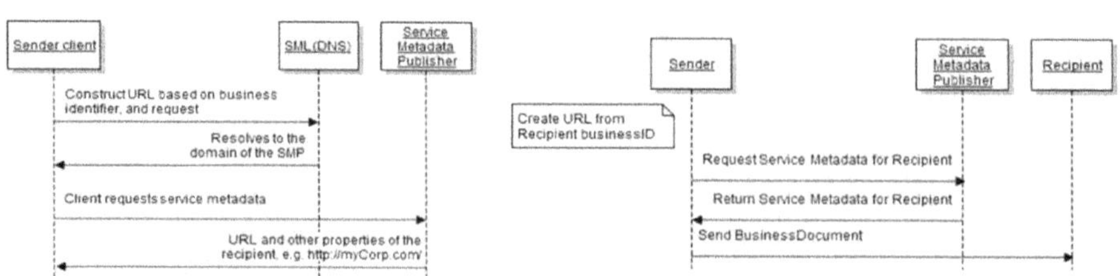

Electronic Identification

The mechanisms of identification of patients, health professionals and healthcare providers have to follow the eIDAS Regulation (European Parliament, 2014), which provides with legal grounds for the mutual recognition of eIDs across borders. The patient must be uniquely and securely identified at national level (by the national infrastructure in the country of affiliation), while the HP in the country of treatment must verify, by the available means, the identity of the patient. Secure eID is an important enabler for cases where patients and health providers need to rely on trustworthy data, in full respect of existing data protection legislation. Little information is more sensitive than that concerning one's health. Member states in the EU have different models around eID and are at various stages of implementation, therefore any solution has to respect, and be in a position to interconnect national infrastructures that will perform mutual recognition of electronic identities. In addition, any solution must be in a position to accommodate countries with either health specific or cross-sectoral means for identification.

Strong eID within the eHealth domain is motivated by two primary goals: patient safety as well as protection against illegitimate disclosure of medical data. Almost every national health system features one or more types of eID and the relevant national regulation and norms effectively govern its appropriate regional application. This, however, yields a pan-European eID landscape of various fairly isolated and incompatible eID solutions.

The means for establishing patient identification within epSOS was based on several technological and organizational prerequisites originally designed to accommodate national specialties, unavailability of suitable technology, and the absence of procedures for patient identification and authentication in a cross-border scenario. E-SENS considered several business stages for patient identification. They are depicted in Table 1.

Depending on the adopted scenario, patients can either be identified by brokered authentication via the HP during a care encounter (traditional epSOS) or strong self-authentication of the patient with digital signature when patient is requesting access to own health data. Legitimacy of the HP request is asserted by on site specific patient consent and using the certificate material of the patient's eID as evidence of the care relationship.

The initial incorporation of the e-SENS BBs to support stages I-III (smartcard integration), was first presented and tested during the Expandathon event in Lisbon, Dec 9-11 2015 (https://gazelle.ihe.net/content/expandathon-lisbon-december-2015). Patients can now sign electronically their consent to provide data access through this mechanism.

Table 1. Business stages considered for consolidating eID in eHealth use cases

Stage	Name	Description
0	Basic stage	Requires the manual entry of the patient's identity into the system. This is the approach used in epSOS to accommodate emergency cases where no other method of identification and authentication is available.
I	Local Attribute Retrieval and Mapping Service	Requires the existence of an eID token, like e.g. a smartcard, which can be read passively. Provides a safer environment for the extraction of publicly available identity attributes from the carrier to provide unauthenticated token for form filling and process, bypassing manual entry.
II	Local Authentication Modules (LAM)	Requires, on top of the previous one, patient authentication by means of a personal identification number. Provides an even safer environment through authentication to carrier, for protected attribute release and supports the signing of a patient's consent.
III	Local Authentication Modules and DSS (LAM+)	Requires, on top of the previous ones, network connectivity to a PKI for real time validation of the authentication of identification and patient's consent.
IV	Virtual pan-European authentication schemes	Distributed, cross-border authentication is introduced, leveraged by means of the eIDAS/ STORK 2.0 infrastructure. All authentication and authorization activities are fulfilled outside the local environment. This stage allows cross-border authentication, in a secure, reliable and trusted way, by making existing national eID systems interoperable.
V	Virtual or mobile eID	Leverages on top of the previous by giving the possibility of authentication and authorization without the need of a physical eID token, by means of a mobile app with a virtual token, specifically developed for this.

It is important to note that a smartcard is a form of eID card that can be used onsite for both online as well as offline personal identification and authentication. The goal is to allow business, citizens and government employees to use the presently widespread (national) identities in cross-border public and private services (Leitold et al., 2014). Foreseen benefits include automated entry of identity traits, removing the need for different middleware, drivers, and software installation for smart card reading, and the transformation and mapping of smart card data onto a singular virtual ISO 24727-3 compliant middleware (Hühnlein et al., 2007) for standard interfaces that can be installed on demand, runs in the doctor's web browser, and is discarded after concluding the workflow.

No further developments for this technology were anticipated to yield critical improvements towards usability or security in particular in reference to mobile applications. Consequently, the e-SENS project evaluated other upcoming candidate technologies in order to virtualize the eID token itself for a more streamlined, user-friendly, and universally deployable solution. The CEF eID BB, or eIDAS eID (https://ec.europa.eu/cefdigital/wiki/display/CEFDIGITAL/eID), was quickly identified as the most promising solution component, not only because of the standardized way of transporting authentications between the relevant parties but in particular due to the stable legal framework encompassing the eIDAS eID service. The latter enabled the eHealth domain to shed the entirely redundant maintenance of a separate eID ecosystem with the heavyweight overhead of governing the legal stability of highly-regulated exchanges between mutually dependent parties and eID solutions as well as their pending national constraints in favor of the eIDAS regulation.

As described in (Katehakis et al., 2017a) the two major obstacles identified during the e-SENS project were the premature termination of an eIDAS eID workflow and the lack of injecting an additional attribute into the eIDAS minimum data set benefitting of all routine protection means of eIDAS eID. For eIDAS eID, the authentication workflow terminates after a patient has been successfully authenticated in the country of treatment, while the eHealth domain relies on this authentication being send back to the patients' country of affiliation to serve as an authenticated supporting token for the national access control systems in the determination of whether the disclosure request for protected health information is indeed legitimate and authorized. The other issue relates to the mandatory expressiveness of the eIDAS data structure to perform an identification.

While patient mapping services naturally exist, an authenticated patient identifier needs to be available at a very early point in the workflow – the initial patient registration in the foreign country – and at the very late point of authorizing a medical data disclosure in the patients' country of affiliation. Consequently, the inclusion of the patient identifier in the eIDAS eID SAML assertion has been documented as being of utmost importance for the eHealth domain.

Finally, the e-SENS project developed an eIDAS Connector that bridged the requirements of the eHealth domain with the capabilities of eIDAS eID and integrated a technology demonstrator into the NCPeH to enable production-level piloting between Austria, Italy, and Greece (Stasis et al., 2018).

SOLUTIONS AND RECOMMENDATIONS

Work presented in the previous section addressed issues relevant to non-repudiation, capability lookup, dynamic service location, and eID, to enable and support efficiently the delivery of cross-border healthcare. E-SENS enhanced epSOS and ensured the successful integration of LSP BBs in the European Interoperability Reference Architecture (EIRA, https://ec.europa.eu/digital-single-market/en/news/new-version-european-interoperability-reference-architecture-available) for cross-border service interoperability, ensuring their maturation, as well as adding value to them.

As far as non-repudiation is concerned the evidence emitter has already been agreed and implemented by the current eHealth DSI solution (evidence recording service) in order to effectively support non-repudiation by electronic means. Evidence makes principals accountable for their actions, creates irrefutable evidence about events/ actions, and is set to settle disputes about the occurrence or non-occurrence of an event. Work done does not provide a complete non-repudiation mechanism, and therefore further work needs to be conducted in respect to, indicatively, dispute resolution and evidence exchange among the NCPeH.

As far as capability lookup and dynamic service location are concerned, work conducted solves the issue of having a single point of failure by providing the means to support end point detection. Each NCPeH provide its public configuration in an SMP record and pushes it to an SMP server. To retrieve a remote configuration, the NCPeH performs DNS-based queries to the location lookup service to obtain a reference to the SMP server. Distributed mechanism to store and locate public configuration information using the OASIS standards SMP and BDXL. The eDelivery SMP (DIGIT Connecting Europe Facility, 2018a) profile is an open specification for publishing service metadata within a four corner network, such as the one of Figure 2. The eDelivery SMP profile describes the request/ response exchanges between an SMP and a client wishing to discover access point metadata. In addition, SML is the other key component that enables dynamic discovery of participants in message exchange infrastructures (DG SANTE & CEF eHealth DSI, 2018e; DIGIT Connecting Europe Facility, 2018a). The SML is used to create or update the resource records in the DNS so that the access points can discover the SMP of the receiving participant. As a result, these infrastructures can scale up without being affected by the management of an increasing number of participants. Instead of having to centrally manage a list of access points (static discovery), the discovery of participants becomes dynamic and possibly fully distributed and consequently much more scalable. No major issues have been found regarding the adoption of these standards in eHealth.

As far as eID is concerned, e-SENS considered several business cases for patient identification. Since patient identifiers need to be available at a very early point in the workflow, a patient, and the assigned medical records, are usually exclusively identified by the patient identifier instead of general demographics. Piloting confirmed the general fitness for use of eIDAS eID for the eHealth domain for real-world cross-border eHealth services. The patient consent is the fundamental instrument legitimating any medical data disclosure and includes specific provisions for technology that is used to regulate the disclosure. EIDAS mandates the citizen to explicitly select all attributes that are authorized to be disclosed. This strained the piloting efforts since every eIDAS-activated eHealth identification required two independent consents to be issued in close proximity. Succeeding in merging both legal instruments into one would streamline the eID process, critically increase usability without eroding any patient right to confidentiality and disclosure control, while benefitting from the general legal stability and security of the eIDAS framework. Some room for mutual improvement, especially regarding the usability of the solution, has been identified (Katehakis, 2017a).

By mutualizing cross-sectorial assets, e-SENS not only has paved the way to a robust and sustainable way for the secure data exchange between EU national eHealth systems, but has also created a reference for BB integration for other sectors. Outcomes of this work have already become part of the CEF eHealth DSI.

FUTURE RESEARCH DIRECTIONS

The work presented addressed reliability and quality challenges and introduced security improvements for better and safer cross-border eHealth services. Prospects for operational services is high, and outcomes of the work presented succeeded in making the IT infrastructure inherited by epSOS more sustainable and more stable. Outcomes of this work (a set of mature eHealth assets) have already become part of the CEF eHealth DSI interoperability specifications.

Developing safe and high quality cross border services in the EU requires coordinated work by several member states at multiple levels (technical, semantic, organizational, legal and political). Non-repudiation, SMP/ SML and basic eID scenarios have already been integrated within the latest versions of OpenNCP and operation in waves has started.

Large-scale deployment of eP/ PS is expected to actively refine and improve already available software infrastructures in order to support effectively patients' rights in cross-border healthcare. In the case of PS, both patient and health professional may have access to the person's PS and other relevant EHR documents as smoothly as at home. In the case of eP dispensation of ePs across the EU may be allowed and support the documentation of dispensed drugs. Using dispensation data from the dispensing pharmacy in the country of temporary stay, the health services in the home country can update the medication record of the patient, making health care and prescriptions safer.

Ongoing work seeks to create a common set of standards across the EU that are expected to embrace the national diversity and facilitate interoperability, thus respecting subsidiarity. The eHealth domain is expected to benefit by adopting solution BBs that have already proved their value in other domains. These BBs will comprise the foundation for a networked infrastructure for cross-border services in the EU, while their sustainability will be secured through handover to the CEF. Sustainability and long-term governance of the LSP BBs and their usage and interoperability within all the EU is an objective tightly coupled with the success and follow-up of the described work. The results of this work will be handed over directly to the eHealth DSI and their implementation by member states will be funded by current and future Generic Services Calls. On the other hand, member states need to be open and flexible in the design of joint solutions, and to be able to ensure the implementation of the decided solutions nationally.

The cross-border healthcare Directive has a large potential to improve and facilitate patients' access to cross-border healthcare and most importantly ensure the best quality of care for all patients. Nevertheless, for the Directive to succeed it is crucial that patients, health care professionals and other stakeholders are well informed about the Directive in all its aspects.

Seven Member States (Finland, Estonia, Czechia, Luxembourg, Portugal, Croatia and Malta) are progressively launching these exchanges by the end of 2019, and more than two thousand Finnish patients have already been able to get their medicines in Estonia during the first half of 2019. Finnish citizens can now retrieve in Croatian pharmacies the medicines prescribed electronically by their doctor in Finland. Soon doctors in Luxembourg will be able to receive digital PSs of travellers coming from Czechia.

Twenty two EU member states are part of the eHealth DSI and are expected to exchange ePs and PSs by 2022. From 21 June, the first health records of patients were able to be exchanged in the EU thanks to the cross-border electronic health services.

Foreseen challenges include supporting dynamic discovery without human intervention, incorporating BBs into end-user applications, and expanding to other cross-border services requiring more complex solutions like e.g. patient access service, medication reimbursement, etc.

CONCLUSION

When one's health is under concern, especially in a life threatening situation, the risk of having a brisk in security poses legal implications. In that sense, risk reduction and improved quality is a goal well set, in parallel with reduced costs. Other considerations are related to cooperation, European level compatibility and sustainability of the underlying national infrastructures required to support the reliable and secure exchange of medical data, as well as the readiness to address the continuously evolving interoperability, legal and safety requirements in a cross-border setting.

What is needed work towards sustainable economic and social benefits of European eHealth systems and services and interoperable applications, to achieve a high level of trust and security, to improve the continuity of care and to ensure access to safer, high quality healthcare.

The incorporation of well-standardized and mature BBs, like the ones presented for non-repudiation, capability lookup, dynamic service location, and eID within the NCPeH reference implementation, is considered extremely important for the introduction of safer, better quality, cross-border eHealth services in Europe. When such interventions are aligned with the EU and national policies, BBs can deliver reliable access to trustworthy information to further support the implementation of the Directive on the application of patients' rights in cross-border healthcare in the most efficient manner.

ACKNOWLEDGMENT

The European Commission, and more specifically the Information and Communication Technologies Policy Support Programme (ICT-PSP) of the Competitiveness and Innovation Framework Programme (CIP), partially supported work reported, under the e-SENS project (contract number 325211). This research was supported by Foundation for Research and Technology – Hellas, Aristotle University of Thessaloniki, and University of Piraeus. Any opinions, results, conclusions, and recommendations expressed in this material are those of the authors and do not necessarily reflect the views of e-SENS or the European Commission.

REFERENCES

Asokan, N. (1998). *Fairness in electronic commerce.* Retrieved from https://www.researchgate.net/publication/2281851_Fairness_in_Electronic_Commerce

Connecting Europe Facility, D. I. G. I. T. (2018a). *eDelivery SMP Profile. Test Assertions Description. Version 1.06. Date 01/06/2018.* Retrieved from https://ec.europa.eu/cefdigital/wiki/display/CEFDIGITAL/SMP+specifications?preview=/82773307/82796300/(CEFeDelivery).(eDelivery_SMP).(TAD).(v1.06).pdf

Connecting Europe Facility, D. I. G. I. T. (2018b). *SML Service Offering Description. Version 1.08. Date 25/09/2018.* Retrieved from https://ec.europa.eu/cefdigital/wiki/display/CEFDIGITAL/SML+service?preview=/82773318/82798522/(eDelivery)(SML)(SOD)(1.08).pdf

DG SANTE & CEF eHealth DSI. (2018a). *Audit Trail Profiles, Document Version 2.2.0, Date 08/06/2018, Wave 2 – Operation Ready*. Retrieved from https://ec.europa.eu/cefdigital/wiki/download/attachments/37752869/eHDSI_Audit_Trail_Profiles_v2.2.0.pdf?version=2&modificationDate=1535471342356&api=v2

DG SANTE & CEF eHealth DSI. (2018c). *ePrescription Functional requirements, Document Version 2.2.3, Date 01/08/2018, Wave 2 – Operation Ready*. Retrieved from https://ec.europa.eu/cefdigital/wiki/download/attachments/35210463/eP%20functional%20requirements_v2.2.3.pdf?version=1&modificationDate=1533135470667&api=v2

DG SANTE & CEF eHealth DSI. (2018d). *PS Functional requirements, Document Version 2.2.2, Date 01/08/2018, Wave 2 – Operation Ready*. Retrieved from https://ec.europa.eu/cefdigital/wiki/download/attachments/35210463/PS%20functional%20requirements_v2.2.2.pdf?version=1&modificationDate=1533135456275&api=v2

DG SANTE & CEF eHealth DSI. (2018e). *Service Location and Capability Lookup Profile, Document Version 2.1.0, Date 01/06/2017, Wave 1 Operation Ready*. Retrieved from https://ec.europa.eu/cefdigital/wiki/display/EHOPERATIONS/Specifications?preview=/35210463/47187054/Service%20Location%20and%20Capability%20Lookup%20Profile_v2.1.0.pdf

eHealth Network. (2013). *Guidelines on minimum/ non-exhaustive patient summary dataset for electronic exchange in accordance with the cross-border Directive 2011/ 24/ EU. Release 1.0*. Retrieved from https://ec.europa.eu/health//sites/health/files/ehealth/docs/guidelines_patient_summary_en.pdf

eHealth Network. (2014). *Guidelines on ePrescriptions dataset for electronic exchange under Cross-Border Directive 2011/24/EU. European Commission*. Release 1. Retrieved from http://ec.europa.eu/health/ehealth/docs/eprescription_guidelines_en.pdf

eHealth Network. (2015). *Guideline on an Organisational Framework for eHealth National Contact Point*. Brussels, Retrieved from http://ec.europa.eu/health/ehealth/docs/ev_20151123_co01_en.pdf

eHealth Network. (2016a). *Guideline on the electronic exchange of health data under Cross-Border Directive 2011/ 24/ EU. Release 2. EPrescriptions and eDispensations*. Retrieved from https://ec.europa.eu/health/sites/health/files/ehealth/docs/ev_20161121_co091_en.pdf

eHealth Network. (2016b). *Guideline on the electronic exchange of health data under Cross-Border Directive 2011/ 24/ EU. Release 2. Patient Summary for unscheduled care.* Retrieved from https://ec.europa.eu/health/sites/health/files/ehealth/docs/ev_20161121_co10_en.pdf

European Commission. (2017). *New European Interoperability Framework. Promoting seamless services and data flows for European public administrations.* Retrieved from https://ec.europa.eu/isa2/sites/isa/files/eif_brochure_final.pdf

European Commission. (2018). *Communication from the Commission to the European Parliament, the Council, the European Economic and Social Committee and the Committee of the Regions on enabling the digital transformation of health and care in the Digital Single Market; empowering citizens and building a healthier society,* COM(2018) 233 final {SWD(2018) 126 final}. Retrieved from https://ec.europa.eu/digital-single-market/en/news/communication-enabling-digital-transformation-health-and-care-digital-single-market-empowering

European Commission. (2019). *Commission Recommendation of 6.2.2019 on a European Electronic Health Record exchange format (Text with EEA relevance),* C(2019) 800 final. Retrieved from https://ec.europa.eu/digital-single-market/en/news/recommendation-european-electronic-health-record-exchange-format

European Court of Auditors. (2019). *EU actions for cross-border healthcare: significant ambitions but improved management required (pursuant to Article 287(4), second subparagraph, TFEU).* Special Report No 7. Retrieved from https://www.eca.europa.eu/Lists/ECADocuments/SR19_07/SR_HEALTH_CARE_EN.pdf

European Parliament. (2011). *Directive 2011/24/EU of the European Parliament and of the Council of 9 March 2011 on the application of patients' rights in cross-border healthcare.* Retrieved from https://eur-lex.europa.eu/legal-content/EN/TXT/?uri=CELEX%3A32011L0024

European Parliament. (2014). *Regulation (EU) No 910/2014 of the European Parliament and of the Council of 23 July 2014 on electronic identification and trust services for electronic transactions in the internal market and repealing Directive 1999/93/EC.* Retrieved from https://eur-lex.europa.eu/legal-content/EN/TXT/?uri=uriserv%3AOJ.L_.2014.257.01.0073.01.ENG

Fonseca, M., Karkaletsis, K., Cruz, I. A., Berler, A., & Oliveira, I. C. (2015, May). *OpenNCP: a novel framework to foster cross-border e-Health services.* MIE.

Haren, V. (2011). *TOGAF Version 9.1 A Pocket Guide.* Van Haren Publishing.

Hollingworth, W., Devine, E. B., Hansen, R. N., Lawless, N. M., Comstock, B. A., Wilson-Norton, J. L., ... Sullivan, S. D. (2007). The impact of e-prescribing on prescriber and staff time in ambulatory care clinics: A time–motion study. *Journal of the American Medical Informatics Association*, *14*(6), 722–730. doi:10.1197/jamia.M2377 PMID:17712088

Hühnlein, D., & Bach, M. (2007). How to use iso/iec 24727-3 with arbitrary smart cards. In *International Conference on Trust, Privacy and Security in Digital Business* (pp. 280-289). Springer. 10.1007/978-3-540-74409-2_30

Iglezakis, I. (2015). *Legal Issues of Identity Management in eGovernment*. Available at SSRN 2690374.

IHE. (2018). *Audit Trail and Node Authentication*. Retrieved from https://wiki.ihe.net/index.php/Audit_Trail_and_Node_Authentication

ISO/IEC .(2009). *Information Technology – Security techniques – Non-repudiation – Part 3: Non-Repudiation mechanisms using asymmetric techniques*. ISO/IEC13888-3:2009.

Katehakis, D. G., Gonçalves, J., Masi, M., & Bittins, S. (2017a). Interoperability Infrastructure Services to enable Secure, Cross-Border, Operational eHealth Services in Europe. *Proceedings of the 17th International HL7 Interoperability Conference IHIC 2017 "Re-shaping healthcare systems"*, 40-51. Retrieved from http://www.ics.forth.gr/~katehaki/publications/ihic2017-2.pdf

Katehakis, D. G., Pangalos, G., & Prentza, A. (2015). Creating a European eHealth Space for cross-border ePrescription and Patient Summary Services. *Proceedings of the 12th European, Mediterranean & Middle Eastern Conference on Information Systems (EMCIS 2015)*.

Katehakis, D. G., Pangalos, G., & Prentza, A. (2017b). Security Improvements for Better and Safer Cross-Border ePrescription and Patient Summary Services. *International Journal of Reliable and Quality E-Healthcare*, *6*(1), 18–28. doi:10.4018/IJRQEH.2017010102

Kierkegaard, P. (2013). E-prescription across Europe. *Health and Technology*, *3*(3), 205–219. doi:10.100712553-012-0037-0

Leitold, H., Lioy, A., & Ribeiro, C. (2014). Stork 2.0: Breaking new grounds on eid and mandates. In *Proceedings of ID World International Congress* (pp. 1-8). Academic Press.

Lovell, M., & Foy, M. A. (2018). General Data Protection Regulation May 2018 (GDPR) How does it affect us? *Bone & Joint 360, 7*(4), 41-42.

Melin, U., Axelsson, K., & Söderström, F. (2016). Managing the development of e-ID in a public e-service context: Challenges and path dependencies from a life-cycle perspective. *Transforming Government: People. Process and Policy, 10*(1), 72–98.

Michels, J. D., & Walden, I. (2018). How Safe is Safe Enough? Improving Cybersecurity in Europe's Critical Infrastructure Under the NIS Directive. *Improving Cybersecurity in Europe's Critical Infrastructure Under the NIS Directive (December 7, 2018). Queen Mary School of Law Legal Studies Research Paper*, (291).

Milieu Ltd & time.lex. (2014). *Overview of the national laws on electronic health records in the EU Member States and their interaction with the provision of cross-border eHealth services. Final report and* recommendations. Brussels. Retrieved from http://ec.europa.eu/health/ehealth/docs/laws_report_recommendations_en.pdf

Mondorf, A., & Wimmer, M. A. (2016). Requirements for an architecture framework for Pan-European e-Government Services. In *International Conference on Electronic Government* (pp. 135-150). Springer. 10.1007/978-3-319-44421-5_11

Nalin, M., Baroni, I., Faiella, G., Romano, M., Matrisciano, F., Gelenbe, E., ... Koutkias, V. (2019). The European cross-border health data exchange roadmap: Case study in the Italian setting. *Journal of Biomedical Informatics, 94*, 103183. doi:10.1016/j.jbi.2019.103183 PMID:31009760

OASIS. (2017a). *Business Document Metadata Service Location Version 1.0.* OASIS Standard. Retrieved from http://docs.oasis-open.org/bdxr/BDX-Location/v1.0/BDX-Location-v1.0.html

OASIS. (2017b). *Service Metadata Publishing (SMP) Version 1.0.* OASIS Standard. Retrieved from http://docs.oasis-open.org/bdxr/bdx-smp/v1.0/bdx-smp-v1.0.html

Pangalos, G., Asimakopoulos, D., & Pagkalos, I. (2013). The new Greek national e-prescription system: An effective tool for improving quality of care and containing medication costs. *Studies in Health Technology and Informatics, 190*, 13–17. PMID:23823360

Pernice, I. (2016). *E-Government and E-Democracy: overcoming legitimacy deficits in a digital Europe.* HIIG Discussion Paper Series No. 2016-01. Retrieved from https://ssrn.com/abstract=2723231

Ruggieri, F. (2010). ETSI specifications for registered e-mail REM. In ISSE 2009 Securing Electronic Business Processes (pp. 242-254). Vieweg+ Teubner. doi:10.1007/978-3-8348-9363-5_24

Staffa, M., Sgaglione, L., Mazzeo, G., Coppolino, L., D'Antonio, S., Romano, L., ... Campegiani, P. (2018). An OpenNCP-based solution for secure eHealth data exchange. *Journal of Network and Computer Applications*, *116*, 65–85. doi:10.1016/j.jnca.2018.05.012

Stasis, A. C., Demiri, L., & Chaniotaki, E. (2018). eIDAS-Electronic Identification for Cross Border eHealth. *International Journal of Reliable and Quality E-Healthcare*, *7*(2), 51–67. doi:10.4018/IJRQEH.2018040104

Stroetmann, K. A., Artmann, J., Stroetmann, V. N., Protti, D., Dumortier, J., Giest, S., ... & Whitehouse, D. (2011). *European countries on their journey towards national eHealth infrastructures*. Luxembourg: Office for Official Publications of the European Communities.

Tinholt, D., Carrara, W., Tol, T., Foley, P., Graux, H., & Erdogan, E. (2013). Study on analysis of the needs for cross-border services and assessment of the organisational, legal, technical and semantic barriers. *European Commission–Directorate-General of Communications Networks, Content & Technology*.

Wang, C. J., Patel, M. H., Schueth, A. J., Bradley, M., Wu, S., Crosson, J. C., ... Bell, D. S. (2009). Perceptions of standards-based electronic prescribing systems as implemented in outpatient primary care: A physician survey. *Journal of the American Medical Informatics Association*, *16*(4), 493–502. doi:10.1197/jamia.M2998 PMID:19390106

Wisniewski, F., Katehakis, D. G., Masi, M., & Bittins, S. (2016). Improving Cross-Border European ePrescription and Patient Summary Services through e-SENS Cross-Sectorial Building Blocks. *Global Telemedicine and eHealth Updates. Knowledge Resources*, *9*, 234–238.

Zadeh, P. E., & Tremblay, M. C. (2016). A review of the literature and proposed classification on e-prescribing: Functions, assimilation stages, benefits, concerns, and risks. *Research in Social & Administrative Pharmacy*, *12*(1), 1–19. doi:10.1016/j.sapharm.2015.03.001 PMID:25847858

ADDITIONAL READING

DG SANTE, & CEF eHealth DSI (2019). *eHealth DSI Patient Summary and ePrescription. Identity Management Specification, Document Version 3.0.0, Date 02/07/2019, Wave 3 Operation Ready*. Retrieved from https://ec.europa.eu/cefdigital/wiki/display/EHOPERATIONS/Identity+Management+Specification?preview=/37752823/110494981/eHDSI_Identity_Management_Specification_v3.0.0_OR.pdf

Dobrev, A., Jones, T., Stroetmann, V., Stroetmann, K., Vatter, Y., & Peng, K. (2010). Interoperable eHealth is Worth it: Securing Benefits from Electronic Health Records and e-prescribing. European Commission. *Information Society and Media Study Report*. Retrieved from http://www.ifap.ru/library/book476.pdf

eHealth DSI Interoperability Specifications. Retrieved from https://ec.europa.eu/cefdigital/wiki/display/EHOPERATIONS/Specifications

ETSI. (2011). ETSI TS 102 640-2 V2. 2.1, *Electronic Signatures and Infrastructures (ESI); Registered Electronic Mail (REM); Part 2: Data requirements, Formats and Signatures for REM*. Retrieved from https://www.etsi.org/deliver/etsi_ts/102600_102699/10264002/02.02.01_60/ts_10264002v020201p.pdf

Kouroubali, A., & Katehakis, D. G. (2019). The new European interoperability framework as a facilitator of digital transformation for citizen empowerment. *Journal of Biomedical Informatics*, *94*, 103166. doi:10.1016/j.jbi.2019.103166 PMID:30978512

Moharra, M., Almazán, C., Decool, M., Nilsson, A. L., Allegretti, N., & Seven, M. (2015). Implementation of a cross-border health service: Physician and pharmacists' opinions from the epSOS project. *Family Practice*, *32*(5), 564–567. doi:10.1093/fampra/cmv052 PMID:26148726

Onieva, J. A., & Zhou, J. (2008). *Secure multi-party non-repudiation protocols and applications* (Vol. 43). Springer Science & Business Media.

Prey, J. E., Polubriaginof, F., Kuperman, G. J., Tiase, V., Collins, S. A., & Vawdrey, D. K. (2016). International perspectives on sharing clinical data with patients. *International Journal of Medical Informatics*, *86*, 135–141. doi:10.1016/j.ijmedinf.2015.11.007 PMID:26631956

Quinn, P., & De Hert, P. (2011). The Patients' Rights Directive (2011/24/EU)–Providing (some) rights to EU residents seeking healthcare in other Member States. *Computer Law & Security Review*, *27*(5), 497–502. doi:10.1016/j.clsr.2011.07.010

KEY TERMS AND DEFINITIONS

Connecting Europe Facility: A European Union fund for pan-European infrastructure investment in transport, energy and digital projects, which aim at a greater connectivity between European Union member states. It operates through grants, financial guarantees, and project bonds.

eHealth DSI: The initial deployment and operation of services for cross-border health data exchange under the Connecting Europe Facility (CEF).

Electronic Identification: The process of using person identification data in electronic form uniquely representing either a natural or legal person, or a natural person representing a legal person.

Electronic Prescription: A medicinal prescription issued and transmitted electronically. The ePrescription service is made up of electronic prescribing and electronic dispensing: ePrescribing is defined as prescribing of medicines in software by a health care professional legally authorized to do so, for dispensing once it has been electronically transmitted, at the pharmacy. eDispensing is defined as the act of electronically retrieving a prescription and giving out the medicine to the patient as indicated in the corresponding ePrescription.

Interoperability: Interoperability, within the context of European public service delivery, is the ability of disparate and diverse organisations to interact towards mutually beneficial and agreed common goals, involving the sharing of information and knowledge between the organisations, through the business processes they support, by means of the exchange of data between their respective ICT systems.

National Contact Point for eHealth: National Contact Point for eHealth, which may act as an organisational and technical gateway for the provision of eHealth Cross-Border Information Services.

Non-Repudiation: The security service by which the entities involved in a communication cannot deny having participated. Specifically the sending entity cannot deny having sent a message (non-repudiation with proof of origin) and the receiving entity cannot deny having received a message (non-repudiation with proof of delivery).

Patient Summary: An identifiable dataset of essential and understandable health information that is made available at the point of care to deliver safe patient care during unscheduled care [and planned care] with its maximal impact in the unscheduled care.

Service Metadata Locator/Dynamic Service Location: The key component that enables dynamic discovery of participants in message exchange networks. As a result, these networks can scale up without being affected by the management of an increasing number of participants. Instead of having participants managed by a central node, address resolution becomes fully distributed and consequently much more scalable.

Service Metadata Publisher/Capability Lookup: Enables the participants of an eDelivery Messaging Infrastructure to dynamically discover each other's capabilities (legal, organisational, and technical). For this to happen, each participant must publish its capabilities and settings in an SMP.

Compilation of References

ACOG. (2005). ACOG practice bulletin, clinical management guidelines for obstetrician-gynecologists, number 65, August 2005: Management of endometrial cancer. *Obstetrics and Gynecology*, *106*(2), 413–425. PMID:16055605

Adams, L. J., Bello, G., & Dumancas, G. G. (2015). Development and Application of a Genetic Algorithm for Variable Optimization and Predictive Modeling of Five-Year Mortality Using Questionnaire Data. *Bioinformatics and Biology Insights*, *9*(Suppl 3), 31–41. doi:10.4137/BBI.S29469 PMID:26604716

Adeli, K., Raizman, J. E., Chen, Y., Higgins, V., Nieuwesteeg, M., Abdelhaleem, M., ... Blais, D. (2015). Complex biological profile of hematological markers across pediatric, adult, and geriatric ages: Establishment of robust pediatric and adult reference intervals based on the Canadian Health Measures Survey. *Clinical Chemistry*, *61*(8), 1075–1086. doi:10.1373/clinchem.2015.240531 PMID:26044509

Afrifa, J., Gyekye, S. A., Owiredu, W. K., Ephraim, R. K., Essien-Baidoo, S., Amoah, S., ... Arthur, A. R. (2015). Application of sigma metrics for the assessment of quality control in clinical chemistry laboratory in Ghana: A pilot study. *Nigerian Medical Journal*, *56*(1), 54–58. doi:10.4103/0300-1652.149172 PMID:25657495

AHA (American Heart Association). (2018). *Heart-Check Meal Certification Program Nutrition Requirements.* Retrieved May 1, 2008, from: https://www.heart.org/en/healthy-living/company-collaboration/heart-check-certification/heart-check-meal-certification-program-foodservice/heart-check-meal-certification-program-nutrition-requirements

Ajami, S., & Bagheri-Tadi, T. (2013). Barriers for adopting electronic health records (EHRs) by physicians. *Acta Informatica Medica*, *21*(2), 129. doi:10.5455/aim.2013.21.129-134 PMID:24058254

Akinbo, S. R., Sokunbi, O., & Ogunbameru, T. (2008). Factors contributing to possession of walking aids among persons with osteoarthritis of the knee. *Nigerian Quarterly Journal of Hospital Medicine*, *18*(2), 64–68. PMID:19068554

Al Juboury, M. I. A., & Al Debag, Z. G. T. (2012). *The Effect Of Critical To Quality Factors In Identification Excellence Strategic Dimensions.* Paper presented at the International Conference on Business Intelligence and Knowledge Economy.

Almeida, J. S., & Noble, P. A. (2000). Neural computing in microbiology. *Journal of Microbiological Methods, 43*(1), 1–2. doi:10.1016/S0167-7012(00)00200-1 PMID:11084224

Altman, D. G., & Bland, J. M. (1994). Statistics Notes: Diagnostic tests 1: sensitivity and specificity. BMJ (Clinical Research Ed.). doi:10.1136/bmj.308.6943.1552

American Cancer Society. (2005). *Detailed Guide: Endometrial Cancer: What are the Risk Factors for Endometrial Cancer?* Retrieved 20 March 2015, 2015, from http://www.cancer.org/cancer/endometrialcancer/detailedguide/endometrial-uterine-cancer-risk-factors

Aminudin, O., & Zainol, M. (2014). Implementation of Six Sigma in Service Industry. *Journal of Quality Measurement and Analysis, 10*(2), 77–86.

Anastasi, A. (1937). *Differential psychology: Individual and group differences in behavior.* New York, NY: Macmillan.

Arbabshirani, M. R., Plis, S., Sui, J., & Calhoun, V. D. (2017). Single subject prediction of brain disorders in neuroimaging: Promises and pitfalls. [PubMed]. *NeuroImage, 145*, 137–165. doi:10.1016/j.neuroimage.2016.02.079

Archondakis, S., Pouliakis, A., Margari, N., & Karakitsos, P. (2014). The Implementation of Cloud-Based Telemedical Applications for External Quality Control Purposes in the Field of Cytopathology. *International Journal of Reliable and Quality E-Healthcare, 3*(3), 22–36. doi:10.4018/ijrqeh.2014070102

Aribisala, B. S., Cowie, C. J. A., He, J., Wood, J., Mendelow, A. D., Mitchell, P., & Blamire, A. M. (2010). Multi-parametric Classification of Traumatic Brain Injury Patients Using Automatic Analysis of Quantitative MRI Scans. Medical Imaging and Augmented Reality: 5th International Workshop, MIAR 2010, Beijing, China, September 19-20, 2010. Proceedings, 51–59. 10.1007/978-3-642-15699-1_6

Aslam, M., & Srinivasa Rao, G. (2019). Control Charts for Monitoring Process Capability Index Using Median Absolute Deviation for Some Popular Distributions. *Processes, 7*(5), 287. Doi.org/10.3390/pr7050287. doi:10.3390/pr7050287

Asokan, N. (1998). *Fairness in electronic commerce.* Retrieved from https://www.researchgate.net/publication/2281851_Fairness_in_Electronic_Commerce

Awasthi, A. K., Wang, M., Wang, Z., Awasthi, M. K., & Li, J. (2018). E-waste management in India: A mini-review. *Waste Management & Research, 36*(5), 408–414. doi:10.1177/0734242X18767038 PMID:29732961

Baak, J. P. A. (1991). *Manual of quantitative pathology in cancer diagnosis and prognosis.* Berlin: Springer-Verlag.

Baak, J. P., Kurver, P. H., Overdiep, S. H., Delemarre, J. F., Boon, M. E., Lindeman, J., & Diegenbach, P. C. (1981). Quantitative, microscopical, computer-aided diagnosis of endometrial hyperplasia or carcinoma in individual patients. *Histopathology*, *5*(6), 689–695. doi:10.1111/j.1365-2559.1981.tb01835.x PMID:7033100

Baer, T. (2019). *Understand, Manage, and Prevent Algorithmic Bias. Understand, Manage, and Prevent Algorithmic Bias*. Berkeley, CA: Apress; doi:10.1007/978-1-4842-4885-0

Balasubramanian, K., Balraj, A., Kumar, J., & Jaykumar. (2015). Customer Preferences to Select a Restaurant Through Smart Phone Applications: An Exploratory Study. *Advanced Science Letters*, *21*(5), 1489–1493. doi:10.1166/asl.2015.6081

Banitsas, K. A., Perakis, K., Tachakra, S., & Koutsouris, D. (2006). Use of 3G mobile phone links for teleconsultation between a moving ambulance and a hospital base station. *Journal of Telemedicine and Telecare*, *12*(1), 23–26. doi:10.1258/135763306775321335 PMID:16438775

Banitsas, K., Perakis, K., Koutsouris, D., Konis, G., & Tachakra, S. (2005). Ambulance 3G. *Conference Proceedings; ... Annual International Conference of the IEEE Engineering in Medicine and Biology Society. IEEE Engineering in Medicine and Biology Society. Conference*, *1*, 371–374. doi:10.1109/IEMBS.2005.1616422 PMID:17282191

Barak, M., & Jaschek, R. (2013). A new and effective way for preventing preanalytical laboratory errors. *Clinical Chemistry and Laboratory Medicine*, *50*(4), 1–4. doi:10.1515/cclm-2013-0597

Bardsley, M. (2016). *Understanding analytical capability in health care: Do we have more data than insight?* The Health Foundation.

Barham, M. P., Clark, G. M., Hayden, M. J., Enticott, P. G., Conduit, R., & Lum, J. A. G. (2017). Acquiring research-grade ERPs on a shoestring budget: A comparison of a modified Emotiv and commercial SynAmps EEG system. *Psychophysiology*, *54*(9), 1393–1404. doi:10.1111/psyp.12888 PMID:28497557

Barth, J. H. (2012). Clinical quality indicators in laboratory medicine. *Annals of Clinical Biochemistry*, *49*(1), 9–16. doi:10.1258/acb.2011.011126 PMID:22042979

Bateni, H., & Maki, B. E. (2005). Assistive Devices for Balance and Mobility: Benefits, Demands, and Adverse Consequences. *Archives of Physical Medicine and Rehabilitation*, *86*(1), 134–145. doi:10.1016/j.apmr.2004.04.023 PMID:15641004

Baxes, G. A. (1994). *Digital image processing: principles and applications* (1st ed.). New York: Wiley.

Bayer, R., & Galea, S. (2015). Public health in the precision-medicine era. *The New England Journal of Medicine*, *373*(6), 499–501. doi:10.1056/NEJMp1506241 PMID:26244305

Beaupre, L., Jones, C., Johnston, D., Wilson, D., & Majumdar, S. (2012). Recovery of function following a hip fracture in geriatric ambulatory persons living in nursing homes: Prospective cohort study. *Journal of the American Geriatrics Society*, *60*(7), 1268–1273. doi:10.1111/j.1532-5415.2012.04033.x PMID:22702238

Beckmann, J. S., & Lew, D. (2016). Reconciling evidence-based medicine and precision medicine in the era of big data: Challenges and opportunities. *Genome Medicine*, *8*(1), 134. doi:10.118613073-016-0388-7 PMID:27993174

Benedetti, F. (2011). *The Patient's Brain: The neuroscience behind the doctor-patient relationship*. Oxford, UK: Oxford University Press.

Bengtsson, E., & Malm, P. (2014). Screening for Cervical Cancer Using Automated Analysis of PAP-Smears. *Computational and Mathematical Methods in Medicine*, *12*. doi:10.1155/2014/842037 PMID:24772188

Bennett, G. G., Steinberg, D. M., Lanpher, M. G., Askew, S., Lane, I. B., Levine, E. L., ... Foley, P. B. (2013). Availability of and ease of access to calorie information on restaurant websites. *PLoS One*, *8*(8), e72009. doi:10.1371/journal.pone.0072009 PMID:23977193

Berg, M. (2001). Implementing information systems in health care organizations: Myths and challenges. *International Journal of Medical Informatics*, *64*(2-3), 143–156. doi:10.1016/S1386-5056(01)00200-3 PMID:11734382

Berg, M., & Mol, A. (Eds.). (1998). *Difference in Medicine; Unravelling Practices, Techniques, and Bodies*. Durham, NC: Duke University Press.

Bergman, L. R., & Vargha, A. (2013). Matching method to problem: A developmental science perspective. *European Journal of Developmental Psychology*, *10*(1), 9–28. doi:10.1080/17405629.2012.732920

Berte, L. M. (2007). Improvement of Clinical Laboratory Services through Quality. *Clinics in Laboratory Medicine*, *27*(4), 771–790. doi:10.1016/j.cll.2007.07.008 PMID:17950897

Bezerra, I. N., Curioni, C., & Sichieri, R. (2012). Association between eating out of home and body weight. *Nutrition Reviews*, *70*(2), 65–79. doi:10.1111/j.1753-4887.2011.00459.x PMID:22300594

Bibbo, M., Bartels, P. H., Galera-Davidson, H., Dytch, H. E., & Wied, G. L. (1986). Markers for malignancy in the nuclear texture of histologically normal tissue from patients with thyroid tumors. *Analytical and Quantitative Cytology and Histology*, *8*(2), 168–176. PMID:2425826

Black, A. D., Car, J., Pagliari, C., Anandan, C., Cresswell, K., Bokun, T., ... Sheikh, A. (2011). The impact of eHealth on the quality and safety of health care: A systematic overview. *PLoS Medicine*, *8*(1), e1000387. doi:10.1371/journal.pmed.1000387 PMID:21267058

Blau, C. A., & Liakopoulou, E. (2013). Can we deconstruct cancer, one patient at a time? *Trends in Genetics*, *29*(1), 6–10. doi:10.1016/j.tig.2012.09.004 PMID:23102584

Blaustein, A., & Kurman, R. J. (2011). *Blaustein's pathology of the female genital tract* (6th ed.). New York, NY: Springer.

Blobel, B. (2018). Interoperable EHR Systems–Challenges, Standards and Solutions. *European Journal for Biomedical Informatics*, *14*(2), 10–19. doi:10.24105/ejbi.2018.14.2.3

Bowens, F. M., Frye, P. A., & Jones, W. A. (2010). Health information technology: integration of clinical workflow into meaningful use of electronic health records. *Perspectives in Health Information Management/AHIMA, American Health Information Management Association, 7.*

Bowman, S. A., & Vinyard, B. T. (2004). Fast Food Consumption of U.S. Adults: Impact on Energy and Nutrient Intakes and Overweight Status. *Journal of the American College of Nutrition, 23*(2), 163–168. doi:10.1080/07315724.2004.10719357 PMID:15047683

Brandt, A., Iwarsson, S., & Ståhl, A. (2003). Satisfaction with rollators among community-living users: A follow-up study. *Disability and Rehabilitation, 25*(7), 343–353. doi:10.1080/0963828021000058495 PMID:12745958

Breiman, L., Friedman, J. H., Olshen, R. A., & Stone, C. J. (1984). Classification and Regression Trees. In The Wadsworth statisticsprobability series (Vol. 19). doi:10.1371/journal.pone.0015807

Brooks, R. (1996). EuroQol: The current state of play. *Health Policy (Amsterdam), 37*(1), 53–72. doi:10.1016/0168-8510(96)00822-6 PMID:10158943

Brouwer, R. M., Schnack, H. G., Nieuwenhuis, M., van Haren, N. E. M., Abramovic, L., Scheewe, T. W., ... Kahn, R. S. (2014). Can structural MRI aid in clinical classification? A machine learning study in two independent samples of patients with schizophrenia, bipolar disorder and healthy subjects. [PubMed]. *NeuroImage, 84*(January), 299–306. doi:10.1016/j.neuroimage.2013.08.053

Bubshait, A., & Al-Dosary, A. (2014).Application of Lean Six-Sigma Methodology to Reduce the Failure Rate of Valves at Oil Field. *Proceedings of the World Congress on Engineering and Computer Science WCECS, 2.*

Buccoliero, A. M., Castiglione, F., Gheri, C. F., Garbini, F., Fambrini, M., Bargelli, G., ... Taddei, G. L. (2007). Liquid-based endometrial cytology: Its possible value in postmenopausal asymptomatic women. *International Journal of Gynecological Cancer, 17*(1), 182–187. doi:10.1111/j.1525-1438.2006.00757.x PMID:17291251

Buccoliero, A. M., Gheri, C. F., Castiglione, F., Garbini, F., Barbetti, A., Fambrini, M., ... Taddei, G. L. (2007). Liquid-based endometrial cytology: Cyto-histological correlation in a population of 917 women. *Cytopathology, 18*(4), 241–249. doi:10.1111/j.1365-2303.2007.00463.x PMID:17559564

Bzdok, D., & Meyer-Lindenberg, A. (2017). Machine learning for precision psychiatry, 1–16. Retrieved from http://arxiv.org/abs/1705.10553

Campbell, C. A., & Horvath, A. R. (2014). Harmonization of critical result management in laboratory medicine. *Clinica Chimica Acta, 432*, 135–147. doi:10.1016/j.cca.2013.11.004

Cantalejo, R. F. (2010). Evaluación de métodos y validez de pruebasdiagnósticas. Estudio de las característicasmetrológicas de un test. In *CursoIVCongresoNacionaldel LaboratorioClinico*. CAPCollege of American Pathologists. Retrieved from http://www.cap.org/

Cardol, M., de Jong, B., & Ward, C. (2001). *On autonomy and participation in rehabilitation*. Amsterdam: Academic Press.

Cardol, M., de Haan, R. J., de Jong, B. A., van den Bos, G. A., & de Groot, I. J. (2001). Psychometric properties of the Impact on Participation and Autonomy Questionnaire. *Archives of Physical Medicine and Rehabilitation, 82*(2), 210–216. doi:10.1053/apmr.2001.18218 PMID:11239312

Cardol, M., de Haan, R., van den Bos, G., de Jong, B., & de Groot, I. (1999). The development of a handicap assessment questionnaire: The Impact on Participation and Autonomy (IPA). *Clinical Rehabilitation, 13*(5), 411–419. doi:10.1191/026921599668601325 PMID:10498348

Care Continuum Alliance. (2012). *Advancing the Population Health Improvement Model.* Retrieved from http://www.fiercehealthit.com/story/hennepin-health-project-looks-build-countywide-ehr-program-national-implica/2012-01-10

CDC Center of Disease Control and Prevention. (n.d.). Retrieved from http://www.cdc.gov/

Ceriotti, F. (2016). Harmonization initiatives in Europe. *EJIFCC, 27*, 5–14. PMID:27683503

Ceriotti, F., Brugnoni, D., & Mattioli, S. (2015). How to define a significant deviation from the expected internal quality control result. *Clinical Chemistry and Laboratory Medicine, 53*(6), 913–918. doi:10.1515/cclm-2014-1149 PMID:25870962

Cetin, E., Muzembo, J., Pardessus, V., Puisieux, F., & Thevenon, A. (2010). Impact of different types of walking aids on the physiological energy cost during gait for elderly individuals with several pathologies and dependent on a technical aid for walking. *Annals of Physical and Rehabilitation Medicine, 53*(6-7), 399–405. doi:10.1016/j.rehab.2010.06.003 PMID:20674533

Chacko, A., & Hayajneh, T. (2018). Security and Privacy Issues with IoT in Healthcare. *EAI Endorsed Transactions on Pervasive Health and Technology, 4*(14).

Chakrabarty, A., & Tan, K. C. (2008). *Case study analysis of Six Sigma in Singapore service organizations.* Paper presented at the 2008 International Conference on Service Systems and Service Management.

Chakraborty, A., & Tan, K. C. (2012). Case study analysis of Six Sigma implementation inservice organisations. *Business Process Management Journal, 18*(6), 992–1019. doi:10.1108/14637151211283384

Charron, P., Kirby, R., & MacLeod, D. (1995). Epidemiology of walker-related injuries and deaths in the united states. *American Journal of Physical Medicine & Rehabilitation, 74*(3), 237–239. doi:10.1097/00002060-199505000-00011 PMID:7779337

Chen, M. S., Wu, M. H., & Lin, M. C. (2014). Application of Indices Cp and Cpk to Improve Quality Control Capability in Clinical Biochemistry Laboratories. *The Chinese Journal of Physiology, 57*(2), 63–68. doi:10.4077/CJP.2014.BAB170 PMID:24694196

Chen, R., Mias, G. I., Li-Pook-Than, J., Jiang, L., Lam, H. Y., Chen, R., ... Snyder, M. (2012). Personal omics profiling reveals dynamic molecular and medical phenotypes. *Cell, 148*(6), 1293–1307. doi:10.1016/j.cell.2012.02.009 PMID:22424236

Chen, T., & Chefd'hotel, C. (2014). Deep Learning Based Automatic Immune Cell Detection for Immunohistochemistry Images. In G. Wu, D. Zhang, & L. Zhou (Eds.), *Machine Learning in Medical Imaging* (Vol. 8679, pp. 17–24). Springer International Publishing. doi:10.1007/978-3-319-10581-9_3

Chetney, R. (2003). The Cardiac Connection Program. *Home Healthcare Nurse*, *21*(10), 680–686. doi:10.1097/00004045-200310000-00007 PMID:14557707

Chlamtac, I., Conti, M., & Liu, J. J. N. (2003). Mobile ad hoc networking: Imperatives and challenges. *Ad Hoc Networks*, *1*(1), 13–64. doi:10.1016/S1570-8705(03)00013-1

Choi, S., Muizelaar, J., & Barnes, T. (1991). Prediction tree for severely head-injured patients. [PubMed]. *Journalism*, *75*, 251–255. doi:10.3171/jns.1991.75.2.0251

Chomsky, N. (1957). *Syntactic structures*. The Hague, The Netherlands: Mouton.

Choudhri, A. F., Carr, T. M. III, Ho, C. P., Stone, J. R., Gay, S. B., & Lambert, D. L. (2012). Handheld device review of abdominal CT for the evaluation of acute appendicitis. *Journal of Digital Imaging*, *25*(4), 492–496. doi:10.100710278-011-9431-9 PMID:22146833

Choudhri, A. F., Norton, P. T., Carr, T. M. III, Stone, J. R., Hagspiel, K. D., & Dake, M. D. (2013). Diagnosis and treatment planning of acute aortic emergencies using a handheld DICOM viewer. *Emergency Radiology*, *20*(4), 267–272. doi:10.100710140-013-1118-8 PMID:23525945

Ciresan, D. C., Giusti, A., Gambardella, L. M., & Schmidhuber, J. (2013). Mitosis detection in breast cancer histology images with deep neural networks. *Med Image Comput Comput Assist Interv*, *16*(Pt 2), 411–418. PMID:24579167

Clarke, J., Proudfoot, J., Birch, M. R., Whitton, A. E., Parker, G., Manicavasagar, V., ... Hadzi-Pavlovic, D. (2014). Effects of mental health self-efficacy on outcomes of a mobile phone and web intervention for mild-to-moderate depression, anxiety and stress: Secondary analysis of a randomised controlled trial. *BMC Psychiatry*, *14*(1), 272. doi:10.118612888-014-0272-1 PMID:25252853

Claustres, M., Kožich, V., Dequeker, E., Fowler, B., Hehir-Kwa, J. Y., Miller, K., ... Barton, D. E. (2014). Recommendations for reporting results of diagnostic genetic testing (biochemical, cytogenetic and molecular genetic). *European Journal of Human Genetics*, *22*(2), 160–170. doi:10.1038/ejhg.2013.125 PMID:23942201

CLIA Clinical Laboratory Improvement Amendments. (n.d.). Retrieved from https://www.cms.gov/Regulations-and uidance/Legislation/CLIA/index.html?redirect

Cloete, B. C., & Bester, A. (2012). A Lean Six Sigma approach to the improvement of the selenium analysis method. *The Onderstepoort Journal of Veterinary Research*, *79*(1), E1–E13. doi:10.4102/ojvr.v79i1.407 PMID:23327320

Cochand-Priollet, B., Koutroumbas, K., Megalopoulou, T. M., Pouliakis, A., Sivolapenko, G., & Karakitsos, P. (2006). Discriminating benign from malignant thyroid lesions using artificial intelligence and statistical selection of morphometric features. *Oncology Reports*, *15*(Spec no), 1023–1026. PMID:16525694

COLA Commission on Office Laboratory Accreditation. (n.d.). Retrieved from http://www.ama-assn.org/ama/pub/physician-resources/clinical-practice-improvement/clinical-quality/accreditation-collaboration/cola.page

Colombo, N., Preti, E., Landoni, F., Carinelli, S., Colombo, A., Marini, C., & Sessa, C. (2013). Endometrial cancer: ESMO Clinical Practice Guidelines for diagnosis, treatment and follow-up. *Annals of Oncology: Official Journal of the European Society for Medical Oncology*, *24*(Suppl 6), vi33–vi38. doi:10.1093/annonc/mdt353 PMID:24078661

Connecting Europe Facility, D. I. G. I. T. (2018a). *eDelivery SMP Profile. Test Assertions Description. Version 1.06. Date 01/06/2018.* Retrieved from https://ec.europa.eu/cefdigital/wiki/display/CEFDIGITAL/SMP+specifications?preview=/82773307/82796300/(CEFeDelivery).(eDelivery_SMP).(TAD).(v1.06).pdf

Connecting Europe Facility, D. I. G. I. T. (2018b). *SML Service Offering Description. Version 1.08. Date 25/09/2018.* Retrieved from https://ec.europa.eu/cefdigital/wiki/display/CEFDIGITAL/SML+service?preview=/82773318/82798522/(eDelivery)(SML)(SOD)(1.08).pdf

Cortes, C., & Vapnik, V. (1995). Support-vector networks. *Machine Learning*, *20*(3), 273–297. doi:10.1007/BF00994018

Coughlin, S., Whitehead, M., Sheats, J., Mastromonico, J., Hardy, D., & Smith, S. (2015). Smartphone Applications for Promoting Healthy Diet and Nutrition: A Literature Review. *Jacobs Journal of Food and Nutrition, 2*(3), 21.

Coughlin, J. F., Pope, J. E., & Leedle, B. R. Jr. (2006). Old Age, New Technology, and Future Innovations in Disease Management and Home Health Care. *Home Health Care Management & Practice*, *18*(3), 196–207. doi:10.1177/1084822305281955

Cruz, J. A., & Wishart, D. S. (2006). Applications of machine learning in cancer prediction and prognosis. *Cancer Informatics*, *2*, 59–77. doi:10.1177/117693510600200030 PMID:19458758

Cunha, A. (2013). Understanding the Ergodic Hypothesis Via Analogies. *Physica E, Low-Dimensional Systems and Nanostructures*, *10*, 9–12.

Cusack, C. M., Knudson, A. D., Kronstadt, J. L., Singer, R. F., & Brown, A. L. (2010). *Practice-Based Population Health: Information Technology to Support Transformation to Proactive Primary Care* (pp. 44). Retrieved from https://pcmh.ahrq.gov/sites/default/files/attachments/Information%20Technology%20to%20Support%20Transformation%20to%20Proactive%20Primary%20Care.pdf

Dallas Jones, G. R. (2015). Analytical performance specifications for EQA schemes –need for harmonization. *Clinical Chemistry and Laboratory Medicine, 53*(6), 919–924. doi:10.1515/cclm-2014-1268

Darcy, A. M., Louie, A. K., & Roberts, L. W. (2016). Machine Learning and the Profession of Medicine. *Journal of the American Medical Association, 315*(6), 551–552. doi:10.1001/jama.2015.18421 PMID:26864406

David, R. E., & Dobreanu, M. (2015). Risk Management in Clinical Laboratory: From Theory to Practice. *Acta Medica Marisiensis, 61*(4), 372–377. doi:10.1515/amma-2015-0086

Dawson, P. S. S. (1988). The 'average cell'— A handicap in bioscience and biotechnology. *Trends in Biotechnology, 6*(5), 87–90. doi:10.1016/0167-7799(88)90063-7

De Smedt, D., Clays, E., Doyle, F., Kotseva, K., Prugger, C., Pająk, A., ... De Bacquer, D. (2013). Validity and reliability of three commonly used quality of life measures in a large European population of coronary heart disease patients. *International Journal of Cardiology, 167*(5), 2294–2299. doi:10.1016/j.ijcard.2012.06.025 PMID:22748284

Deetz, C. O., Nolan, D. K., & Scott, M. G. (2012). An examination of the usefulness of repeat testing practices in a large hospital clinical chemistry laboratory. *American Journal of Clinical Pathology, 137*(1), 20–25. doi:10.1309/AJCPWPBF62YGEFOR PMID:22180474

Dehnavieh, R., Ebrahimipour, H., Molavi-Taleghani, Y., Vafaee-Najar, A., Noori Hekmat, S., & Esmailzdeh, H. (2014). Proactive risk assessment of blood transfusion process, in pediatric emergency, using the Health Care Failure Mode and Effects Analysis (HFMEA). *Global Journal of Health Science, 7*(1), 322–331. doi:10.5539/gjhs.v7n1p322 PMID:25560332

Demers, L., Monette, M., LaPierre, Y., Arnold, D. L., & Wolfson, C. (2002). Reliability, validity, and applicability of the Quebec User Evaluation of Satisfaction with assistive Technology (QUEST 2.0) for adults with multiple sclerosis. *Disability And Rehabilitation, 24*(1/2/3), 21-30.

Demers, L., Weiss-Lambrou, R., & Bernadette, S. (2002). The Quebec User Evaluation os Satisfaction with Assistive Technology (QUEST 2.0): An overview and recent progress. *Technology and Disability, 14*(3), 101–105. doi:10.3233/TAD-2002-14304

Demers, L., Weiss-Lambrou, R., & Ska, B. (2000). *Quebec User Evaluation of Satisfaction with Assistive Technology (QUEST Version 2.0). An Outcome Measure for Assistive Technology Devices.* Webster: The Institute for Matching Person & Technology.

Dennison, L., Morrison, L., Conway, G., & Yardley, L. (2013). Opportunities and challenges for smartphone applications in supporting health behavior change: Qualitative study. *Journal of Medical Internet Research, 15*(4), e86. doi:10.2196/jmir.2583 PMID:23598614

Deo, R. C. (2015). Machine Learning in Medicine. [PubMed]. *Circulation, 132*(20), 1920–1930. doi:10.1161/CIRCULATIONAHA.115.001593

Devgun, M. S., Chan, M. K., El-Nujumi, A. M., Abara, R., Armbruster, D., & Adeli, K. (2015). Clinical decision limits for interpretation of direct bilirubin— A CALIPER study of healthy multiethnic children and case report reviews. *Clinical Biochemistry*, *48*(1-2), 93–96. doi:10.1016/j.clinbiochem.2014.10.011 PMID:25445233

DG SANTE & CEF eHealth DSI. (2018a). *Audit Trail Profiles, Document Version 2.2.0, Date 08/06/2018, Wave 2 – Operation Ready*. Retrieved from https://ec.europa.eu/cefdigital/wiki/download/attachments/37752869/eHDSI_Audit_Trail_Profiles_v2.2.0.pdf?version=2&modificationDate=1535471342356&api=v2

DG SANTE & CEF eHealth DSI. (2018c). *ePrescription Functional requirements, Document Version 2.2.3, Date 01/08/2018, Wave 2 – Operation Ready*. Retrieved from https://ec.europa.eu/cefdigital/wiki/download/attachments/35210463/eP%20functional%20requirements_v2.2.3.pdf?version=1&modificationDate=1533135470667&api=v2

DG SANTE & CEF eHealth DSI. (2018d). *PS Functional requirements, Document Version 2.2.2, Date 01/08/2018, Wave 2 – Operation Ready*. Retrieved from https://ec.europa.eu/cefdigital/wiki/download/attachments/35210463/PS%20functional%20requirements_v2.2.2.pdf?version=1&modificationDate=1533135456275&api=v2

DG SANTE & CEF eHealth DSI. (2018e). *Service Location and Capability Lookup Profile, Document Version 2.1.0, Date 01/06/2017, Wave 1 Operation Ready*. Retrieved from https://ec.europa.eu/cefdigital/wiki/display/EHOPERATIONS/Specifications?preview=/35210463/47187054/Service%20Location%20and%20Capability%20Lookup%20Profile_v2.1.0.pdf

Diamantis, A., Magiorkinis, E., & Koutselini, H. (2014). 50 years after the death of George Nicholas Papanicolaou (1883-1962): Evaluation of his scientific work. *Acta Medico-Historica Adriatica: AMHA*, *12*(1), 181–188. PMID:25310617

Dimitriou, M., Giazitzi, K., Stavridi, E., Palisidis, G., Karathanos, V., & Boskou, G. (2017). Evaluation of an Electronic Application for Nutritional Information in Food Service Outlets: A Pilot mHealth Application. *International Journal of Reliable and Quality E-Healthcare*, *6*(1), 46–58. doi:10.4018/IJRQEH.2017010104

Donnelly, K. P. (2015). *Adolphe Quetelet, Social Physics and the Average Men of Science, 1796–1874*. London: Pickering & Chatto. doi:10.4324/9781315653662

Drosos, D., Tsotsolas, N., Chalikias, M., Skordoulis, M., & Koniordos, M. (2015). A survey on the use of social networking sites in Greece. In A. Kravets, M. Shcherbakov, M. Kultsova, & O. Shabalina (Eds.), *Creativity in Intelligent, Technologies and Data Science, Communications in Computer and Information Science* (pp. 556–570). Cham, Switzerland: Springer.

Duda, R. O., Hart, P. E., & Stork, D. G. (2001). *Pattern classification* (2nd ed.). New York: Wiley.

Efthimiou, E., Fotinea, S., Goulas, T., Koutsombogera, M., Karioris, P., Vacalopoulou, A., & ... . (2016). The MOBOT rollator human-robot interaction model and user evaluation process. *2016 IEEE Symposium Series On Computational Intelligence (SSCI)*. 10.1109/SSCI.2016.7850061 eHealth Network. (2013). *Guidelines on minimum/ non-exhaustive patient summary dataset for electronic exchange in accordance with the cross-border Directive 2011/ 24/ EU. Release 1.0.* Retrieved from https://ec.europa.eu/health//sites/health/files/ehealth/docs/guidelines_patient_summary_en.pdf

eHealth Network. (2014). *Guidelines on ePrescriptions dataset for electronic exchange under Cross-Border Directive 2011/24/EU. European Commission.* Release 1. Retrieved from http://ec.europa.eu/health/ehealth/docs/eprescription_guidelines_en.pdf

eHealth Network. (2015). *Guideline on an Organisational Framework for eHealth National Contact Point.* Brussels, Retrieved from http://ec.europa.eu/health/ehealth/docs/ev_20151123_co01_en.pdf

eHealth Network. (2016a). *Guideline on the electronic exchange of health data under Cross-Border Directive 2011/ 24/ EU. Release 2. EPrescriptions and eDispensations.* Retrieved from https://ec.europa.eu/health/sites/health/files/ehealth/docs/ev_20161121_co091_en.pdf

eHealth Network. (2016b). *Guideline on the electronic exchange of health data under Cross-Border Directive 2011/ 24/ EU. Release 2. Patient Summary for unscheduled care.* Retrieved from https://ec.europa.eu/health/sites/health/files/ehealth/docs/ev_20161121_co10_en.pdf

El-Gilany, A. H., El-Shaer, S., Khashaba, E., El-Dakroory, S. A., & Omar, N. (2017). Knowledge, attitude, and practice (KAP) of 'teaching laboratory' technicianstowards laboratory safety and waste management: A pilot interventional study. *The Journal of Hospital Infection, 96*(2), 192–194. doi:10.1016/j.jhin.2017.02.007 PMID:28268025

El-Hashmi, K., & Gnieber, O. K. (2014). Applying Process Capability Analysis in Measuring Clinical Laboratory Quality - A Six Sigma Project. *Proceedings of the 2014 International Conference on Industrial Engineering and Operations Management Bali, Indonesia. Abstract Book*, 1780-1789.

EMOTIV. (2017). *Emotiv insight Brainware®.* Retrieved 2 Sept., 2017, from https://www.emotiv.com/insight/

ENISA. (2015). *Security and Resilience in eHealth Infrastructures and Services.* Retrieved from https://www.enisa.europa.eu/publications/security-and-resilience-in-ehealth-infrastructures-and-services

ENISA. (2016). *Cyber security and resilience for Smart Hospitals.* Retrieved from https://www.enisa.europa.eu/publications/cyber-security-and-resilience-for-smart-hospitals

Espino, J. U., Wagner, M. M., Tsui, F.-C., Su, H.-D., Olszewski, R. T., Lie, Z., ... Dara, J. (2004). The RODS Open Source Project: Removing a barrier to syndromic surveillance. *Studies in Health Technology and Informatics, 107*(Pt 2), 1192–1196.

Esterle, L., & Kouroubali, A. (2010), Political and organizational factors influencing large scale implementation of electronic health records: Recommendations for a realistic plan. *Report of the European Project EHR-Implement.* Retrieved from http://www.eurorec.org/files/filesPublic/EHR-I%20%20Recommendations.pdf

EU Directorate-General for Health and Food Safety. (2014). *Overview of the national laws on electronic health records in the EU Member States and their interaction with the provision of cross-border eHealth services.* Retrieved from http://ec.europa.eu/health/ehealth/docs/laws_report_recommendations_en.pdf

EU Regulation No 1169/2011 of the European Parliament and of the Council of 25 October 2011 on the provision of food information to consumers, OJ L 304 22.11.2011

Eugster, M. J., Schmid, M., Binder, H., & Schmidberger, M. (2013). Grid and cloud computing methods in biomedical research. *Methods of Information in Medicine*, *52*(1), 62–64. doi:10.1055-0038-1627052 PMID:23318694

European Commission (2018). *Communication from the Commission to the European Parliament, the Council, the European Economic and Social Committee and the Committee of the Regions on enabling the digital transformation of health and care in the Digital Single Market; empowering citizens and building a healthier society*, COM(2018) 233 final {SWD(2018) 126 final}.

European Commission (2019). *Commission Recommendation of 6.2.2019 on a European Electronic Health Record exchange format* (Text with EEA relevance), C(2019) 800 final.

European Commission. (2017). *New European Interoperability Framework, Promoting seamless services and data flows for European public administrations.* Belgium: European Union.

European Commission. (2017). *New European Interoperability Framework. Promoting seamless services and data flows for European public administrations.* Retrieved from https://ec.europa.eu/isa2/sites/isa/files/eif_brochure_final.pdf

European Commission. (2018). *Communication from the Commission to the European Parliament, the Council, the European Economic and Social Committee and the Committee of the Regions on enabling the digital transformation of health and care in the Digital Single Market; empowering citizens and building a healthier society*, COM(2018) 233 final {SWD(2018) 126 final}. Retrieved from https://ec.europa.eu/digital-single-market/en/news/communication-enabling-digital-transformation-health-and-care-digital-single-market-empowering

European Commission. (2019). *Commission Recommendation of 6.2.2019 on a European Electronic Health Record exchange format (Text with EEA relevance)*, C(2019) 800 final. Retrieved from https://ec.europa.eu/digital-single-market/en/news/recommendation-european-electronic-health-record-exchange-format

European Court of Auditors. (2019). *EU actions for cross-border healthcare: significant ambitions but improved management required (pursuant to Article 287(4), second subparagraph, TFEU).* Special Report No 7. Retrieved from https://www.eca.europa.eu/Lists/ECADocuments/SR19_07/SR_HEALTH_CARE_EN.pdf

European Parliament. (2011). *Directive 2011/24/EU of the European Parliament and of the Council of 9 March 2011 on the application of patients' rights in cross-border healthcare.* Retrieved from https://eur-lex.europa.eu/legal-content/EN/TXT/?uri=CELEX%3A32011L0024

European Parliament. (2014). *Regulation (EU) No 910/2014 of the European Parliament and of the Council of 23 July 2014 on electronic identification and trust services for electronic transactions in the internal market and repealing Directive 1999/93/EC*. Retrieved from https://eur-lex.europa.eu/legal-content/EN/TXT/?uri=uriserv%3AOJ.L_.2014.257.01.0073.01.ENG

EuroQol. (1990). EuroQol—A new facility for the measurement of health related quality of life. *Health Policy (Amsterdam)*, *16*(3), 199–208. doi:10.1016/0168-8510(90)90421-9

EuroQol. (2007). *EQ5D Value Sets-inventory, comparative review and user guide. EuroQol group Monographs*. Springer.

Evans, H. (2018). *Does the public see tax rises as the answer to NHS funding pressures?* London: The King's Fund.

Fambrini, M., Buccoliero, A. M., Bargelli, G., Cioni, R., Piciocchi, L., Pieralli, A., ... Marchionni, M. (2008). Clinical utility of liquid-based cytology for the characterization and management of endometrial polyps in postmenopausal age. *International Journal of Gynecological Cancer*, *18*(2), 306–311. doi:10.1111/j.1525-1438.2007.01019.x PMID:17624992

Fawcett, T. (2015). Mining the Quantified Self: Personal Knowledge Discovery as a Challenge for Data Science. *Big Data*, *3*(4), 249–266. doi:10.1089/big.2015.0049 PMID:27441406

FDA (Food and Drug Administration). (2018). *Menu Labeling Requirements*. Retrieved August 13, 2019, from: https://www.fda.gov/food/food-labeling-nutrition/menu-labeling-requirements

FDA. (2019a). *Cybersecurity*. Retrieved 20 August, 2019, from https://www.fda.gov/medical-devices/digital-health/cybersecurity

FDA. (2019b). *The FDA'S role in medical device cybersecurity: Dispelling Myths and Understanding Facts*. Retrieved 20 August, 2019, from https://www.fda.gov/media/103696/download

Ferenczy, A., & Bergeron, C. (1992). Endometrial hyperplasia. In D. Lowe & H. Fox (Eds.), *Advances in Gynaecological Pathology* (pp. 207–234). Edinburgh, UK: Churchill Livingstone.

Feroz, A., Perveen, S., & Aftab, W. (2017). Role of mHealth applications for improving antenatal and postnatal care in low and middle income countries: A systematic review. *BMC Health Services Research*, *17*(1), 704. doi:10.118612913-017-2664-7 PMID:29115992

Finkelstein, A., Levy, G. H., Hui, P., Prasad, A., Virk, R., Chhieng, D. C., ... Prasad, M. L. (2012). Papillary thyroid carcinomas with and without BRAF V600E mutations are morphologically distinct. *Histopathology*, *60*(7), 1052–1059. doi:10.1111/j.1365-2559.2011.04149.x PMID:22335197

Finkelstein, E. A., Khavjou, O. A., Thompson, H., Trogdon, J. G., Pan, L., Sherry, B., & Dietz, W. (2011). Obesity and severe obesity forecasts through 2030. *American Journal of Preventive Medicine*, *42*(6), 563–570. doi:10.1016/j.amepre.2011.10.026 PMID:22608371

Finkelstein, J., Hripcsak, G., & Cabrera, M. (1998). Telematic system for monitoring of asthma severity in patients' homes. *Studies in Health Technology and Informatics*, *52*(Pt 1), 272–276. PMID:10384460

Fischer, K. W., & Bidell, T. R. (2006). Dynamic development of action and thought. In W. Damon & R. M. Lerner (Eds.), Theoretical models of human development. Handbook of child psychology (6th ed.; Vol. 1, pp. 313–399). New York, NY: John Wiley & Sons.

Flegar-Meštrić, Z., Perkov, S., Radeljak, A., Kardum Paro, M. M., Prkačin, I., & Devčić-Jeras, A. (2017). Risk analysis of the preanalytical process based on quality indicators data. *Clinical Chemistry and Laboratory Medicine*, *55*(3), 368–377. doi:10.1515/cclm-2016-0235 PMID:27580180

Fodor, J. (1983). *The modularity of mind: An essay on faculty psychology*. Cambridge, MA: MIT Press. doi:10.7551/mitpress/4737.001.0001

Fong, D. Y., Lam, C., Mak, K. K., Lo, S. W., Lai, K. Y., Ho, Y. S., & Lam, T. H. (2010). The Short Form-12 Health Survey was a valid instrument in Chinese adolescents. *Journal of Clinical Epidemiology*, *63*(9), 1020–1029. doi:10.1016/j.jclinepi.2009.11.011 PMID:20189764

Fonseca, M., Karkaletsis, K., Cruz, I. A., Berler, A., & Oliveira, I. C. (2015, May). *OpenNCP: a novel framework to foster cross-border e-Health services*. MIE.

Foran, D. J., Chen, W., & Yang, L. (2011). Automated image interpretation computer-assisted diagnostics. *Analytical Cellular Pathology (Amsterdam)*, *34*(6), 279–300. doi:10.1155/2011/239761 PMID:22082571

Forrest, D. W. (1974). *Francis Galton: The Life and Work of a Victorian Genius*. New York: Taplinger.

Fotinea, S. E., Efthimiou, E., Dimou, A. L., Goulas, T., Karioris, P., Peer, A., ... Stanzyk, B. (2014). Data acquisition towards defining a multimodal interaction model for human - assistive robot communication. In. Lecture Notes in Computer Science: Vol. 8515. *Universal Access in Human-Computer Interaction. Aging and Assistive Environments* (pp. 613–624). Springer International Publishing. doi:10.1007/978-3-319-07446-7_59

Fox, H. (1984). The endometrial hyperplasias. *Obstetrics and Gynecology Annual*, *13*, 197–209. PMID:6371615

Fragidis, L. L., & Chatzoglou, P. D. (2011, September). The use of electronic health record in greece: current status. In *2011 IEEE 11th International Conference on Computer and Information Technology* (pp. 475-480). IEEE. 10.1109/CIT.2011.42

Franco, R. Z., Fallaize, R., Lovegrove, J. A., & Hwang, F. (2016). Popular Nutrition-Related Mobile Apps: A Feature Assessment. *JMIR mHealth and uHealth*, *4*(3), e85. doi:10.2196/mhealth.5846 PMID:27480144

Frey, C. B., & Osborne, M. A. (2017). The Future of Employment: How susceptible are jobs to computerisation? *Technological Forecasting and Social Change*, *114*, 254–280. doi:10.1016/j.techfore.2016.08.019

Frizera, A., Ceres, R., Pons, J., Abellanas, A., & Raya, R. (2008). The smart walkers as geriatric assistive device. The simbiosis purpose. *Gerontechnology (Valkenswaard)*, *7*(2). doi:10.4017/gt.2008.07.02.045.00

Fulciniti, F., Yanoh, K., Karakitsos, P., Watanabe, J., Di Lorito, A., Margari, N., ... Hirai, Y. (2018). The Yokohama system for reporting directly sampled endometrial cytology: The quest to develop a standardized terminology. *Diagnostic Cytopathology*, *46*(5), 400–412. doi:10.1002/dc.23916 PMID:29479846

Fursule, N.V., Bansod, S.V., & Fursule, N.S. (2012). Understanding the benefits and limitations of Six Sigma Methodology. *International Journal of Scientific and Research Publications, 2*(1), 1-9.

Galatzer-Levy, I. R., Ma, S., Statnikov, A., Yehuda, R., & Shalev, A. Y. (2017). Utilization of machine learning for prediction of post-traumatic stress: A re-examination of cortisol in the prediction and pathways to non-remitting PTSD. [PubMed]. *Translational Psychiatry*, *7*(3), e0. doi:10.1038/tp.2017.38

Gandek, B., Ware, J. E., Aaronson, N. K., Apolone, G., Bjorner, J. B., Brazier, J. E., ... Sullivan, M. (1998). Cross-Validation of Item Selection and Scoring for the SF-12 Health Survey in Nine Countries. *Journal of Clinical Epidemiology*, *15*(11), 1171–1178. doi:10.1016/S0895-4356(98)00109-7 PMID:9817135

Gani, A., Li, X., Yang, L., & Zakaria, O. (2008). Radio frequency combination for TCP/IP suite protocol improvement in 4G mobile internet networks. *International Journal of Communication*, *2*(1), 27–36.

Garcia, F., Barker, B., Davis, J., Shelton, T., Harrigill, K., Schalk, N., ... Hatch, K. (2003). Thin-layer cytology and histopathology in the evaluation of abnormal uterine bleeding. *The Journal of Reproductive Medicine*, *48*(11), 882–888. PMID:14686021

Garcia-Gomez, J. M., de la Torre-Diez, I., Vicente, J., Robles, M., Lopez-Coronado, M., & Rodrigues, J. J. (2014). Analysis of mobile health applications for a broad spectrum of consumers: A user experience approach. *Health Informatics Journal*, *20*(1), 74–84. doi:10.1177/1460458213479598 PMID:24550566

García-Lario, J. V., & Boned Juliani, B. (2012). Control de la CalidadInterno: Una PrácticaMuyActual. *EdCont Lab Clín*, *15*, 97–111.

Garrett, D. D., Samanez-Larkin, G. R., MacDonald, S. W., Lindenberger, U., McIntosh, A. R., & Grady, C. L. (2013). Moment-to-moment brain signal variability: A next frontier in human brain mapping? *Neuroscience and Biobehavioral Reviews*, *37*(4), 610–624. doi:10.1016/j.neubiorev.2013.02.015 PMID:23458776

Gaston, C. M., & Mitchell, G. (2005). Information giving and decision-making in patients with advanced cancer: A systematic review. *Social Science & Medicine*, *61*(10), 2252–2264. doi:10.1016/j.socscimed.2005.04.015 PMID:15922501

Georgoulakis, J., Pouliakis, A., Koutroumbas, K., Megalopoulou, T. M., Archontakis, S., Kataitianos, I. G., ... Karakitsos, P. (2008). Discrimination of benign from malignant breast lesions using statistical clasifiers. *Archives of the Balkan Medical Union*, *43*(3), 149–153.

Gerostamoulos, D. (2013). Urinary drug screening. *Australian Prescriber, 36*(2), 62–64. doi:10.18773/austprescr.2013.025

Geunho, L., Jung, E.-J., Ohnuma, T., Chong, N. Y., & Yi, B.-J. (2011). JAIST Robotic Walker Control Based on a Two-Layered Kalman Filter. *2011 IEEE International Conference on Robotics and Automation*, 3682-3687.

Ghorai, K., Akter, S., Khatun, F., & Ray, P. (2014). mHealth for Smoking Cessation Programs: A Systematic Review. *Journal of Personalized Medicine, 4*(3), 412–423. doi:10.3390/jpm4030412 PMID:25563359

Giacomini, M., Ruggiero, C., Calegari, L., & Bertone, S. (2000). Artificial neural network based identification of environmental bacteria by gas-chromatographic and electrophoretic data. *Journal of Microbiological Methods, 43*(1), 45–54. doi:10.1016/S0167-7012(00)00203-7 PMID:11084227

Gimenez-Marin, A., Rivas-Ruiz, F., Perez-Hidalgo, M. M., & Molina-Mendoza, P. (2014). Preanalytical errors management in the clinical laboratory: A five-year study. *Biochemical Medicine, 24*(2), 248–257. doi:10.11613/BM.2014.027 PMID:24969918

Glaser, J. (2011). Cloud computing can simplify HIT infrastructure management. *Healthcare Financial Management, 65*(8), 52–55. PMID:21866720

Gleick, F. (1997). *Chaos: the Amazing Science of the Unpredictable*. London: Minerva.

Globe, D., Levin, S., Chang, T., Mackenzie, P., & Azen, S. (2002). Validity of the SF-12 Quality of Life Instrument in Patients with Retinal Diseases. *Ophthalmology, 109*(10), 1793–1798. doi:10.1016/S0161-6420(02)01124-7 PMID:12359596

Goodman, A., & Hutchinson, M. L. (1996). Cell surplus on sampling devices after routine cervical cytologic smears. A study of residual cell populations. *The Journal of Reproductive Medicine, 41*(4), 239–241. PMID:8728075

Grabe, N., Lahrmann, B., Pommerencke, T., von Knebel Doeberitz, M., Reuschenbach, M., & Wentzensen, N. (2010). A virtual microscopy system to scan, evaluate and archive biomarker enhanced cervical cytology slides. *Cellular Oncology, 32*(1-2), 109–119. doi:10.3233/CLO-2009-0508 PMID:20208139

Graf, B., Hans, M., & Schraft, R. (2004). Care-O-bot II—Development of a Next Generation Robotic Home Assistant. *Autonomous Robots, 16*(2), 193–205. doi:10.1023/B:AURO.0000016865.35796.e9

Grami, A., & Schell, B. H. (2004). *Future trends in mobile commerce: Service offerings, technological advances and security challenges*. Paper presented at the the Second Annual Conference on Privacy, Security and Trust.

Greenhalgh, T., Wherton, J., Papoutsi, C., Lynch, J., Hughes, J., A'Court, C., ... Shaw, S. (2017). Beyond Adoption: A New Framework for Theorizing and Evaluating Nonadoption, Abandonment, and Challenges to the Scale-Up, Spread, and Sustainability of Health and Care Technologies. *Journal of Medical Internet Research, 19*(11), e367. doi:10.2196/jmir.8775 PMID:29092808

Gupta, S., Chang, P., Anyigbo, N., & Sabharwal, A. (2011). mobileSpiro: accurate mobile spirometry for self-management of asthma. *Proceedings of the First ACM Workshop on Mobile Systems, Applications, and Services for Healthcare*. 10.1145/2064942.2064944

Gustavsson, A., Svensson, M., Jacobi, F., Allgulander, C., Alonso, J., Beghi, E., ... Olesen, J. (2011). Cost of disorders of the brain in Europe 2010. [PubMed]. *European Neuropsychopharmacology, 21*(10), 718–779. doi:10.1016/j.euroneuro.2011.08.008

Habib, J. L. (2010). EHRs, meaningful use, and a model EMR. *Drug Benefit Trends, 22*(4), 99–101.

Hallén, K., Orrenius, U., & Rose, L. (2006). *Ergonomical evaluation of the rollator prototype Walker*. ERAK report 2006-02.

Hammerling, J. A. (2012). A Review of MedicalErrors in Laboratory Diagnostics and WhereWe Are Today. *Laboratory Medicine, 43*(2), 41–44. Doi.org/10.1309/LM6ER9WJR1IHQAUY. doi:10.1309/LM6ER9WJR1IHQAUY

Handel, M. J. (2011). mHealth (mobile health)-using Apps for health and wellness. *Explore (New York, N.Y.), 7*(4), 256–261. doi:10.1016/j.explore.2011.04.011 PMID:21724160

Haralick, R. M., Shanmugam, K., & Dinstein, I. H. (1973). Textural Features for Image Classification. *Systems, Man and Cybernetics. IEEE Transactions on, 3*(6), 610–621.

Haren, V. (2011). *TOGAF Version 9.1 A Pocket Guide*. Van Haren Publishing.

Hawkins, R. (2012). Managing the pre- and post-analytical phases of the total testing process. *Annals of Laboratory Medicine, 32*(1), 5–16. doi:10.3343/alm.2012.32.1.5 PMID:22259773

Haykin, S. S. (1999). *Neural networks: a comprehensive foundation* (2nd ed.). Upper Saddle River, NJ: Prentice Hall.

Health Service Executive. (2015). *Guidance for calorie posting implementation*. Retrieved from: https://www.hse.ie/eng/health/hl/calorieposting/

Heart, T., Ben-Assuli, O., & Shabtai, I. (2017). A review of PHR, EMR and EHR integration: A more personalized healthcare and public health policy. *Health Policy and Technology, 6*(1), 20–25. doi:10.1016/j.hlpt.2016.08.002

Hebden, L., Cook, A., Van der Ploeg, H., & Allman-Farinelli, M. (2012). Development of Smartphone Applications for Nutrition and Physical Activity Behavior Change. *JMIR Research Protocols, 1(2), e9*. doi:10.2196/resprot.2205

Hekmatpanah, M., Ravichandran, N., Shahin, A., & Ahmadi, H. (2013). Investigating the Application of Six Sigma Methodology and Quality Control Tools and Techniques in Sepanhan Oil Company. *The Global eLearning Journal, 2*(3), 1-24.

Herrmann, M., Boehme, P., Mondritzki, T., Ehlers, J. P., Kavadias, S., & Truebel, H. (2018). Digital transformation and disruption of the health care sector: Internet-based observational study. *Journal of Medical Internet Research, 20*(3), e104. doi:10.2196/jmir.9498 PMID:29588274

Higgins, J. (2002). Nonlinear Systems in Medicine. *The Yale Journal of Biology and Medicine*, *75*, 247–260. PMID:14580107

Hill, K., Goldstein, R., Gartner, E. J., & Brooks, D. (2008). Daily Utility and Satisfaction With Rollators Among Persons With Chronic Obstructive Pulmonary Disease. *Archives of Physical Medicine and Rehabilitation*, *89*(6), 1108–1113. doi:10.1016/j.apmr.2007.11.032 PMID:18503807

Hillman, M. (2002). *Testimony before the Subcommittee on Health of the House Committee on Ways and Means, Hearing on Promoting Disease Management in Medicare*. Retrieved 10 June, 2015, from http://waysandmeans.house.gov/Legacy/health/107cong/4-16-02/4-16hill.htm

HiMSS Analytics. (2019). *EMRAM: A strategic roadmap for effective EMR adoption and maturity*. Retrieved from: http://www.himssanalytics.org/emram

HiMSS. (2011). *Electronic Health Records*. Retrieved from http://www.himss.org/library/ehr

HL7 International. (2014). *Personal Health Record System Functional Model, Release 1*. Retrieved from http://www.hl7.org/implement/standards/product_brief.cfm?product_id=88

Hochreiter, S., & Schmidhuber, J. (1997). Long Short-Term Memory. [PubMed]. *Neural Computation*, *9*(8), 1735–1780. doi:10.1162/neco.1997.9.8.1735

Hoffmann, C., McFarland, B., Kinzie, J., Bresler, L., Rakhlin, D., Wolf, S., & Kovas, A. E. (2005). Psychometric properties of a Russian version of the SF-12 Health Survey in a refugee population. *Comprehensive Psychiatry*, *46*(5), 390–397. doi:10.1016/j.comppsych.2004.12.002 PMID:16122541

Hollingworth, W., Devine, E. B., Hansen, R. N., Lawless, N. M., Comstock, B. A., Wilson-Norton, J. L., ... Sullivan, S. D. (2007). The impact of e-prescribing on prescriber and staff time in ambulatory care clinics: A time–motion study. *Journal of the American Medical Informatics Association*, *14*(6), 722–730. doi:10.1197/jamia.M2377 PMID:17712088

Holt-Lunstad, J., Smith, T. B., Baker, M., Harris, T., & Stephenson, J. (2015). Loneliness and Social Isolation as Risk Factors for Mortality: A Meta-Analytic Review. *Perspectives on Psychological Science*, *10*(2), 227–237. doi:10.1177/1745691614568352 PMID:25910392

Horwitz, R. I., Feinstein, A. R., Horwitz, S. M., & Robboy, S. J. (1981). Necropsy diagnosis of endometrial cancer and detection-bias in case/control studies. *Lancet*, *2*(8237), 66–68. doi:10.1016/S0140-6736(81)90412-8 PMID:6113441

Howe, R., & Spence, C. (2004). *Population Health Management: Healthways. In PopWorks* (Vol. 2, pp. 291–297). HCT Project. Retrieved from http://mthink.com/article/population-health-management-healthways-popworks/

Howlader, N., Noone, A. M., Krapcho, M., Neyman, N., Aminou, R., Waldron, W., … Edwards, B. K. (2011). *SEER Cancer Statistics Review, 1975-2008*. Retrieved 10 January 2015, 2015, from http://seer.cancer.gov/archive/csr/1975_2008/

Hsieh, Y. J., Huang, L. Y., & Wang, C. T. (2012). A framework for the selection of Six Sigma projects in services: Case studies of banking and health care services in Taiwan. *Service Business*, *6*(2), 243–264. doi:10.100711628-012-0134-1

Hsu, C. H., Lin, C. Y., Ouyang, M., & Guo, Y. K. (2013). Biocloud: Cloud computing for biological, genomics, and drug design. *BioMed Research International*, *909470*. doi:10.1155/2013/909470

Hühnlein, D., & Bach, M. (2007). How to use iso/iec 24727-3 with arbitrary smart cards. In *International Conference on Trust, Privacy and Security in Digital Business* (pp. 280-289). Springer. 10.1007/978-3-540-74409-2_30

Humphrey, N. (2002). *The mind made flesh*. Oxford, UK: Oxford University Press.

Hung, S. H., Wang, P. C., Lin, H. C., Chen, H. Y., & Su, C. T. (2015). Integration of Value Stream Map and Healthcare Failure Mode and Effect Analysis into Six Sigma Methodology to Improve Process of Surgical Specimen Handling. *Journal of Healthcare Engineering*, *6*(3), 377–398. doi:10.1260/2040-2295.6.3.377 PMID:26753440

Hunt, B. R., & York, J. A. (1993). Maxwell on chaos. *Nonlinear Sci. Today*, *3*, 1–4.

Hurst, N., Kind, P., Ruta, D., Hunter, M., & Stubbings, A. (1997). Measuring health related quality of life in rheumatoid arthritis: Validity, responsiveness and reliability of EuroQol (EQ-5D). *British Journal of Rheumatology*, *36*(5), 551–559. doi:10.1093/rheumatology/36.5.551 PMID:9189057

Iakovidis, I. (1998). Towards personal health record: Current situation, obstacles and trends in implementation of electronic healthcare record in Europe. *International Journal of Medical Informatics*, *52*(1-3), 105–115. doi:10.1016/S1386-5056(98)00129-4 PMID:9848407

Iatrakis, G., Diakakis, I., Kourounis, G., Sakellaropoulos, G., Rammos, G., Ladopoulos, J., ... Tzingounis, V. (1997). Postmenopausal uterine bleeding. *Clinical and Experimental Obstetrics & Gynecology*, *24*(3), 157. PMID:9478305

IFCC. (n.d.). Retrieved from http://www.ifcc.org/ifccfiles/docs/fundamentals-for-eqa.pdf

Iglezakis, I. (2015). *Legal Issues of Identity Management in eGovernment*. Available at SSRN 2690374.

IHE. (2018). *Audit Trail and Node Authentication*. Retrieved from https://wiki.ihe.net/index.php/Audit_Trail_and_Node_Authentication

Ilie, G., & Ciocoiu, C. N. (2010). Application of Fishbone Diagram to Determine the Risk of an Event with Multiple Causes. *Management Research and Practice*, *2*(1), 1–20.

Iltifat, H. (2010). Gyromaniac app for iPhone could help gastroenterologists when learning how to perform a colonoscopy. *iMedicalApps*. Retrieved 20 Aug., 2017, from https://www.imedicalapps.com/2010/06/gastroenterologists-iphone-4-medical-spatial-orientation/#

In vitro diagnostic medical devices 98/79 EC.

Indrawati, S., Firmansyah, A., & Sunaryo. (n.d.). *Manufacturing Performance Improvement through Integrated Six Sigma: An Aircraft Industry Case Application*. Retrieved from http://iieng.org/images/proceedings_pdf/7171E0114558.pdf

Institute of Medicine (IOM). (2005). *Performance Measurement: Accelerating Improvement*. Washington, DC: NationalAcademy Press.

ISO 15189:2012. (2012). *Medical laboratories – requirements for quality and competence*. Geneva, Switzerland: International Organization for Standardization.

ISO 17511:2003. (2003). *In vitro diagnostic medical devices -Measurement of quantities in biological samples - Metrological traceability of values assigned to calibrators and control materials*. ISO.

ISO 18153: 2003. (2003). *In vitro diagnostic medical devices – Measurement of quantities in biological samples – metrological traceability of values for catalytic concentration of enzymes assigned to calibrators and control materials*. ISO.

ISO/IEC .(2009). *Information Technology – Security techniques – Non-repudiation – Part 3: Non-Repudiation mechanisms using asymmetric techniques*. ISO/IEC13888-3:2009.

ISO/IEC 17025:2005. (2005). *General requirements for the competence of testing and calibration laboratories*. ISO.

ISO/IEC 17043 (2010). *Conformity assessment—General requirements for proficiency testing*. ISO.

ISO/TS 22367: 2008. (2008). *Medical laboratories—Reduction of error through risk management and continual improvement*. ISO.

Istepanian, R., Laxminarayan, S., & Pattichis, C. (Eds.). (2006). *M-Health: Emerging Mobile Health Systems*. New York: Springer. doi:10.1007/b137697

Itani, W., Kayssi, A., & Chehab, A. (2016). Wireless Body Sensor Networks: Security, Privacy, and Energy Efficiency in the Era of Cloud Computing. *International Journal of Reliable and Quality E-Healthcare*, *5*(2), 1–30. doi:10.4018/IJRQEH.2016040101

Jain, A. K. (1989). *Fundamentals of digital image processing* (1st ed.). Englewood Cliffs, NJ: Prentice Hall.

Janevski, T. (2009). *5G Mobile Phone Concept*. Paper presented at the 2009 6th IEEE Consumer Communications and Networking Conference.

JCAHO Joint Commission. (n.d.). *Accreditation, Health care, certification*. Retrieved from www.jointcommission.org

Jegede, F. E., Mbah, H. A., Aminu, M., Yakubu, T. N., & Torpey, K. (2015). Evaluation of Laboratory Performance withQualityIndicators in Infectious DiseaseHospital, Kano, Nigeria. *Open Journal of Clinical Diagnostics*, *5*(01), 1–9. doi:10.4236/ojcd.2015.51001

Jemal, A., Siegel, R., Ward, E., Murray, T., Xu, J., Smigal, C., & Thun, M. J. (2006). Cancer statistics, 2006. *CA: a Cancer Journal for Clinicians*, *56*(2), 106–130. doi:10.3322/canjclin.56.2.106 PMID:16514137

Johnson, P. T., Zimmerman, S. L., Heath, D., Eng, J., Horton, K. M., Scott, W. W., & Fishman, E. K. (2012). The iPad as a mobile device for CT display and interpretation: Diagnostic accuracy for identification of pulmonary embolism. *Emergency Radiology*, *19*(4), 323–327. doi:10.100710140-012-1037-0 PMID:22450843

Joncich, G. (1968). *The Sane Positivist: A Biography of Edward L. Thorndike*. Middletown: Wesleyan University Press.

Jones, G. R. (2016). Average of delta: A new quality control tool for clinicallaboratories. *Annals of Clinical Biochemistry*, *53*(1), 133–140. doi:10.1177/0004563215581400 PMID:25800407

Jones, G. R., & Koetsia, S. D. (2014). Combinedreferenceintervals and analytical EQA. *The Clinical Biochemist. Reviews / Australian Association of Clinical Biochemists*, *35*(4), 243–250.

Jospe, M. R., Fairbairn, K. A., Green, P., & Perry, T. L. (2015). Diet app use by sports dietitians: A survey in five countries. *JMIR mHealth and uHealth*, *3*(1), e7. doi:10.2196/mhealth.3345 PMID:25616274

Kanigel, R. (2005). *The One Best Way: Frederick Winslow Taylor and the Enigma of Efficiency*. Cambridge, MA: MIT Press Books.

Kant, A. K., & Graubard, B. I. (2004). Eating out in America, 1987-2000: Trends and nutritional correlates. *Preventive Medicine*, *38*(2), 243–249. doi:10.1016/j.ypmed.2003.10.004 PMID:14715218

Kapur, S., Phillips, A. G., & Insel, T. R. (2012). Why has it taken so long for biological psychiatry to develop clinical tests and what to do about it? [PubMed]. *Molecular Psychiatry*, *17*(12), 1174–1179. doi:10.1038/mp.2012.105

Karakitsos, P., Cochand-Priollet, B., Guillausseau, P. J., & Pouliakis, A. (1996). Potential of the back propagation neural network in the morphologic examination of thyroid lesions. *Analytical and Quantitative Cytology and Histology*, *18*(6), 494–500. PMID:8978873

Karakitsos, P., Cochand-Priollet, B., Pouliakis, A., Guillausseau, P. J., & Ioakim-Liossi, A. (1999). Learning vector quantizer in the investigation of thyroid lesions. *Analytical and Quantitative Cytology and Histology*, *21*(3), 201–208. PMID:10560492

Karakitsos, P., Ioakim-Liossi, A., Pouliakis, A., Botsoli-Stergiou, E. M., Tzivras, M., Archimandritis, A., & Kyrkou, K. (1998). A comparative study of three variations of the learning vector quantizer in the discrimination of benign from malignant gastric cells. *Cytopathology*, *9*(2), 114–125. doi:10.1046/j.1365-2303.1998.00063.x PMID:9577738

Karakitsos, P., Kyroudes, A., Pouliakis, A., Stergiou, E. B., Voulgaris, Z., & Kittas, C. (2002). Potential of the learning vector quantizer in the cell classification of endometrial lesions in postmenopausal women. *Analytical and Quantitative Cytology and Histology*, *24*(1), 30–38. PMID:11865947

Karakitsos, P., Megalopoulou, T. M., Pouliakis, A., Tzivras, M., Archimandritis, A., & Kyroudes, A. (2004). Application of discriminant analysis and quantitative cytologic examination to gastric lesions. *Analytical and Quantitative Cytology and Histology*, *26*(6), 314–322. PMID:15678613

Karakitsos, P., Pouliakis, A., Kordalis, G., Georgoulakis, J., Kittas, C., & Kyroudes, A. (2005). Potential of radial basis function neural networks in discriminating benign from malignant lesions of the lower urinary tract. *Analytical and Quantitative Cytology and Histology*, *27*(1), 35–42. PMID:15794450

Karakitsos, P., Pouliakis, A., Koutroumbas, K., Stergiou, E. B., Tzivras, M., Archimandritis, A., & Liossi, A. I. (2000). Neural network application in the discrimination of benign from malignant gastric cells. *Analytical and Quantitative Cytology and Histology*, *22*(1), 63–69. PMID:10696462

Karakitsos, P., Stergiou, E. B., Pouliakis, A., Tzivras, M., Archimandritis, A., Liossi, A. I., & Kyrkou, K. (1996). Potential of the back propagation neural network in the discrimination of benign from malignant gastric cells. *Analytical and Quantitative Cytology and Histology*, *18*(3), 245–250. PMID:8790840

Karakitsos, P., Stergiou, E. B., Pouliakis, A., Tzivras, M., Archimandritis, A., Liossi, A., & Kyrkou, K. (1997). Comparative study of artificial neural networks in the discrimination between benign from malignant gastric cells. *Analytical and Quantitative Cytology and Histology*, *19*(2), 145–152. PMID:9113307

Karar, M. E., & El-Brawany, M. A. (2011). Automated Cardiac Drug Infusion System Using Adaptive Fuzzy Neural Networks Controller. *Biomedical Engineering and Computational Biology*, *3*, 1-11. doi:10.4137/BECB.S6495

Karkalousos, P., & Evangelopoulos, A. (2011). *Quality Control in Clinical Laboratories, Applications and Experiences of Quality Control*. In Tech. Retrieved from http://www.intechopen.com/books/applications-and-experiences-of-quality-control/quality-control-in clinical-laboratories.

Kastania, A. N., & Moumtzoglou, A. (2012). Quality Implications of the Medical Applications for 4G Mobile Phones. *International Journal of Reliable and Quality E-Healthcare*, *1*(1), 58–67. doi:10.4018/ijrqeh.2012010106

Kastania, A., & Moumtzoglou, A. (2012). Is there a Quality linkage of E-health? *International Journal of Reliable and Quality E-Healthcare*, *1*(1), i–iv.

Katehakis, D. G., Gonçalves, J., Masi, M., & Bittins, S. (2017a). Interoperability Infrastructure Services to enable Secure, Cross-Border, Operational eHealth Services in Europe. *Proceedings of the 17th International HL7 Interoperability Conference IHIC 2017 "Re-shaping healthcare systems"*, 40-51. Retrieved from http://www.ics.forth.gr/~katehaki/publications/ihic2017-2.pdf

Katehakis, D. G. (2018). Electronic Medical Record Implementation Challenges for the National Health System in Greece. *International Journal of Reliable and Quality E-Healthcare*, *7*(1), 16–30. doi:10.4018/IJRQEH.2018010102

Katehakis, D. G., Halkiotis, S., & Kouroubali, A. (2011). Materialization of Regional Health Information Networks in Greece: Electronic Health Record Barriers & Enablers. *Journal of Healthcare Engineering*, *2*(3), 389–403. doi:10.1260/2040-2295.2.3.389

Katehakis, D. G., Kondylakis, H., Koumakis, L., Kouroubali, A., & Marias, K. (2017a). Integrated care solutions for the citizen: Personal health record functional models to support interoperability. *EJBI*, *13*(1), 41–56. doi:10.24105/ejbi.2017.13.1.8

Katehakis, D. G., & Kouroubali, A. (2019). A Framework for the Consistent Management of eHealth Interoperability in Greece. *Proceedings of the 21st International Conference on Enterprise Information Systems (ICEIS 2019)*, 2, 689-695. 10.5220/0007796906890695

Katehakis, D. G., Pangalos, G., & Prentza, A. (2015). Creating a European eHealth Space for cross-border ePrescription and Patient Summary Services. *Proceedings of the 12th European, Mediterranean & Middle Eastern Conference on Information Systems (EMCIS 2015).*

Katehakis, D. G., Pangalos, G., & Prentza, A. (2017b). Security Improvements for Better and Safer Cross-Border ePrescription and Patient Summary Services. *International Journal of Reliable and Quality E-Healthcare*, *6*(1), 18–28. doi:10.4018/IJRQEH.2017010102

Katehakis, D. G., & Tsiknakis, M. (2006). *Electronic health record.* Wiley Encyclopedia of Biomedical Engineering.

Kaur, N., Chahal, J. S., Bandlish, U., Kaul, R., Mardi, K., & Kaur, H. (2014). Correlation between cytological and histopathological examination of the endometrium in abnormal uterine bleeding. *Journal of Cytology / Indian Academy of Cytologists*, *31*(3), 144–148. doi:10.4103/0970-9371.145645 PMID:25538383

Kavakiotis, I., Tsave, O., Salifoglou, A., Maglaveras, N., Vlahavas, I., & Chouvarda, I. (2017). Machine Learning and Data Mining Methods in Diabetes Research. [PubMed]. *Computational and Structural Biotechnology Journal*, *15*, 104–116. doi:10.1016/j.csbj.2016.12.005

Kemp, G. M., Bird, C. E., & Barth, J. H. (2012). Short-term interventions on wards fail to Reducepreanalytical errors: Results of two prospective controlled trials. *Annals of Clinical Biochemistry*, *49*(2), 166–169. doi:10.1258/acb.2011.011133 PMID:22169099

Kenwothy, H. W. (2004). *Critical to quality-Aligning Improvement/Design efforts with customer requirements.* Retrieved 11 Sep., 2019, from https://www.slideshare.net/Vijay_Bijaj/critical-to-quality-aligning-improvement-design-efforts-with-customer-requirements

Kersten, P., Cardol, M., George, S., Ward, C., Sibley, A., & White, B. (2007). Validity of the impact on participation and autonomy questionnaire: A comparison between two countries. *Disability and Rehabilitation*, *29*(19), 1502–1509. doi:10.1080/09638280601030066 PMID:17852246

Kharbanda, V. C. J., Bohlin, N., Sehlstedt, U., & Treutiger, J. (2017). *Building the Smart Hospital Agenda*. Retrieved from https://www.adlittle.com/sites/default/files/viewpoints/ADL_Smart%20 Hospital.pdf

Kierkegaard, P. (2011). Electronic health record: Wiring Europe's healthcare. *Computer Law & Security Review*, *27*(5), 503–515. doi:10.1016/j.clsr.2011.07.013

Kierkegaard, P. (2013). E-prescription across Europe. *Health and Technology*, *3*(3), 205–219. doi:10.100712553-012-0037-0

Kindig, D. A. (2007). Understanding population health terminology. *The Milbank Quarterly*, *85*(1), 139–161. doi:10.1111/j.1468-0009.2007.00479.x PMID:17319809

King, G. (2011). Ensuring the data-rich future of the social sciences. *Science*, *331*(6018), 719–721. doi:10.1126cience.1197872 PMID:21311013

Kipp, B. R., Medeiros, F., Campion, M. B., Distad, T. J., Peterson, L. M., Keeney, G. L., ... Clayton, A. C. (2008). Direct uterine sampling with the Tao brush sampler using a liquid-based preparation method for the detection of endometrial cancer and atypical hyperplasia: A feasibility study. *Cancer*, *114*(4), 228–235. doi:10.1002/cncr.23636 PMID:18548528

Kiselev, A. R., Gridnev, V. I., Shvartz, V. A., Posnenkova, O. M., & Dovgalevsky, P. Y. (2012). Active ambulatory care management supported by short message services and mobile phone technology in patients with arterial hypertension. *Journal of the American Society of Hypertension*, *6*(5), 346–355. doi:10.1016/j.jash.2012.08.001 PMID:22995803

Kitanov, S., Monteiro, E., & Janevski, T. (2016). *5G and the Fog — Survey of related technologies and research directions*. Paper presented at the 2016 18th Mediterranean Electrotechnical Conference (MELECON).

Knop, K. (2016). Using a QFD method and CTQ Tree to identify the areas needing Improvement in the Product-Farm Truck Trailer. Academic Press.

Ko, C., & Agrawal, S. (2010). *Walk-Assist Robot: A Novel Approach to Gain Selection of a Braking Controller using Differential Flatness*. In 2010 American Control Conference. Marriott Waterfront, Baltimore, MD.

Koerbin, G., Sikaris, K. A., Jones, G. R., Ryan, J., Reed, M., & Tate, J. (2014). Evidence-based approach to harmonized reference intervals. *Clinica Chimica Acta*, *432*, 99–107. doi:10.1016/j.cca.2013.10.021 PMID:24183842

Kohonen, T., Kangas, J., Laaksonen, J., & Torkkola, K. (1992). *LVQPAK: A software package for the correct application of Learning Vector Quantization algorithms*. Paper presented at the Neural Networks, 1992. IJCNN., International Joint Conference on.

Kohonen, T. (1989). *Self-organization and associative memory* (3rd ed.). Berlin: Springer-Verlag. doi:10.1007/978-3-642-88163-3

Kontodimopoulos, N., Pappa, E., Niakas, D., & Tountas, Y. (2007). Validity of SF-12 summary scores in a Greek general population. *Health and Quality of Life Outcomes*, *5*(1), 55. doi:10.1186/1477-7525-5-55 PMID:17900374

Kontodimopoulos, N., Pappa, E., Niakas, D., Yfantopoulos, J., Dimitrakaki, C., & Tountas, Y. (2008). Validity of the EuroQoL (EQ-5D) instrument in a Greek General Population. *Value in Health*, 11. PMID:18489492

Kopcinovic, L. M., Trifunović, J., Pavosevic, T., & Nikolac, N. (2015). Croatian survey on critical results reporting. *Biochemia Medica*, *25*(2), 193–202. doi:10.11613/BM.2015.019 PMID:26110031

Koumpouros, Y. (2015). Big Data in Healthcare. In A. Information Resources Management (Ed.), Healthcare Administration: Concepts, Methodologies, Tools, and Applications (pp. 23-46). Hershey, PA: IGI Global. doi:10.4018/978-1-4666-6339-8.ch002

Koumpouros, Y., Karavasili, A., Efthimiou, E., Fotinea, S., Goulas, T., & Vacalopoulou, A. (2017b). User Evaluation of the MOBOT rollator type robotic mobility assistive device. *Proceedings Of The 10Th International Conference On Pervasive Technologies Related To Assistive Environments - PETRA '17*. 10.1145/3056540.3076183

Koumpouros, Y., Papageorgiou, E., & Karavasili, A. (2016). Development of a new psychometric scale (PYTHEIA) to assess the satisfaction of users with any assistive technology. *7th International Conference on Applied Human Factors and Ergonomics, AHFE 2016. Florida, USA: IEEE Proceedings.*

Koumpouros, Y. (2016). A Systematic Review on Existing Measures for the Subjective Assessment of Rehabilitation and Assistive Robot Devices. *Journal of Healthcare Engineering*, *2016*, 1–10. doi:10.1155/2016/1048964 PMID:27196802

Koumpouros, Y., Karavasili, A., Efthimiou, E., Fotinea, S., Goulas, T., & Vacalopoulou, A. (2017a). User Evaluation of the MOBOT Rollator Type Robotic Mobility Assistive Device. *Technologies*, *5*(4), 73. doi:10.3390/technologies5040073

Koumpouros, Y., Karavasili, A., Papageorgiou, E., & Siavelis, P. (2016). Validation of the Greek version of the device subscale of the Quebec User Evaluation of Satisfaction with Assistive Technology 2.0 (QUEST 2.0). *Assistive Technology*, *28*(3), 152–158. doi:10.1080/10400435.2015.1131758 PMID:26854178

Koumpouros, Y., Papageorgiou, E., Karavasili, A., & Koureta, F. (2016). PYTHEIA: A Scale for Assessing Rehabilitation and Assistive Robotics. *International Journal of Medical, Health, Biomedical, Bioengineering and Pharmaceutical Engineering*, *10*(11), 522–526.

Kouroubali, A., & Katehakis, D. G. (2019). The new European interoperability framework as a facilitator of digital transformation for citizen empowerment. *Journal of Biomedical Informatics*, *94*, 103166. doi:10.1016/j.jbi.2019.103166 PMID:30978512

Kourou, K., Exarchos, T. P., Exarchos, K. P., Karamouzis, M. V., & Fotiadis, D. I. (2015). Machine learning applications in cancer prognosis and prediction. [PubMed]. *Computational and Structural Biotechnology Journal*, *13*, 8–17. doi:10.1016/j.csbj.2014.11.005

Koutroumbas, K., Pouliakis, A., Megalopoulou, T., Georgoulakis, J., Giachnaki, A.-E., & Karakitsos, P. (2006). Discrimination of Benign from Malignant Breast Lesions Using Statistical Classifiers. In G. Antoniou, G. Potamias, C. Spyropoulos, & D. Plexousakis (Eds.), *Advances in Artificial Intelligence* (Vol. 3955, pp. 543–546). Springer Berlin Heidelberg. doi:10.1007/11752912_64

Kredo, T., Bernhardsson, S., Machingaidze, S., Young, T., Louw, Q., Ochodo, E., & Grimmer, K. (2016). Guide to clinical practice guidelines: The current state of play. *International Journal for Quality in Health Care*, *28*(1), 122–128. doi:10.1093/intqhc/mzv115 PMID:26796486

Krzysztof, W., & Krzysztof, P. M. (2016). Translation of Medical Texts using Neural Networks. *International Journal of Reliable and Quality E-Healthcare*, *5*(4), 51–66. doi:10.4018/IJRQEH.2016100104

Kulyukin, V. A., Kutiyanawala, A., LoPresti, E., Matthews, J. T., & Simpson, R. (2008). iWalker: Toward a Rollator-Mounted Wayfinding System for the Elderly. *2008 IEEE International Conference on RFID*, 303-311.

Kumar, N. S., & Ray, L. (2013). Application of Sigma Metrics in Medical Biochemistry. *Journal of Clinical and Diagnostic Research: JCDR*, *7*(12), 2689–2691. doi:10.7860/JCDR/2013/7292.3700 PMID:24551613

Kumar, S., Nilsen, W. J., Abernethy, A., Atienza, A., Patrick, K., Pavel, M., ... Swendeman, D. (2013). Mobile health technology evaluation: The mHealth evidence workshop. *American Journal of Preventive Medicine*, *45*(2), 228–236. doi:10.1016/j.amepre.2013.03.017 PMID:23867031

Kuo, A. M. (2011). Opportunities and challenges of cloud computing to improve health care services. *Journal of Medical Internet Research*, *13*(3), e67. doi:10.2196/jmir.1867 PMID:21937354

Kyroudi, A., Paefthimiou, M., Symiakaki, H., Mentzelopoulou, P., Voulgaris, Z., & Karakitsos, P. (2006). Increasing diagnostic accuracy with a cell block preparation from thin-layer endometrial cytology: A feasibility study. *Acta Cytologica*, *50*(1), 63–69. doi:10.1159/000325896 PMID:16514842

Lai, M. (2015). *Deep Learning for Medical Image Segmentation.* preprint arXiv, arXiv:1505.02000.

Lakshman, M., Ravindra Reddy, B., & Bhulaxmi, P. (2015). Evaluation of sigma metrics in a Medical Biochemistry lab. *International Journal of Biomedical Research*, *6*(03), 164–171. doi:10.7439/ijbr.v6i3.1709

Lam, Q., Ajzner, E., Campbell, C. A., & Young, A. (2016). Critical risk results – an update on international initiatives. *EJIFCC*, *27*(1), 66–76. PMID:27683507

Lao, E.G., García, A.S., Figuerola, M.B., Ester Moreno, E., & Paraire, A.H. (2017). Errors of Clinical Laboratory and Its Impact on Patient Safety. *Open Journal of Social Sciences, 5*, 243-253.

Laugesen, K., Baggesen, L. M., Schmidt, S. L. J., Glymour, M. M., Mathias, L., Arnold, M., & … . (2018). Social isolation and all-cause mortality:a population-based cohort study in Denmark. *Scientific Reports*, *8*(1), 4731. doi:10.103841598-018-22963-w PMID:29549355

Leitold, H., Lioy, A., & Ribeiro, C. (2014). Stork 2.0: Breaking new grounds on eid and mandates. In *Proceedings of ID World International Congress* (pp. 1-8). Academic Press.

Lesko, L. J. (2007). Personalized Medicine: Elusive Dream or Imminent Reality? *Clinical Pharmacology and Therapeutics*, *81*(6), 807–816. doi:10.1038j.clpt.6100204 PMID:17505496

Levsky, J. M., & Singer, R. H. (2003). Gene expression and the myth of the average cell. *Trends in Cell Biology*, *13*(1), 4–6. doi:10.1016/S0962-8924(02)00002-8 PMID:12480334

Lewin, R. (1999). *Complexity: Life at the Edge of Chaos*. Chicago: The University of Chicago Press.

Lezzoni, L. I., Rao, S. R., & Kinkel, R. P. (2009). Patterns of mobility aid use among working-age persons with multiple sclerosis living in the community in the United States. *Disability and Health Journal*, *2*(2), 67–76. doi:10.1016/j.dhjo.2008.12.001 PMID:21122745

Liebow, E. B., Derzon, J. H., Fontanesi, J., Favoretto, A. M., Baetz, R. A., Shaw, C., ... Epner, P. (2012). Effectiveness of Automated Notification and CustomerServiceCallCenters for Timely and Accurate Reporting of Critical Values: A Laboratory Medicine Best Practices Systematic Review and Meta-Analysis. *Clinical Biochemistry*, *45*(13-14), 979–987. doi:10.1016/j.clinbiochem.2012.06.023 PMID:22750773

Lim, L., & Fisher, J. (1999). Use of the 12-item short-form (SF-12) health survey in an Australian heart and stroke population. *Quality of Life Research: An International Journal of Quality of Life Aspects of Treatment, Care and Rehabilitation*, *8*(1-2), 1–8. doi:10.1023/A:1026409226544 PMID:10457733

Linder, J. A., Schnipper, J. L., Tsurikova, R., Melnikas, A. J., Volk, L. A., & Middleton, B. (2006). Barriers to electronic health record use during patient visits. *AMIA ... Annual Symposium Proceedings - AMIA Symposium. AMIA Symposium*, *2006*, 499. PMID:17238391

Lippi, G., Baird, G. S., Banfi, G., Bölenius, K., Cadamuro, J., Church, S., ... Simundic, A.-M. (2017). Improving quality in the preanalytical phase through innovation, on behalf of the European Federation for Clinical Chemistry and Laboratory Medicine (EFLM) Working Group for Preanalytical Phase (WG-PRE). *Clinical Chemistry and Laboratory Medicine*, *55*(4), 489–500. doi:10.1515/cclm-2017-0107 PMID:28231060

Lippi, G., Becan-McBride, K., Behúlová, D., Bowen, R. A., Church, S., Delanghe, J., ... Simundic, A.-M. (2013). Preanalytical quality improvement: In quality we trust. *Clinical Chemistry and Laboratory Medicine*, *51*(1), 229–241. doi:10.1515/cclm-2012-0597 PMID:23072858

Lippi, G., Betsou, F., Cadamuro, J., Cornes, M., Fleischhacker, M., Neumaier, M., & … . (2019). Working Group for Preanalytical Phase (WG-PRE), European Federation of Clinical Chemistry and Laboratory Medicine (EFLM).Preanalytical challenges - time for solutions. *Clinical Chemistry and Laboratory Medicine*, *57*(7), 974–981. doi:10.1515/cclm-2018-1334 PMID:30710481

Lippi, G., & Cadamuro, J. (2017). Novel opportunities for improving the quality of preanalytical phase. A glimpse to the future? *Journal of Medical Biochemistry*, *36*(4), 1–6. doi:10.1515/jomb-2017-0029 PMID:30581325

Lippi, G., Chance, J. J., Church, S., Dazzi, P., Fontana, R., Giavarina, D., ... Simundic, A.-M. (2011). Preanalytical quality improvement: From dream to reality. *Clinical Chemistry and Laboratory Medicine*, *49*(7), 1113–1126. doi:10.1515/CCLM.2011.600 PMID:21517699

Lippi, G., Mattiuzzi, C., & Favaloro, E. J. (2015). Pre-analytical variability and quality of diagnostic testing. Looking at the moon and gazing beyond the finger. *N Z J Med Lab Sci*, *69*, 4–8.

Lippi, G., & Plebani, M. (2018). A Six-Sigma approach for comparing diagnostic errors in healthcare-where does laboratory medicine stand? *Annals of Translational Medicine*, *6*(10), 180. doi:10.21037/atm.2018.04.02 PMID:29951502

Lippi, G., Plebani, M., & Graber, M. L. (2016). Building a bridge to safe diagnosis in health care. The role of the clinical laboratory. *Clinical Chemistry and Laboratory Medicine*, *54*(1), 1–3. doi:10.1515/cclm-2015-1135 PMID:26630697

Lippi, G., von Meyer, A., Cadamuro, J., & Simundic, A. M. (2019). Blood sample quality. *Diagnosis (Berl)*, *6*(1), 25–31. doi:10.1515/dx-2018-0018 PMID:29794250

Li, T., & Yorke, J. A. (1975). Period three implies chaos. *The American Mathematical Monthly*, *82*(10), 985–992. doi:10.1080/00029890.1975.11994008

Liu, Q., Cui, X., Abbod, M. F., Huang, S.-J., Han, Y.-Y., & Shieh, J. (2011). Brain death prediction based on ensembled artificial neural networks in neurosurgical intensive care unit. *Journal of the Taiwan Institute of Chemical Engineers*, *42*(1), 97–107. doi:10.1016/j.jtice.2010.05.006

Longford, N. T. (1987). A fast scoring algorithm for maximum likelihood estimation in unbalanced mixed models with nested random effects. *Biometrika*, *74*(4), 817–827. doi:10.1093/biomet/74.4.817

Lovell, M., & Foy, M. A. (2018). General Data Protection Regulation May 2018 (GDPR) How does it affect us? *Bone & Joint 360, 7*(4), 41-42.

Lovell, N., & Bibby, J. (2018). *What makes us healthy? An introduction to the social determinants of health*. London: The Health Foundation.

Low, D., Kuralmani, V., Ng, S. K., Lee, K. K., Ng, I., & Ang, B. T. (2009). Prediction of Outcome Utilizing Both Physiological and Biochemical Parameters in Severe Head Injury. [PubMed]. *Journal of Neurotrauma*, *26*(8), 1177–1182. doi:10.1089/neu.2008.0841

Lu, J., Yao, J. E., & Yu, C.-S. (2005). Personal innovativeness, social influences and adoption of wireless Internet services via mobile technology. *The Journal of Strategic Information Systems*, *14*(3), 245–268. doi:10.1016/j.jsis.2005.07.003

Lund, F., Petersen, P. H., Fraser, C. G., & Sölétormos, G. (2015). Calculation of limits for significant bidirectional changes in two or more serial results of a biomarker based on a computer simulation model. *Annals of Clinical Biochemistry*, *52*(4), 434–440. doi:10.1177/0004563214555163 PMID:25249664

Luo, H., Ye, H., Ng, H. W., Shi, L., Tong, W., Mendrick, D. L., & Hong, H. (2015). Machine Learning Methods for Predicting HLA-Peptide Binding Activity. *Bioinformatics and Biology Insights*, *9*(Suppl 3), 21–29. doi:10.4137/BBI.S29466 PMID:26512199

Lupse, O. S., Vida, M., & Stoicu-Tivadar, L. (2012). Cloud computing technology applied in healthcare for developing large scale flexible solutions. *Studies in Health Technology and Informatics*, *174*, 94–99. PMID:22491119

Mack, C. A. (2011). Fifty Years of Moore's Law. *IEEE Transactions on Semiconductor Manufacturing*, *24*(2), 202–207. doi:10.1109/TSM.2010.2096437

Maksem, J. A., Meiers, I., & Robboy, S. J. (2007). A primer of endometrial cytology with histological correlation. *Diagnostic Cytopathology*, *35*(12), 817–844. doi:10.1002/dc.20745 PMID:18008351

Maksem, J. A., Robboy, S. J., Bishop, J. W., & Meiers, I. (2009). *Endometrial Cytology with Tissue Correlations*. New York: Springer US.

Malone, R. E. (2003). Distal nursing. *Social Science & Medicine*, *56*(11), 2317–2326. doi:10.1016/S0277-9536(02)00230-7 PMID:12719184

Mandelbrot, B. B. (1983). The fractal geometry of nature (Updated and augm. ed.). New York: W.H. Freeman.

Marasinghe, J. P., Chintana, H. D., Karunananda, S. A., & Amarasinghe, A. A. (2007). Liquid-based endometrial cytology: its possible value in postmenopausal asymptomatic women. *Int J Gynecol Cancer, 17*(4), 934; author reply 935. doi:10.1111/j.1525-1438.2007.00918.x

Margari, N., Pouliakis, A., Anoinos, D., Terzakis, E., Koureas, N., Chrelias, C., ... Karakitsos, P. (2016). A reporting system for endometrial cytology: Cytomorphologic criteria-Implied risk of malignancy. *Diagnostic Cytopathology*, *44*(11), 888–901. doi:10.1002/dc.23605 PMID:27653446

Margari, N., Pouliakis, A., Spathis, A., Mastorakis, E., Karakostas, E. S. S., Panayiotides, I., & Karakitsos, P. (2015). Quality Control and Telemedicine for BRAF V600E Mutations in Papillary Thyroid Carcinomas: Image Analysis and Classification and Regression Trees. *International Journal of Reliable and Quality E-Healthcare*, *4*(2), 12–30. doi:10.4018/IJRQEH.2015040102

Market Research Future. (2017). *Global Big Data in Healthcare Market Promises a Striking Revenue of USD 35 Billion By 2021*. Retrieved 27 Aug., 2017, from http://www.prnewswire.com/news-releases/global-big-data-in-healthcare-market-promises-a-striking-revenue-of-usd-35-billion-by-2021-300472980.html

Markets and Markets. (2017). *Healthcare Analytics Market worth 24.55 Billion USD by 2021.* Retrieved 25 Aug., 2017, from http://www.marketsandmarkets.com/PressReleases/healthcare-data-analytics.asp

Markoff, J., & Lohr, S. (2016). The Race Is On to Control Artificial Intelligence, and Tech's Future. The New York Times. Retrieved April 3, 2017, from https://www.nytimes.com/2016/03/26/technology/the-race-is-on-to-control-artificial-intelligence-and-techs-future.html?_r=0

Markopoulos, C., Karakitsos, P., Botsoli-Stergiou, E., Pouliakis, A., Gogas, J., Ioakim-Liossi, A., & Kyrkou, K. (1997). Application of back propagation to the diagnosis of breast lesions by fine needle aspiration. *The Breast*, *6*(5), 293–298. doi:10.1016/S0960-9776(97)90008-4

Markopoulos, C., Karakitsos, P., Botsoli-Stergiou, E., Pouliakis, A., Ioakim-Liossi, A., Kyrkou, K., & Gogas, J. (1997). Application of the learning vector quantizer to the classification of breast lesions. *Analytical and Quantitative Cytology and Histology*, *19*(5), 453–460. PMID:9349906

Martins, M., Frizera-Neto, A., Urendes, E., dos Santos, C., Ceres, R., & Bastos-Filho, T. (2012). A novel human-machine interface for guiding: The neoasas smart walker. *Biosignals and Biorobotics Conference (BRC).* 10.1109/BRC.2012.6222195

Martins, M., Santos, C., Frizera-Neto, A., & Ceres, R. (2012). Assistive mobility devices focusing on Smart Walkers: Classification and review. *Robotics and Autonomous Systems*, *60*(4), 548–562. doi:10.1016/j.robot.2011.11.015

Martin, T. (2012). Assessing mHealth: Opportunities and barriers to patient engagement. *Journal of Health Care for the Poor and Underserved*, *23*(3), 935–941. doi:10.1353/hpu.2012.0087 PMID:24212144

Masalski, M., Kipiński, L., Grysiński, T., & Kręcicki, T. (2016). Hearing Tests on Mobile Devices: Evaluation of the Reference Sound Level by Means of Biological Calibration. *Journal of Medical Internet Research*, *18*(5), e130. doi:10.2196/jmir.4987 PMID:27241793

May, R. M. (1974). Biological populations with nonoverlapping generations: Stable points,stable cycles, and chaos. *Science*, *186*(4164), 645–647. doi:10.1126cience.186.4164.645 PMID:4412202

Mazziotta, J. C., Woods, R., Iacoboni, M., Sicotte, N., Yaden, K., Tran, M., ... Toga, A. W. (2009). The myth of the normal, average human brain--the ICBM experience: (1) subject screening and eligibility. *NeuroImage*, *44*(3), 914–922. doi:10.1016/j.neuroimage.2008.07.062 PMID:18775497

Medical Design. (2013). *Platform makes possible remote fetal monitoring and cardiac care.* Retrieved 10 Aug., 2017, from http://medicaldesign.com/business/platform-makes-possible-remote-fetal-monitoring-and-cardiac-care

Megalopoulou, T. M., Koutroumbas, K., Pouliakis, A., Sivolapenko, G., & Karakitsos, P. (2006). The potential of feature selection by statistical techniques and the use of statistical classifiers in the discrimination of benign from malignant gastric lesions. *Oncology Reports*, *15*(Spec no), 1033–1036. PMID:16525696

Melin, U., Axelsson, K., & Söderström, F. (2016). Managing the development of e-ID in a public e-service context – challenges and path dependencies from a life-cycle perspective. *Transforming Government: People. Process and Policy*, *10*(1), 77–98.

Melin, U., Axelsson, K., & Söderström, F. (2016). Managing the development of e-ID in a public e-service context: Challenges and path dependencies from a life-cycle perspective. *Transforming Government: People. Process and Policy*, *10*(1), 72–98.

Mellors, R. C., & Silver, R. (1951). A micro-fluorometric scanner for the differential detection of cells; application of exfoliative cytology. *Science*, *114*(2962), 356–360. doi:10.1126cience.114.2962.356 PMID:14883859

Menachemi, N., & Collum, T. H. (2011). Benefits and drawbacks of electronic health record systems. *Risk Management and Healthcare Policy*, *4*, 47. doi:10.2147/RMHP.S12985 PMID:22312227

Mendes, M. E., Ebner, P. R., Romano, P., Neto, M. P., Sant'anna, A., & Sumita, N. M. (2013). Practical aspects of the use of FMEA tool in clinical laboratory risk management. *Jornal Brasileiro de Patologia e Medicina Laboratorial*, *49*(3), 174–181. doi:10.1590/S1676-24442013000300004

Metelmann, C., & Metelmann, B. (2017). Can a Mobile Video Communication Improve Patient Safety in Prehospital Emergency Medicine? *International Journal of Reliable and Quality E-Healthcare*, *6*(4), 27–36. doi:10.4018/IJRQEH.2017100104

Michels, J. D., & Walden, I. (2018). How Safe is Safe Enough? Improving Cybersecurity in Europe's Critical Infrastructure Under the NIS Directive. *Improving Cybersecurity in Europe's Critical Infrastructure Under the NIS Directive (December 7, 2018). Queen Mary School of Law Legal Studies Research Paper*, (291).

Mikulecky, D. C. (1996). Complexity, communication between cells, and identifying the functional components of living systems: Some observations. *Acta Biotheoretica*, *44*(3-4), 179–208. doi:10.1007/BF00046527 PMID:8953209

Milieu Ltd & time.lex. (2014). *Overview of the national laws on electronic health records in the EU Member States and their interaction with the provision of cross-border eHealth services. Final report and* recommendations. Brussels. Retrieved from http://ec.europa.eu/health/ehealth/docs/laws_report_recommendations_en.pdf

Milieu Ltd and Time.lex. (2013). *Overview of the national laws on electronic health records in the EU Member States, National Report for Greece*. Retrieved from http://ec.europa.eu/health//sites/health/files/ehealth/docs/laws_greece_en.pdf

Mindell, D. A. (2015). *Our robots, ourselves: robotics and the myths of autonomy*. Viking.

Ministers in charge of eGovernment policy and coordination from 32 countries of the EU and EFTA. (2017). *Tallinn Declaration on eGovernment at the ministerial meeting during Estonian Presidency of the Council of the EU on 6 October 2017*. Retrieved from https://ec.europa.eu/newsroom/document.cfm?doc_id=47559

Minor, M., & Minor, S. (2013). *Patient care skills* (7th ed.). Pearson.

Miri-Dashe, T., Osawe, S., Tokdung, M., Daniel, N., Choji, R. P., Mamman, I., ... Abimiku, A. (2014). ComprehensiveReferenceRanges for Hematology and Clinical Chemistry Laboratory Parameters Derived from Normal Nigerian Adults. *PLoS One*, *9*(5), e93919. doi:10.1371/journal.pone.0093919 PMID:24832127

Mirza, H., & El-Masri, S. (2013). National Electronic Medical Records integration on Cloud Computing System. *Studies in Health Technology and Informatics*, *192*, 1219. PMID:23920993

Mischel, W. (1973). Toward a cognitive social learning reconceptualization of personality. *Psychological Review*, *80*(4), 252–283. doi:10.1037/h0035002 PMID:4721473

Mitchell, C., Hobcraft, J., McLanahan, S. S., Siegel, S. R., Berg, A., Brooks-Gunn, J., ... Notterman, D. (2014). Social disadvantage, genetic sensitivity,and children's telomere length. *Proceedings of the National Academy of Sciences of the United States of America*, *111*(16), 5944–5949. doi:10.1073/pnas.1404293111 PMID:24711381

Mitchell, T. M. (1997). *Machine Learning*. McGraw-Hill.

Mobisante Inc. (2017). *MobiSante Inc. web site*. Retrieved 19 Aug., 2017, from http://www.mobisante.com

Molenaar, P. (2007). On the Implications of the Classical Ergodic Theorems: Analysis of Developmental Processes Has to Focus on Intra-Individual Variation. *Developmental Psychobiology*, *50*(1), 60–69. doi:10.1002/dev.20262 PMID:18085558

Molenaar, P. C. M. (2013). On the necessity to use person-specific data analysis approaches in psychology. *European Journal of Developmental Psychology*, *10*(1), 29–39. doi:10.1080/17405629.2012.747435

Mondorf, A., & Wimmer, M. A. (2016). Requirements for an architecture framework for Pan-European e-Government Services. In *International Conference on Electronic Government* (pp. 135-150). Springer. 10.1007/978-3-319-44421-5_11

Montfort, A.P.W.P., & van der Helm, M.H.J. (2006). Telemonitoring of Patients with Chronic Heart Failure. *Disease Management & Health Outcomes*, *14*(1), 33–35.

Moore, G. E. (1965). Cramming More Components Onto Integrated Circuits, Electronics, April 19, 1965. *Electronics (Basel)*, *38*(8), 82–85. doi:10.1109/JPROC.1998.658762

Morris, M. E., & Aguilera, A. (2012). Mobile, Social, and Wearable Computing and the Evolution of Psychological Practice. *Professional Psychology, Research and Practice*, *43*(6), 622–626. doi:10.1037/a0029041 PMID:25587207

Moses, R. E., & Feld, A. D. (2008). Legal risks of clinical practice guidelines. *The American Journal of Gastroenterology*, *103*(1), 7–11. doi:10.1111/j.1572-0241.2007.01399.x PMID:18184116

Moumtzoglou, A. (2014). Demystifying Quality of Healthcare in the Cloud. In M. Anastasius & N. K. Anastasia (Eds.), *Cloud Computing Applications for Quality Health Care Delivery* (pp. 284–301). Hershey, PA: IGI Global. doi:10.4018/978-1-4666-6118-9.ch015

Moumtzoglou, A. (Ed.). (2016). *M-Health Innovations for Patient-Centered Care*. Hershey, PA: IGI Global. doi:10.4018/978-1-4666-9861-1

Moumtzoglou, A., & Kastania, A. (Eds.). (2014). *Cloud computing applications for quality health care delivery*. Hershey, PA: IGI Global. doi:10.4018/978-1-4666-6118-9

Moumtzoglou, A., & Pouliakis, A. (2015). Mapping Population Health Management Roadmap into Cervical Cancer Screening Programs. *International Journal of Reliable and Quality E-Healthcare*, *4*(3), 1–18. doi:10.4018/IJRQEH.2015070101

Moumtzoglou, A., & Pouliakis, A. (2018). Populatin health Management & the Science of Individuality. *International Journal of Reliable and Quality E-Healthcare*, *7*(2), 1–25. doi:10.4018/IJRQEH.2018040101

Mourtzikou, A., Stamouli, M., & Athanasiadi, E. (2013). Article. *International Journal of Reliable and Quality E-Healthcare, 2*(2), 38-46. Doi: 104018/ijrqeh.2013040103

Mourtzikou, A., & Stamouli, M. (2017). An Update On Best Practices and Regulatory Requirements for the Improvement of Clinical Laboratory Services through Quality. *International Journal of Reliable and Quality E-Healthcare*, *6*(1), 1–17. doi:10.4018/IJRQEH.2017010101

Mouwen, D. J., Capita, R., Alonso-Calleja, C., Prieto-Gomez, J., & Prieto, M. (2006). Artificial neural network based identification of Campylobacter species by Fourier transform infrared spectroscopy. *Journal of Microbiological Methods*, *67*(1), 131–140. doi:10.1016/j.mimet.2006.03.012 PMID:16632003

Murphy, L. J., Murphy, L. C., & Friesen, H. G. (1987). Estrogen induces insulin-like growth factor-I expression in the rat uterus. *Molecular Endocrinology (Baltimore, Md.)*, *1*(7), 445–450. doi:10.1210/mend-1-7-445 PMID:2484720

Murray, E., Burns, J., See Tai, S., Lai, R., & Nazareth, I. (2005). Interactive Health Communication Applications for people with chronic disease. *Cochrane Database of Systematic Reviews*, *CD004274*(4). PMID:16235356

Murray, H. A. (1938). *Explorations in personality:Aclinical and experimental study of fifty men of college age Press*. New York, NY: Oxford University.

Myers, G. L., & Miller, W. G. (2016). The International Consortium for Harmonization of Clinical Laboratory Results (ICHCLR) – A pathway for harmonization. *EJIFCC*, *27*(1), 30–36. PMID:27683504

Nalin, M., Baroni, I., Faiella, G., Romano, M., Matrisciano, F., Gelenbe, E., ... Koutkias, V. (2019). The European cross-border health data exchange roadmap: Case study in the Italian setting. *Journal of Biomedical Informatics*, *94*, 103183. doi:10.1016/j.jbi.2019.103183 PMID:31009760

Nesselroade, J. R., Gerstorf, D., Hardy, S. A., & Ram, N. (2007). Focus Article: Idiographic Filters for Psychological Constructs. *Measurement: Interdisciplinary Research and Perspectives*, *5*(4), 217–235. doi:10.1080/15366360701741807

Neuburger, J., Walker, K., Sherlaw-Johnson, C., van der Meulen, J., & Cromwell, D. A. (2017). Comparison of control charts for monitoring clinical performance using binary data. *BMJ Quality & Safety*, *26*(11), 919–928. doi:10.1136/bmjqs-2016-005526 PMID:28947635

Nguyen, K. (2018). Certification of eIDAS trust services and new global transparency trends. *Datenschutz und Datensicherheit-DuD*, *42*(7), 424–428. doi:10.100711623-018-0972-7

Nilsson, E., Wenemark, M., Bendtsen, P., & Kristenson, M. (2007). Respondent satisfaction regarding SF-36 and EQ-5D, and patients' perspectives concerning health outcome assessment within routine health care. *Quality of Life Research: An International Journal of Quality of Life Aspects of Treatment, Care and Rehabilitation*, *16*(10), 1647–1654. doi:10.100711136-007-9263-8 PMID:17922304

Njoroge, W. S., & Nichols, H. J. (2014). Risk Management in the Clinical Laboratory. *Annals of Laboratory Medicine*, *34*(4), 274–278. doi:10.3343/alm.2014.34.4.274 PMID:24982831

Noble, M. (2009). *Quality Management for the Medical Laboratory*. Retrieved from www.polqm.ca/.../qmformedlab2008

Nollen, N. L., Mayo, M. S., Carlson, S. E., Rapoff, M. A., Goggin, K. J., & Ellerbeck, E. F. (2014). Mobile technology for obesity prevention: A randomized pilot study in racial- and ethnic-minority girls. *American Journal of Preventive Medicine*, *46*(4), 404–408. doi:10.1016/j.amepre.2013.12.011 PMID:24650843

Nordin, G. (2015). Before defining performance criteria we must agree on what a "qualitative test procedure" is. *Clinical Chemistry and Laboratory Medicine*, *53*(6), 939–941. doi:10.1515/cclm-2015-0005 PMID:25879322

Norimatsu, Y., Yanoh, K., & Kobayashi, T. K. (2013). The role of liquid-based preparation in the evaluation of endometrial cytology. *Acta Cytologica*, *57*(5), 423–435. doi:10.1159/000353148 PMID:24021666

Notterman, D. A., & Mitchell, C. (2015). Epigenetics and understanding the impact of social determinants of health. *Pediatric Clinics of North America*, *62*(5), 1227–1240. doi:10.1016/j.pcl.2015.05.012 PMID:26318949

O'Connor, Y., Heavin, C., & O'Donoghue, J. (2015). Review of Key Stakeholders for an mHealth Pilot Study in Malawi Motivations and Expectations. *International Journal of Reliable and Quality E-Healthcare*, *4*(2), 51–66. doi:10.4018/IJRQEH.2015040105

OASIS. (2017a). *Business Document Metadata Service Location Version 1.0*. OASIS Standard. Retrieved from http://docs.oasis-open.org/bdxr/BDX-Location/v1.0/BDX-Location-v1.0.html

OASIS. (2017b). *Service Metadata Publishing (SMP) Version 1.0*. OASIS Standard. Retrieved from http://docs.oasis-open.org/bdxr/bdx-smp/v1.0/bdx-smp-v1.0.html

Obesity Policy Coalition. (2018). *Policy brief: Menu kilojoule labelling in chain food outlets in Australia*. Retrieved January, 2018 from: http://www.opc.org.au/downloads/policy-briefs/menu-kj-labelling-in-chain-food-outlets-in-australia.pdf

Office for National Statistics. (n.d.). *Which occupations are at highest risk of being automated?* Retrieved June 3, 2019, from www.ons.gov.uk/employmentandlabourmarket/peopleinwork/employmentandemployeetypes/articles/whichoccupationsareathighestriskofbeingautomated/2019-03-25

Okumus, B., Ali, F., Bilgihan, A., & Ozturk, A. B. (2018). Psychological factors influencing customers' acceptance of smartphone diet apps when ordering food at restaurants. *International Journal of Hospitality Management*, *72*, 67–77. doi:10.1016/j.ijhm.2018.01.001

Okumus, B., & Bilgihan, A. (2014). Proposing a model to test smartphone users' intention to use smart applications when ordering food in restaurants. *Journal of Hospitality and Tourism Technology*, *5*(1), 31–49. doi:10.1108/JHTT-01-2013-0003

Okumus, B., Bilgihan, A., & Ozturk, A. B. (2016). Factors Affecting the Acceptance of Smartphone Diet Applications. *Journal of Hospitality Marketing & Management*, *25*(6), 726–747. doi:10.1080/19368623.2016.1082454

Orfanos, P., Naska, A., Trichopoulos, D., Slimani, N., Ferrari, P., van Bakel, M., ... Trichopoulou, A. (2007). Eating out of home and its correlates in 10 European countries. The European Prospective Investigation into Cancer and Nutrition (EPIC) study. *Public Health Nutrition*, *10*(12), 1515–1525. doi:10.1017/S1368980007000171 PMID:17582244

Oudshoorn, N. (2009). Physical and digital proximity: Emerging ways of health care in face-to-face and telemonitoring of heart-failure patients. *Sociology of Health & Illness*, *31*(3), 390–405. doi:10.1111/j.1467-9566.2008.01141.x PMID:19144084

Padoan, A., Antonelli, G., Aita, A., Sciacovelli, L., & Plebani, M. (2017). Issues and challenges in applicability of measurement uncertainty estimation in medical laboratories. *Journal of Laboratory and Precision Medicine*, *2*, 69–72. doi:10.21037/jlpm.2017.08.10

Palisidis, G., Giazitzi, K., Karathanos, V. T., & Boskou, G. (2016). Nutritional application software for restaurants: The tool of customer satisfaction and behavior. *International Journal of Electronic Customer Relationship Management*, *10*(2-4).

Pandher, P. S., & Bhullar, K. K. (2014). Smartphone applications for seizure management. *Health Informatics Journal*. doi:10.1177/1460458214540906 PMID:25038202

Pangalos, G., Asimakopoulos, D., & Pagkalos, I. (2013). The new Greek national e-prescription system: An effective tool for improving quality of care and containing medication costs. *Studies in Health Technology and Informatics*, *190*, 13–17. PMID:23823360

Pantazopoulos, D., Karakitsos, P., Iokim-Liossi, A., Pouliakis, A., Botsoli-Stergiou, E., & Dimopoulos, C. (1998). Back propagation neural network in the discrimination of benign from malignant lower urinary tract lesions. *The Journal of Urology*, *159*(5), 1619–1623. doi:10.1097/00005392-199805000-00057 PMID:9554366

Pantazopoulos, D., Karakitsos, P., Iokim-Liossi, A., Pouliakis, A., & Dimopoulos, K. (1998). Comparing neural networks in the discrimination of benign from malignant lower urinary tract lesions. *British Journal of Urology*, *81*(4), 574–579. doi:10.1046/j.1464-410x.1998.00587.x PMID:9598630

Pantazopoulos, D., Karakitsos, P., Pouliakis, A., Iokim-Liossi, A., & Dimopoulos, M. A. (1998). Static cytometry and neural networks in the discrimination of lower urinary system lesions. *Urology*, *51*(6), 946–950. doi:10.1016/S0090-4295(98)00024-7 PMID:9609631

Panteghini, M., Ceriotti, F., Jones, G., Oosterhuis, W., Plebani, M., & Sandberg, S. (2017). Strategies to define performance specifications in laboratory medicine: 3 years on from the Milan Strategic Conference. *Clinical Chemistry and Laboratory Medicine*, *55*(12), 1849–1856. doi:10.1515/cclm-2017-0772 PMID:29031018

Pantell, M., Rehkopf, D., Jutte, D., Syme, S. L., Balmes, J., & Adler, N. (2013). Social isolation: A predictor of mortality comparable to traditional clinical risk factors. *American Journal of Public Health*, *103*(11), 2056–2062. doi:10.2105/AJPH.2013.301261 PMID:24028260

Papadopoulos, A., Ikonomakis, E., Kontodimopoulos, N., Frydas, A., & Niakas, D. (2007). Assessment of health-related quality of life for diabetic patients type 2. *Archives of Hellenic Medicine*, *24*(1), 66–74.

Papaefthimiou, M., Symiakaki, H., Mentzelopoulou, P., Giahnaki, A. E., Voulgaris, Z., Diakomanolis, E., ... Karakitsos, P. (2005). The role of liquid-based cytology associated with curettage in the investigation of endometrial lesions from postmenopausal women. *Cytopathology*, *16*(1), 32–39. doi:10.1111/j.1365-2303.2004.00224.x PMID:15859313

Papaefthimiou, M., Symiakaki, H., Mentzelopoulou, P., Tsiveleka, A., Kyroudes, A., Voulgaris, Z., ... Karakitsos, P. (2005). Study on the morphology and reproducibility of the diagnosis of endometrial lesions utilizing liquid-based cytology. *Cancer*, *105*(2), 56–64. doi:10.1002/cncr.21025 PMID:15751019

Papanicolaou, G., & Traut, H. (1941). The diagnostic value of vaginal smears in carcinoma of the uterus. *American Journal of Obstetrics and Gynecology*, *42*(2), 193–206. doi:10.1016/S0002-9378(16)40621-6

Parazzini, F., La Vecchia, C., Bocciolone, L., & Franceschi, S. (1991). The epidemiology of endometrial cancer. *Gynecologic Oncology*, *41*(1), 1–16. doi:10.1016/0090-8258(91)90246-2 PMID:2026352

Patel, R. P. (2012). Cloud computing and virtualization technology in radiology. *Clinical Radiology*, *67*(11), 1095–1100. doi:10.1016/j.crad.2012.03.010 PMID:22607956

Patrick, K., Raab, F., Adams, M. A., Dillon, L., Zabinski, M., Rock, C. L., ... Norman, G. J. (2009). A text message-based intervention for weight loss: Randomized controlled trial. *Journal of Medical Internet Research*, *11*(1), e1. doi:10.2196/jmir.1100 PMID:19141433

Pavlopoulos, S., Kyriacou, E., Berler, A., Dembeyiotis, S., & Koutsouris, D. (1998). A novel emergency telemedicine system based on wireless communication technology--AMBULANCE. *IEEE Transactions on Information Technology in Biomedicine*, *2*(4), 261–267. doi:10.1109/4233.737581 PMID:10719536

Pelletier, S. (2012). *Explosive growth in health care apps raises oversight questions*. Retrieved October, 2012, from: http://www.aamc.org/newsroom/reporter/october2012/308516/health-care-apps.html

Pergialiotis, V., Pouliakis, A., Parthenis, C., Damaskou, V., Chrelias, C., Papantoniou, N., & Panayiotides, I. (2018). The utility of artificial neural networks and classification and regression trees for the prediction of endometrial cancer in postmenopausal women. *Public Health*, *164*, 1–6. doi:10.1016/j.puhe.2018.07.012 PMID:30149185

Pernice, I. (2016). *E-Government and E-Democracy: overcoming legitimacy deficits in a digital Europe.* HIIG Discussion Paper Series No. 2016-01. Retrieved from https://ssrn.com/abstract=2723231

Perroti, R., Pouliakis, A., Margari, N., Panopoulou, E., Karakitsou, E., Iliopoulou, D., ... Koutsouris, D. D. (2018). CytoNet, A Versatile Web-Based System for Accessing Advisory Cytology Services: Application of Artificial Intelligence. *International Journal of Reliable and Quality E-Healthcare*, *7*(3), 37–56. doi:10.4018/IJRQEH.2018070103

Persson, P. B., & Wagner, C. D. (1996). General principles of chaotic dynamics. *Cardiovascular Research*, *31*(3), 332–341. doi:10.1016/S0008-6363(96)00006-5 PMID:8681321

Peterson, S. K., Shinn, E. H., Basen-Engquist, K., Demark-Wahnefried, W., Prokhorov, A. V., Baru, C., ... Patrick, K. (2013). Identifying early dehydration risk with home-based sensors during radiation treatment: A feasibility study on patients with head and neck cancer. *Journal of the National Cancer Institute. Monographs*, *2013*(47), 162–168. doi:10.1093/jncimonographs/lgt016 PMID:24395986

Petru, R. (2016). How to use EHRs to improve the quality of care? Interview included in "eHealth Trends & Talks". *Polish Healthcare Journal*, 69-72. Retrieved from https://www.osoz.pl/static_files/osoz/eHealth_2016.pdf

Pezzilli, R., Morselli-Labate, A., Frulloni, L., Cavestro, G., Ferri, B., Comparato, G., & .... (2006). The quality of life in patients with chronic pancreatitis evaluated using the SF-12 questionnaire: A comparative study with the SF-36 questionnaire. *Digestive and Liver Disease*, *38*, 109–111. PMID:16243011

Philippe, P., & Mansi, O. (1998). Author. *Theoretical Medicine and Bioethics*, *19*(6), 591–607. doi:10.1023/A:1009979306346 PMID:10051792

Pitas, I. (2000). *Digital image processing algorithms and applications* (1st ed.). New York: Wiley.

Pitoglou, S. (2018). Machine Learning in Healthcare, Introduction and Real World Application Considerations. *International Journal of Reliable and Quality E-Healthcare*, *7*(2), 27–36. doi:10.4018/IJRQEH.2018040102

Pitsch, M. (2016). Dormant digitization. Interview included in "eHealth Trends & Talks". *Polish Healthcare Journal*, 62-64. Retrieved from https://www.osoz.pl/static_files/osoz/eHealth_2016.pdf

Plebani, M. (2016). Harmonization of clinical laboratory information – current and future strategies. *EJIFCC*, *27*(1), 15–22. PMID:27683502

Plebani, M., Astion, M. L., Barth, J. H., Chen, W., de Oliveira Galoro, C. A., Escuer, M. I., ... Sumarac, Z. (2014). Harmonization of quality indicators in laboratory medicine. A preliminary consensus. *Clinical Chemistry and Laboratory Medicine*, *52*(7), 951–958. doi:10.1515/cclm-2014-0142 PMID:24622792

Plebani, M., Laposata, M., & Lippi, G. (2019). Driving the route of laboratory medicine: A manifesto for the future. *Internal and Emergency Medicine*, *14*(3), 337–340. doi:10.100711739-019-02053-z PMID:30783946

Plebani, M., Sciacovelli, L., & Aita, A. (2017). Quality Indicators for the Total Testing Process. *Clinics in Laboratory Medicine*, *37*(1), 187–205. doi:10.1016/j.cll.2016.09.015 PMID:28153366

Plebani, M., Sciacovelli, L., Aita, A., Pelloso, M., & Chiozza, M. L. (2015). Performance criteria and quality indicators for the pre-analytical phase. *Clinical Chemistry and Laboratory Medicine*, *53*(6), 943–948. doi:10.1515/cclm-2014-1124 PMID:25719322

Pohl, M. (2017). *325,000 mobile health apps available in 2017, Android now the leading mHealth platform*. Retrieved from: Research 2 Guidance https://research2guidance.com/325000-mobile-health-apps-available-in-2017/

Porter, M., & Teisberg, E. (2006). *Redefining Health Care: Creating Value-Based Competition on Results. Watertown.* Harvard Business School Press.

Pouliakis, A., Archondakis, S., Karakitsou, E., & Karakitsos, P. (2014). Cloud Computing for Cytopathologists. In A. Moumtzoglou & A. Kastania (Eds.), *Cloud computing applications for quality health care delivery* (pp. 250–271). Hershey, PA: IGI Global. doi:10.4018/978-1-4666-6118-9.ch013

Pouliakis, A., Archondakis, S., Margari, N., & Karakitsos, P. (2016). From telecytology to mobile cytopathology: Past, present and future. In A. Moumtzoglou (Ed.), *M-Health Innovations for Patient-Centered Care*. Hershey, PA: IGI Global. doi:10.4018/978-1-4666-9861-1.ch012

Pouliakis, A., Karakitsou, E., & Margari, N. (2019). Cytopathology and the Smartphone: An Update. In M. Anastasius (Ed.), *Mobile Health Applications for Quality Healthcare Delivery* (pp. 136–164). Hershey, PA: IGI Global. doi:10.4018/978-1-5225-8021-8.ch007

Pouliakis, A., Karakitsou, E., Margari, N., Bountris, P., Haritou, M., Panayiotides, J., ... Karakitsos, P. (2016). Artificial Neural Networks as Decision Support Tools in Cytopathology: Past, Present, and Future. *Biomedical Engineering and Computational Biology*, *7*, 1–18. doi:10.4137/BECB.S31601 PMID:26917984

Pouliakis, A., Margari, C., Margari, N., Chrelias, C., Zygouris, D., Meristoudis, C., ... Karakitsos, P. (2014). Using classification and regression trees, liquid-based cytology and nuclear morphometry for the discrimination of endometrial lesions. *Diagnostic Cytopathology*, *42*(7), 582–591. doi:10.1002/dc.23077 PMID:24273089

Pouliakis, A., Margari, N., Archondakis, S., Karakitsou, E., & Karakitsos, P. (2016). Emerging Technologies Serving Cytopathology. Big Data, the Cloud and Mobile Computing. In I. E. Naqa (Ed.), *Handbook of Research on Emerging Developments and Practices in Oncology* (pp. 114–152). Hershey, PA: IGI Global.

Pouliakis, A., Margari, N., Karakitsou, E., Alamanou, E., Koureas, N., Chrelias, G., ... Karakitsos, P. (2018). Artificial Intelligence for the Identification of Endometrial Malignancies: Application of the Learning Vector Quantizer. *International Journal of Reliable and Quality E-Healthcare*, *7*(2), 37–50. doi:10.4018/IJRQEH.2018040103

Pouliakis, A., Margari, N., Karakitsou, E., Valasoulis, G., Koufopoulos, N., Koureas, N., ... Panayiotides, I. G. (2019). Artificial Intelligence via Competitive Learning and Image Analysis for Endometrial Malignancies: Discriminating Endometrial Cells and Lesions. *International Journal of Reliable and Quality E-Healthcare*, *8*(4), 38–54. doi:10.4018/IJRQEH.2019100102

Pouliakis, A., Spathis, A., Kottaridi, C., Mourtzikou, A., Stamouli, M., Archondakis, S., ... Karakitsos, P. (2014). Cloud Computing for BioLabs. In A. Moumtzoglou & A. Kastania (Eds.), *Cloud computing applications for quality health care delivery* (pp. 228–249). Hershey, PA: IGI Global. doi:10.4018/978-1-4666-6118-9.ch012

Prey, J. E., Polubriaginof, F., Kuperman, G. J., Tiase, V., Collins, S. A., & Vawdrey, D. K. (2016). International perspectives on sharing clinical data with patients. *International Journal of Medical Informatics*, *86*, 135–141. doi:10.1016/j.ijmedinf.2015.11.007 PMID:26631956

Que, C. L., Kenyon, C. M., Olivenstein, R., Macklem, P. T., & Maksym, G. N. (2001). Homeokinesis and short-term variability of human airway caliber. *Journal of Applied Physiology (Bethesda, Md.)*, *91*(3), 1131–1141. doi:10.1152/jappl.2001.91.3.1131 PMID:11509508

Quinn, C. C., Shardell, M. D., Terrin, M. L., Barr, E. A., Ballew, S. H., & Gruber-Baldini, A. L. (2011). Cluster-randomized trial of a mobile phone personalized behavioral intervention for blood glucose control. *Diabetes Care*, *34*(9), 1934–1942. doi:10.2337/dc11-0366 PMID:21788632

Rana, A. (2017). The Immense Potential of M-Care in India: Catering Better to Patients Needs in the Context of a Fragmented Healthcare System. *International Journal of Reliable and Quality E-Healthcare*, *6*(4), 1–3. doi:10.4018/IJRQEH.2017100101

Rashid, G., Goldman, J., Weinstein, D., Tohami, T., Neumark, E., & Weiss, E. (2015). Reporting Critical Lab Results, a Challenge for the lab and the Physician - A Summary of Four Years of Experience in Meir Medical Center Laboratories. *Harefuah*, *154*(8), 494–498, 541. PMID:26480612

Reagan, J. W. (1980). Can screening for endometrial cancer be justified? *Acta Cytologica*, *24*(2), 87–89. PMID:6768202

Reason, J. (2000). Human error: Models and management. *British Medical Journal*, *320*(7237), 768–770. doi:10.1136/bmj.320.7237.768 PMID:10720363

Resnik, L., Allen, S., Isenstadt, D., Wasserman, M., & Iezzoni, L. (2009). Perspectives on use of mobility aids in a diverse population of seniors: Implications for intervention. *Disability and Health Journal*, *2*(2), 77–85. doi:10.1016/j.dhjo.2008.12.002 PMID:20160951

Ribu, L., Holmen, H., Torbjornsen, A., Wahl, A. K., Grottland, A., Smastuen, M. C., ... Arsand, E. (2013). Low-intensity self-management intervention for persons with type 2 diabetes using a mobile phone-based diabetes diary, with and without health counseling and motivational interviewing: Protocol for a randomized controlled trial. *JMIR Research Protocols*, *2*(2), e34. doi:10.2196/resprot.2768 PMID:23978690

Rodríguez-Borja, E., Villalba-Martinez, C., & Carratalá–Calvo, A. (2014). Enquiry time as part of turnaround time: When do our clinicians really consult our results? *Journal of Clinical Pathology*, *67*(7), 642–644. doi:10.1136/jclinpath-2013-202102 PMID:24706264

Roehrs, A., Da Costa, C. A., da Rosa Righi, R., & De Oliveira, K. S. F. (2017). Personal health records: A systematic literature review. *Journal of Medical Internet Research*, *19*(1), e13. doi:10.2196/jmir.5876 PMID:28062391

Roman de Mettelinge, T., & Cambier, D. (2015). Understanding the Relationship Between Walking Aids and Falls in Older Adults. *Journal of Geriatric Physical Therapy*, *38*(3), 127–132. doi:10.1519/JPT.0000000000000031 PMID:25594520

Rosales Saurer, B., Mueller-Gorchs, M., & Kunze, C. (2009). Scenario-based design of an ICT platform for mobile information services in ambulatory care nursing. *Studies in Health Technology and Informatics*, *146*, 64–68. PMID:19592810

Rosenblatt, F. (1958). The perceptron: A probabilistic model for information storage and organization in the brain. [PubMed]. *Psychological Review*, *65*(6), 386–408. doi:10.1037/h0042519

Rosenthal, A., Mork, P., Li, M. H., Stanford, J., Koester, D., & Reynolds, P. (2010). Cloud computing: A new business paradigm for biomedical information sharing. *Journal of Biomedical Informatics*, *43*(2), 342–353. doi:10.1016/j.jbi.2009.08.014 PMID:19715773

Rose, T. (2015). *The End of Average: How We Succeed in a World That Values Sameness*. New York, NY: HarperOne.

Rossler, O. E., & Rossler, R. (1994). Chaos in physiology. *Integrative Physiological and Behavioral Science*, *29*(3), 328–333. doi:10.1007/BF02691336 PMID:7811652

Roussos, G., Marsh, A. J., & Maglavera, S. (2005). Enabling pervasive computing with smart phones. *IEEE Pervasive Computing*, *4*(2), 20–27. doi:10.1109/MPRV.2005.30

Rubenach, S., Shadbolt, B., McCallum, J., & Nakamura, T. (2002). Assessing health-related quality of life following myocardial infarction: Is the SF-12 useful? *Journal of Clinical Epidemiology*, *55*(3), 306–309. doi:10.1016/S0895-4356(01)00426-7 PMID:11864802

Ruggieri, F. (2010). ETSI specifications for registered e-mail REM. In ISSE 2009 Securing Electronic Business Processes (pp. 242-254). Vieweg+ Teubner. doi:10.1007/978-3-8348-9363-5_24

Rughani, A. I., Dumont, T. M., Lu, Z., Bongard, J., Horgan, M. A., Penar, P. L., ... Object, V. (2010). Use of an artificial neural network to predict head injury outcome. [PubMed]. *Journal of Neurosurgery*, *113*(3), 585–590. doi:10.3171/2009.11.JNS09857

Rumelhart, D. E., McClelland, J. L., & University of California San Diego. PDP Research Group. (1986). *Parallel distributed processing: explorations in the microstructure of cognition*. Cambridge, MA: MIT Press.

Russ, J. C. (1995). *The image processing handbook* (2nd ed.). Boca Raton, FL: CRC Press.

Ryu, J. H., & Hong Wan, H. (2010). Optimal Design of a CUSUM Chart for a Mean Shift of Unknown Size. *Journal of Quality Technology*, *42*(3), 311–326. doi:10.1080/00224065.2010.11917826

Sadiq, F., Yasmeen, F., Mumtaz, A., Hussain, W., Butt, A. T., Qureshi, S. A., & Ibrahim, M. (2014). Frequency of Errors in Clinical Laboratory Practice. *Iranian Journal of Pathology*, *9*(1), 45–49.

Salamalekis, E., Pouliakis, A., Margari, N., Kottaridi, C., Spathis, A., Karakitsou, E., ... Chrelias, C. (2019). An Artificial Intelligence Approach for the Detection of Cervical Abnormalities: Application of the Self Organizing Map. *International Journal of Reliable and Quality E-Healthcare*, *8*(2), 15–35. doi:10.4018/IJRQEH.2019040102

Salvador, R., Radua, J., Canales-Rodrõâguez, E. J., Solanes, A., Sarroa, S., Goikolea, J. M., ... Pomarol-Clote, E. (2017). Evaluation of machine learning algorithms and structural features for optimal MRI-based diagnostic prediction in psychosis. [PubMed]. *PLoS One*, *12*(4), 1–24. doi:10.1371/journal.pone.0175683

Sama, P. R., Eapen, Z. J., Weinfurt, K. P., Shah, B. R., & Schulman, K. A. (2014). An evaluation of mobile health application tools. *JMIR mHealth and uHealth*, *2*(2), e19. doi:10.2196/mhealth.3088 PMID:25099179

Sams, S. B., Currens, H. S., & Raab, S. S. (2012). Liquid-based Papanicolaou tests in endometrial carcinoma diagnosis. Performance, error root cause analysis, and quality improvement. *American Journal of Clinical Pathology*, *137*(2), 248–254. doi:10.1309/AJCPLFBK1A2XJDQI PMID:22261450

Samuel, A. L. (1959). Some Studies in Machine Learning Using the Game of Checkers. *IBM Journal of Research and Development*, *3*(3), 210–229. doi:10.1147/rd.33.0210

Santo, A., Laizner, A. M., & Shohet, L. (2005). Exploring the value of audiotapes for health literacy: A systematic review. *Patient Education and Counseling*, *58*(3), 235–243. doi:10.1016/j.pec.2004.07.001 PMID:16054796

Schroder, H., Fıto, M., & Covas, M. I. (2007). Association of fast food consumption with energy intake, diet quality, body mass index and the risk of obesity in a representative Mediterranean population. *British Journal of Nutrition*, *98*(6), 1274–1280. doi:10.1017/S0007114507781436 PMID:17625027

Seely, A. J., & Christou, N. V. (2000). Multiple organ dysfunction syndrome: Exploring the paradigm of complex nonlinear systems. *Critical Care Medicine*, *28*(7), 2193–2200. doi:10.1097/00003246-200007000-00003 PMID:10921540

Seffens, W., Evans, C., Minority Health, G. N., & Taylor, H. (2015). Machine Learning Data Imputation and Classification in a Multicohort Hypertension Clinical Study. *Bioinformatics and Biology Insights*, *9*(Suppl 3), 43–54. doi:10.4137/BBI.S29473 PMID:27199552

Shahangian, S., & Snyder, S. R. (2009). Laboratory medicine quality indicators: A review of the literature. *American Journal of Clinical Pathology*, *131*(3), 418–431. doi:10.1309/AJCPJF8JI4ZLDQUE PMID:19228647

Shcolnik, W., de Oliveira, C. A., de São José, A. S., de Oliveira Galoro, C. A., Plebani, M., & Burnett, D. (2012). Brazilian laboratory indicators program. *Clinical Chemistry and Laboratory Medicine*, *50*(11), 1923–1934. doi:10.1515/cclm-2012-0357 PMID:23096110

Shin, J., Rusakov, A., & Meyer, B. (2016). SmartWalker: Towards an Intelligent Robotic Walker for the Elderly. *Journal of Ambient Intelligence and Smart Environments*, *1*, 1–5.

Shoda, Y., Mischel, W., & Wright, J. C. (1994). Intraindividual Stability in the Organization and Patterning of Behavior: Incorporating Psychological Situations into the Idiographic Analysis of Personality. *Journal of Personality and Social Psychology*, *67*(4), 674–687. doi:10.1037/0022-3514.67.4.674 PMID:7965613

Shorey, S., Yang, Y. Y., & Dennis, C. L. (2018). A Mobile Health App-Based Postnatal Educational Program (Home-but not Alone): Descriptive Qualitative Study. *Journal of Medical Internet Research*, *20*(4), e119. doi:10.2196/jmir.9188 PMID:29674314

Shyamala, G., & Ferenczy, A. (1981). The effect of sodium molybdate on the cytoplasmic estrogen and progesterone receptors in human endometrial tissues. *Diagnostic Gynecology and Obstetrics*, *3*(4), 277–282. PMID:7200003

Sibley, A., Kersten, P., Ward, C., White, B., Mehta, R., & George, S. (2006). Measuring autonomy in disabled people: Validation of a new scale in a UK population. *Clinical Rehabilitation*, *20*(9), 793–803. doi:10.1177/0269215506070808 PMID:17005503

Siegler, R. S. (2007). Cognitive variability. *Developmental Science*, *10*(1), 104–109. doi:10.1111/j.1467-7687.2007.00571.x PMID:17181707

Sikaris, K. (2015). Performance criteria of the post-analytical phase. *Clinical Chemistry and Laboratory Medicine*, *53*(6), 949–958. doi:10.1515/cclm-2015-0016 PMID:25894643

Simundic, A.M., Cornes, M., Grankvist, K., Lippi, G.,andNybo, M. (2014).

Simundic, A. M., Kackov, S., Miler, M., Fraser, C. G., & Petersen, P. H. (2015). Terms and symbols used in studies on biological variation: The need for harmonization. *Clinical Chemistry*, *61*(2), 438–439. doi:10.1373/clinchem.2014.233791 PMID:25403815

Sirinukunwattana, K., Raza, S., Tsang, Y. W., Snead, D., Cree, I., & Rajpoot, N. (2016). Locality Sensitive Deep Learning for Detection and Classification of Nuclei in Routine Colon Cancer Histology Images. *IEEE Transactions on Medical Imaging*, *35*(5), 1196–1206. doi:10.1109/TMI.2016.2525803 PMID:26863654

Siristatidis, C., Pouliakis, A., Chrelias, C., & Kassanos, D. (2011). Artificial intelligence in IVF: A need. *Systems Biology in Reproductive Medicine*, *57*(4), 179–185. doi:10.3109/19396368.2011.558607 PMID:21375363

Siristatidis, C., Vogiatzi, P., Pouliakis, A., Trivella, M., Papantoniou, N., & Bettocchi, S. (2016). Predicting IVF Outcome: A Proposed Web-based System Using Artificial Intelligence. *In Vivo (Athens, Greece)*, *30*(4), 507–512. PMID:27381616

Siu, S., Wong, M., Shah, A., Li, H., Soong, A., & Cao, R. (2008). Redesign of the Rollator's (Walker's) Parking Brake System. In *Proceedings of the IASTED International Conference on Telehealth* (pp. 129-132). ACTA Press.

Skinner, J. E. (1994). Low-dimensional chaos in biological systems. *Biotechnology*, *12*, 596–600. PMID:7764948

Skrovseth, S. O., Arsand, E., Godtliebsen, F., & Hartvigsen, G. (2012). Mobile phone-based pattern recognition and data analysis for patients with type 1 diabetes. *Diabetes Technology & Therapeutics*, *14*(12), 1098–1104. doi:10.1089/dia.2012.0160 PMID:23035775

Smith-Bindman, R., Kerlikowske, K., Feldstein, V. A., Subak, L., Scheidler, J., Segal, M., ... Grady, D. (1998). Endovaginal ultrasound to exclude endometrial cancer and other endometrial abnormalities. *Journal of the American Medical Association*, *280*(17), 1510–1517. doi:10.1001/jama.280.17.1510 PMID:9809732

Sniderman, A. D., LaChapelle, K. J., Rachon, N. A., & Furberg, C. D. (2013). The necessity for clinical reasoning in the era of evidence-based medicine. *Mayo Clinic Proceedings*, *88*(10), 1108–1114. doi:10.1016/j.mayocp.2013.07.012 PMID:24079680

Söderberg, J., Brulin, C., Grankvist, K., & Wallin, O. (2009). Preanalytical errors in primary healthcare: A questionnaire study of information search procedures, test request management and test tube labelling. *Clinical Chemistry and Laboratory Medicine*, *47*(2), 195–201. doi:10.1515/CCLM.2009.048 PMID:19191726

Soer, R., Reneman, M. F., Speijer, B. L., Coppes, M. H., & Vroomen, P. C. (2012). Clinimetric properties of the EuroQol-5D in patients with chronic low back pain. *The Spine Journal, 12*(11), 1035–1039. doi:10.1016/j.spinee.2012.10.030 PMID:23199409

Software, M. I. M. (2017). *MIM Software web site*. Retrieved 20 Aug., 2017, from https://www.mimsoftware.com

Soliman, P. T., Oh, J. C., Schmeler, K. M., Sun, C. C., Slomovitz, B. M., Gershenson, D. M., ... Lu, K. H. (2005). Risk factors for young premenopausal women with endometrial cancer. *Obstetrics and Gynecology, 105*(3), 575–580. doi:10.1097/01.AOG.0000154151.14516.f7 PMID:15738027

Solinger, A. B., & Rothman, S. I. (2013). Risks of mortality associated with common laboratory tests: A novel, simple and meaningful way to set decision limits from data available in the Electronic Medical Record. *Clinical Chemistry and Laboratory Medicine, 51*(9), 1803–1813. doi:10.1515/cclm-2013-0167 PMID:23729574

Solway, S., Brooks, D., Lacasse, Y., & Thomas, S. (2001). A Qualitative Systematic Overview of the Measurement Properties of Functional Walk Tests Used in the Cardiorespiratory Domain. *Chest, 119*(1), 256–270. doi:10.1378/chest.119.1.256 PMID:11157613

Soman, A. K. (2011). Cloud-based solutions for healthcare IT. Enfield, NH: Science Publishers. doi:10.1201/b10737

Sonka, M., Hlavac, V., & Boyle, R. (1993). *Image processing, analysis, and machine vision* (1st ed.). London: Chapman & Hall Computing. doi:10.1007/978-1-4899-3216-7

Spat, S., Holl, B., Petritsch, G., Schaupp, L., Beck, P., & Pieber, T. R. (2013). Automatic system testing of a decision support system for insulin dosing using Google Android. *Studies in Health Technology and Informatics, 186*, 187–191. PMID:23542995

Spyra, G., Buchanan, W. J., Cruickshank, P., & Ekonomou, E. (2014). Cloud-Based Identity and Identity Meta-Data: Secure and Control of Data in Globalization Era. *International Journal of Reliable and Quality E-Healthcare, 3*(1), 49–66. doi:10.4018/ijrqeh.2014010105

Srirama, S. (2006). *Publishing and discovery of mobile web services in peer to peer networks.* Paper presented at the First International Workshop on Mobile Services and Personalized Environments.

Srirama, S., Jarke, M., & Prinz, W. (2007). *Mobile web service discovery in peer to peer networks.* Paper presented at the 5th International Workshop on Ubiquitous Mobile Information and Collaboration Systems.

Srirama, S., Jarke, M., Zhu, H., & Prinz, W. (2008). *Scalable Mobile Web Service Discovery in Peer to Peer Networks.* Paper presented at the Third International Conference on Internet and Web Applications and Services. 10.1109/ICIW.2008.52

Staffa, M., Sgaglione, L., Mazzeo, G., Coppolino, L., D'Antonio, S., Romano, L., ... Campegiani, P. (2018). An OpenNCP-based solution for secure eHealth data exchange. *Journal of Network and Computer Applications, 116*, 65–85. doi:10.1016/j.jnca.2018.05.012

Stahl, R. (2003). Customers rarely feel the average performance of a system–instead, they tend to experience the variability. *Six Sigma Forum Magazine*, 17-26. Retrieved from http://asq.org/healthcaresixsigma/pdf/healthcares_horizon.pdf

Stahlberg, A., Kubista, M., & Aman, P. (2011). Single-cell gene-expression profiling and its potential diagnostic applications. *Expert Review of Molecular Diagnostics*, *11*(7), 735–740. doi:10.1586/erm.11.60 PMID:21902535

Stahl, E., Jansson, S., Jonsson, A., Svensson, K., Lundback, B., & Andersson, F. (2003). Health-related quality of life, utility, and productivity outcomes instruments: Ease of completion by subjects with COPD. *Health and Quality of Life Outcomes*, *1*(1), 18–24. doi:10.1186/1477-7525-1-18 PMID:12809558

Stamouli, M., Mourtzikou, A., Karkalousos, P. L., Athanasiadou, Z., Marasidi, E., & Skliris, A. (2019). Application of Failure Modes and Effects Analysis (FMEA) During the Pre-analytical Phase in a Greek Biochemistry Laboratory. *International Journal of Reliable and Quality E-Healthcare*, *4*(3), 22–35. doi:10.4018/IJRQEH.2019070102

Standardization of collection requirements for fasting samples: for the Working Group on Preanalytical Phase (WG-PA) of the European Federation of Clinical Chemistry and Laboratory Medicine (EFLM). (n.d.). *ClinChimActa, 15*(432), 33-7. Doi:10.1016/j.cca.2013.11.008

Stasis, A. C., Demiri, L., & Chaniotaki, E. (2018). eIDAS-Electronic Identification for Cross Border eHealth. *International Journal of Reliable and Quality E-Healthcare*, *7*(2), 51–67. doi:10.4018/IJRQEH.2018040104

Statnikov, A., Aliferis, C. F., Hardin, D. P., & Guyon, I. (2011). A Gentle Introduction To Support Vector Machines. In *Biomedicine*. World Scientific Publishing Co Inc.

Stevens, J., Thomas, K., Teh, L., & Greenspan, A. (2009). Unintentional Fall Injuries Associated with Walkers and Canes in Older Adults Treated in U.S. Emergency Departments. *Journal of the American Geriatrics Society*, *57*(8), 1464–1469. doi:10.1111/j.1532-5415.2009.02365.x PMID:19555423

Stoiljkovic, V., Milosavljevic, P., Mladenovic, S., Pavlovic, D., & Todorovic, M. (2014). Improving the Efficiency of the Center for Medical Biochemistry clinical Center, by Applying Lean Six Sigma Methodology. *Journal of Medical Biochemistry*, *33*(3), 299–307. doi:10.2478/jomb-2014-0012

Stroetmann, K. A., Artmann, J., & Stroetmann, V. (2011). Developing national eHealth infrastructures--results and lessons from Europe. *AMIA ... Annual Symposium proceedings. AMIA Symposium*, 1347–1354.

Stroetmann, K. A., Artmann, J., Stroetmann, V. N., Protti, D., Dumortier, J., Giest, S., ... & Whitehouse, D. (2011). *European countries on their journey towards national eHealth infrastructures*. Luxembourg: Office for Official Publications of the European Communities.

Subversus Interactive. (2011). *Gyromaniac*. Retrieved 16 Aug., 2017, from http://subvers.us

Su, C. J., & Chu, T. W. (2014). A mobile multi-agent information system for ubiquitous fetal monitoring. *International Journal of Environmental Research and Public Health*, *11*(1), 600–625. doi:10.3390/ijerph110100600 PMID:24452256

Su, J., Xu, X., He, Y., & Song, J. (2016). Automatic Detection of Cervical Cancer Cells by a Two-Level Cascade Classification System. *Analytical Cellular Pathology (Amsterdam), 9535027*. doi:10.1155/2016/9535027 PMID:27298758

Tamposis, I., Pouliakis, A., Fezoulidis, I., & Karakitsos, P. (2016). Mobile Platforms Supporting Health Professionals: Need, Technical Requirements and Applications. In A. Moumtzoglou (Ed.), *M-Health Innovations for Patient-Centered Care*. Hershey, PA: IGI Global. doi:10.4018/978-1-4666-9861-1.ch005

Taner, M. T. K., Gamze, C. S., Erbas, E. K., & Kemal, M. (2013). Formation of Six Sigma Infrastructure for the Coronary Stenting Process. *International Review of Management and Marketing*, *3*(4), 232–242.

Tang, P. C., Ash, J. S., Bates, D. W., Overhage, J. M., & Sands, D. Z. (2006). Personal health records: Definitions, benefits, and strategies for overcoming barriers to adoption. *Journal of the American Medical Informatics Association*, *13*(2), 121–126. doi:10.1197/jamia.M2025 PMID:16357345

Taskin, S., Bozaci, E. A., Seval, M. M., & Unlu, C. (2006). Transvaginal sonographic assessment of endometrial thickness and endometrial morphology in postmenopausal bleeding. *International Journal of Gynaecology and Obstetrics: the Official Organ of the International Federation of Gynaecology and Obstetrics*, *92*(2), 155–156. doi:10.1016/j.ijgo.2005.10.023 PMID:16360156

Tate, J. R., Sikaris, K. A., Jones, G. R., Yen, T., Koerbin, G., Ryan, J., ... Graham, P. (2014). Harmonising Adult and Paediatric Reference Intervals in Australia and New Zealand: An Evidence-Based Approach for Establishing a First Panel of Chemistry Analytes. *The Clinical Biochemist. Reviews / Australian Association of Clinical Biochemists*, *35*(4), 213–235. PMID:25678727

Tezuka, F., Namiki, T., & Higashiiwai, H. (1992). Observer variability in endometrial cytology using kappa statistics. *Journal of Clinical Pathology*, *45*(4), 292–294. doi:10.1136/jcp.45.4.292 PMID:1577966

Thelen, E., & Smith, L. B. (2006). Dynamic systems theories. In W. Damon & R. M. Lerner (Eds.), Theoretical models of human development. Handbook of child psychology (6th ed.; Vol. 1, pp. 258–312). New York, NY: John Wiley & Sons.

Theodoridis, S., & Koutroumbas, K. (2009). *Pattern recognition* (4th ed.). London: Academic Press.

Thiel, R., Deimel, L., Schmidtmann, D., Piesche, K., Hüsing, T., Rennoch, J., . . . Stroetmann, K. (2019). In *#SmartHealthSystems International comparison of digital strategies.* Retrieved from https://www.bertelsmann-stiftung.de/en/publications/publication/did/smarthealthsystems-1/

Thomas, S., Halbert, J., Mackintosh, S., Cameron, I. D., Kurrle, S., Whitehead, C., ... Crotty, M. (2010). Walking aid use after discharge following hip fracture is rarely reviewed and often inappropriate: An observational study. *Journal of Physiotherapy*, *56*(4), 267–272. doi:10.1016/S1836-9553(10)70010-2 PMID:21091417

Thompson, M., & Wood, R. (1995). Harmonized guidelines for internal quality control in analytical chemistry laboratories. *Pure and Applied Chemistry*, *67*(4), 649–666. doi:10.1351/pac199567040649

Thordardottir, B., Malmgren Fänge, A., Lethin, C., Rodriguez Gatta, D., & Chiatti, C. (2019). Acceptance and Use of Innovative Assistive Technologies among People with Cognitive Impairment and Their Caregivers: A Systematic Review. *BioMed Research International*, *2019*, 1–18. doi:10.1155/2019/9196729 PMID:30956989

Tinholt, D., Carrara, W., Tol, T., Foley, P., Graux, H., & Erdogan, E. (2013). Study on analysis of the needs for cross-border services and assessment of the organisational, legal, technical and semantic barriers. *European Commission–Directorate-General of Communications Networks, Content & Technology*.

Toomey, R. J., Ryan, J. T., McEntee, M. F., Evanoff, M. G., Chakraborty, D. P., McNulty, J. P., ... Brennan, P. C. (2010). Diagnostic efficacy of handheld devices for emergency radiologic consultation. *AJR. American Journal of Roentgenology*, *194*(2), 469–474. doi:10.2214/AJR.09.3418 PMID:20093611

Topol, E. (2019). High-performance medicine: The convergence of human and artificial intelligence. *Nature Medicine*, *25*(1), 44–56. doi:10.103841591-018-0300-7 PMID:30617339

Topol, E. J. (2012). *The creative destruction of medicine: how the digital revolution will create better health care*. New York: Basic Books.

Toye, E., Sharp, R., Madhavapeddy, A., Scott, D., Upton, E., & Blackwell, A. (2007). Interacting with mobile services: An evaluation of camera-phones and visual tags. *Personal and Ubiquitous Computing*, *11*(2), 97–106. doi:10.100700779-006-0064-9

Trust, W. (2019). *The ethical, social and political challenges of using artificial intelligence in healthcare*. Retrieved June 3, 2019 from https://wellcomeac.uk/funding/ethical-social-and-political-challenges-using-artificial-intelligence-healthcare

Tzivras, M., Megalopoulou, T. M., Pouliakis, A., Giahnaki, A. E., Karaitianos, I. G., Archondakis, S., ... Karakitsos, P. (2008). The potential of tree classifiers on the cytological examination of gastric lesions. *Archives of the Balkan Medical Union*, *43*(4), 239–244.

United Nations, Department of Economic and Social Affairs, Population Division. (2015). *World Population Ageing 2015* (ST/ESA/SER.A/390). Author.

United States Census Bureau. (2019). *Mobility is Most Common Disability Among Older Americans*. Retrieved 11 September 2019, from https://www.census.gov/newsroom/press-releases/2014/cb14-218.html

University of Illinois College of Engineering. (2017). *New handheld spectral analyzer uses power of smartphone to detect disease.* Retrieved 10 Aug., 2017, from https://www.eurekalert.org/pub_releases/2017-08/uoic-nhs081017.php

University of Oxford. (n.d.). *Patient Reported Outcomes Measurement Group.* Retrieved May 24, 2014, from http://phi.uhce.ox.ac.uk/inst_types.php

Usha, S., Adiga, U. S., Preethika, A., & Swathi, K. (2015).Sigma metrics in clinical chemistry laboratory – A guide to quality control. *Al Ameen J Med Sci, 8*(4), 281-287.

Utah Department of Health. (2001). *Interpreting the SF-12.* Utah Health Status Survey, Utah Department of Health.

Vaisanen, O., Makijarvi, M., & Silfvast, T. (2003). Prehospital ECG transmission: Comparison of advanced mobile phone and facsimile devices in an urban Emergency Medical Service System. *Resuscitation, 57*(2), 179–185. doi:10.1016/S0300-9572(03)00028-5 PMID:12745186

van der Graaf, Y., Vooijs, G. P., Gaillard, H. L., & Go, D. M. (1987). Screening errors in cervical cytologic screening. *Acta Cytologica, 31*(4), 434–438. PMID:3604538

Van der Loos, H. M., & Reinkensmeyer, D. J. (2008). Rehabilitation and Health Care Robotics. In B. Siciliano & O. Khatib (Eds.), *Springer Handbook of Robotics.* Berlin: Springer. doi:10.1007/978-3-540-30301-5_54

Van Geert, P. (2011). The Contribution of Complex Dynamic Systems to Development. *Child Development Perspectives, 5*(4), 273–278. doi:10.1111/j.1750-8606.2011.00197.x

van Geert, P., & van Dijk, M. (2002). Focus on variability: New tools to study intra-individual variability in developmental data. *Infant Behavior and Development, 25*(4), 340–374. doi:10.1016/S0163-6383(02)00140-6

Varlatzidou, A., Pouliakis, A., Stamataki, M., Meristoudis, C., Margari, N., Peros, G., ... Karakitsos, P. (2011). Cascaded learning vector quantizer neural networks for the discrimination of thyroid lesions. *Analytical and Quantitative Cytology and Histology, 33*(6), 323–334. PMID:22590810

Vazirinejad, R., Lilley, J., & Ward, C. (2003). The 'Impact on Participation and Autonomy': Acceptability of the English version in a multiple sclerosis outpatient setting. *Multiple Sclerosis Journal, 9*(6), 612–615. doi:10.1191/1352458503ms936oa PMID:14664475

Ventola, C. L. (2014). Mobile devices and apps for health care professionals: Uses and benefits. *P&T, 39*(5), 356–364. PMID:24883008

Vilagut, G., Forero, C., Pinto-Meza, A., Haro, J., de Graaf, R., & Bruffaerts, R. (2013). The Mental Component of the Short-Form 12 Health Survey (SF-12) as a FP7 - MOBOT – 600796 74 Measure of Depressive Disorders in the General Population: Results with Three Alternative Scoring Methods. *Value in Health, 16*, 564–573. doi:10.1016/j.jval.2013.01.006 PMID:23796290

Vilhena, J., Vicente, H., Martins, M. R., Grañeda, J., Caldeira, F., Gusmão, R., ... Neves, J. I. (2017). An Artificial Intelligence Approach to Thrombophilia Risk. *International Journal of Reliable and Quality E-Healthcare*, *6*(2), 49–69. doi:10.4018/IJRQEH.2017040105

Vincent, J. (2017). AI star Andrew Ng announces departure from Chinese tech giant Baidu - The Verge. The Verge. Retrieved from http://www.theverge.com/2017/3/22/15020064/baidu-ai-andrew-ng-resigns

Virk, R. K., Theoharis, C. G., Prasad, A., Chhieng, D., & Prasad, M. L. (2014). Morphology predicts BRAF (V600E) mutation in papillary thyroid carcinoma: An interobserver reproducibility study. *Virchows Archiv*, *464*(4), 435–442. doi:10.100700428-014-1552-3 PMID:24549591

Virk, R. K., Van Dyke, A. L., Finkelstein, A., Prasad, A., Gibson, J., Hui, P., ... Prasad, M. L. (2013). BRAFV600E mutation in papillary thyroid microcarcinoma: A genotype-phenotype correlation. *Modern Pathology*, *26*(1), 62–70. doi:10.1038/modpathol.2012.152 PMID:22918165

Vogiatzi, P., Pouliakis, A., & Siristatidis, C. (2019). An artificial neural network for the prediction of assisted reproduction outcome. *Journal of Assisted Reproduction and Genetics*, *36*(7), 1441–1448. doi:10.100710815-019-01498-7 PMID:31218565

Wagstaff, K. (2012). Machine Learning that Matters. *Journal of the American Medical Informatics Association*, *14*(5), 574–580. Retrieved from http://arxiv.org/abs/1206.4656

Waldrop, M. M. (2016). The chips are down for Moore's law. [PubMed]. *Nature*, *530*(7589), 144–147. doi:10.1038/530144a

Walsh, T., Caraceni, A., Fainsinger, R., Foley, K., Glare, P., & Goh, C. (2009). *Palliative Medicine* (1st ed.). Elsevier.

Wang, C. J., Patel, M. H., Schueth, A. J., Bradley, M., Wu, S., Crosson, J. C., ... Bell, D. S. (2009). Perceptions of standards-based electronic prescribing systems as implemented in outpatient primary care: A physician survey. *Journal of the American Medical Informatics Association*, *16*(4), 493–502. doi:10.1197/jamia.M2998 PMID:19390106

Wang, Q., Egelandsdal, B., Amdam, G. V., Almli, V. L., & Oostindjer, M. (2016). Diet and Physical Activity Apps: Perceived Effectiveness by App Users. *JMIR mHealth and uHealth*, *4*(2), e33. doi:10.2196/mhealth.5114 PMID:27056639

Ware, J. Jr, Kosinski, M., & Keller, S. (1996). A 12-Item Short-Form Health Survey: Construction of scales and preliminary tests of reliability and validity. *Medical Care*, *34*(3), 220–233. doi:10.1097/00005650-199603000-00003 PMID:8628042

Ware, J., Snow, K., Kosinski, M., Gandek, B., & Institute, N. E. (1993). *SF-36 health survey: manual and interpretation guide*. The Health Institute, New England Medical Center.

Watts, N., Amann, M., Arnell, N., Ayeb-Karlsson, S., Belesova, K., Berry, H., ... Costello, A. (2018). The 2018 report of the Lancet Countdown on health and climate change: Shaping the health of nations for centuries to come. *The Lancet Review.*, *392*(10163), 2479–2514. doi:10.1016/S0140-6736(18)32594-7 PMID:30503045

Wavelet Health. (2017). *Wavelet Health web site*. Retrieved 14 Aug., 2017, from https://wavelethealth.com

Waxer, N., Ninan, D., Ma, A., & Dominguez, N. (2013). How cloud computing and social media are changing the face of health care. *The Physician Executive Journal, 39*(2), 58-60, 62.

Webb, G. (2012). Making the cloud work for healthcare: Cloud computing offers incredible opportunities to improve healthcare, reduce costs and accelerate ability to adopt new IT services. *Health Management Technology*, *33*(2), 8–9. PMID:22397112

Webster, A. J. (2002). Innovative health technologies and the social: Redefining health, medicine and the body. *Current Sociology*, *50*(3), 443–457. doi:10.1177/0011392102050003009

Wells, T. S., Ozminkowski, R. J., Hawkins, K., Bhattarai, G. R., & Armstrong, D. G. (2016). Leveraging big data in population health management. *Big Data Analytics*, *1*(1), 1. doi:10.118641044-016-0001-5

Westgard, J. O., Barry, P. L., Quam, E. F., Shermeyer, S. S., Plaut, D., & Statland, B. E. (2002). *Chapter6 in Basic QC Practices, Training in StatisticalQuality Control for Healthcare Laboratories* (2nd ed.). Madison, WI: Westgard QC, Inc.

Wheatley, M. J. (1999). *Leadership and the new science: Discovering order in a chaotic world.* San Fransisco: Berrett-Koehler.Wofford.

White, G. H., Campbell, C. A., & Horvath, A. R. (2014). Is this a critical, panic, alarm, urgent or markedly abnormal result? *Clinical Chemistry*, *60*(12), 1589–70. doi:10.1373/clinchem.2014.227645 PMID:25189694

WHO. (1980). International classification of impairments, disabilities and handicaps: a manual of classification relating to the consequences of disease (ICIDH). Geneva: World Health Organization (WHO).

WHO. (2001). The international classification of functioning, disability and health - ICF. Geneva: World Health Organization (WHO).

WHO. (2015). *Healthy diet*. Retrieved from: http://www.who.int/mediacentre/factsheets/fs394/en/

WHO. (2018). *Obesity and overweight*. Retrieved from: http://www.who.int/en/news-room/fact-sheets/detail/obesity-and-overweight

WHO. (2019). *Ageing and health*. Retrieved 11 September 2019, from https://www.who.int/news-room/fact-sheets/detail/ageing-and-health

Whynes, D., McCahon, R., Ravenscroft, A., Hodgkinson, V., Evley, R., & Hardman, J. (2013). Responsiveness of the EQ-5D Health-Related Quality-of-Life Instrument in Assessing Low Back Pain. *Value in Health*, *16*(1), 124–132. doi:10.1016/j.jval.2012.09.003 PMID:23337223

Willis, M., Duckworth, P., Coulter, A., Meyer, E. T., & Osborne, M. (2019). The Future of Health Care: Protocol for Measuring the Potential of Task Automation Grounded in the National Health Service Primary Care System. *JMIR Research Protocols*, *8*(4), e11232. doi:10.2196/11232 PMID:30964437

Wilson, J. (2006). 3G to Web 2.0? Can Mobile Telephony Become an Architecture of Participation? *Convergence*, *12*(2), 229–242. doi:10.1177/1354856506066122

Wisniewski, F., Katehakis, D. G., Masi, M., & Bittins, S. (2016). Improving Cross-Border European ePrescription and Patient Summary Services through e-SENS Cross-Sectorial Building Blocks. *Global Telemedicine and eHealth Updates. Knowledge Resources*, *9*, 234–238.

Witzke, K., & Specht, O. (2017). M-Health Telemedicine and Telepresence in Oral and Maxillofacial Surgery: An Innovative Prehospital Healthcare Concept in Structurally Weak Areas. *International Journal of Reliable and Quality E-Healthcare*, *6*(4), 37–48. doi:10.4018/IJRQEH.2017100105

Wolfe, B., Evans, W., & Seeman, T. E. (Eds.). (2012). The Biological Consequences of Socioeconomic Inequalities. Russell Sage Foundation.

Woolford, J., Smith, E., & Miller, D. (2005). The multimedia computer for office-based patient education: A systematic review. *Patient Education and Counseling*, *59*(2), 148–157. doi:10.1016/j.pec.2004.10.011 PMID:16257619

World Health Organisation. (2003). *Adherence to long-term therapies. Evidence for action.* Retrieved 23 July, 2019, from https://www.who.int/chp/knowledge/publications/adherence_report/en/

World Health Organization. (2015). *Postnatal Care for Mothers and Newborns Highlights from the World Health Organization 2013 Guidelines*. Retrieved July 25, 2019, from https://www.who.int/maternal_child_adolescent/publications/WHO-MCA-PNC-2014-Briefer_A4.pdf

Yanoh, K., Norimatsu, Y., Hirai, Y., Takeshima, N., Kamimori, A., Nakamura, Y., ... Shiraishi, T. (2009). New diagnostic reporting format for endometrial cytology based on cytoarchitectural criteria. *Cytopathology*, *20*(6), 388–394. doi:10.1111/j.1365-2303.2008.00581.x PMID:18657157

Ybarra, M. L., Holtrop, J. S., Prescott, T. L., & Strong, D. (2014). Process evaluation of a mHealth program: Lessons learned from Stop My Smoking USA, a text messaging-based smoking cessation program for young adults. *Patient Education and Counseling*, *97*(2), 239–243. doi:10.1016/j.pec.2014.07.009 PMID:25103183

Ye, Z. K., Tang, H. L., & Zhai, S. D. (2013). Benefits of therapeutic drug monitoring of vancomycin: A systematic review and meta-analysis. *PLoS One*, *8*(10), e77169. doi:10.1371/journal.pone.0077169 PMID:24204764

Yfantopoulos, J. (2001). The Greek version of the EuroQol (EQ-5D) instrument. *Archives of Hellenic Medicine, 18*(2), 180-191.

Yuh-Shan, H. (2019). Comment on Chen, J.; Su, Y.; Si, H.; Chen, J. Managerial Areas of Construction and Demolition Waste: A Scientometric Review. *Int. J. Environ. Res. Public Health* 2018, *15*, 2350. *International Journal of Environmental Research and Public Health*, *16*(10), 1837. doi:10.3390/ijerph16101837

Yun, E. K., & Chun, K. M. (2008). Critical to quality in telemedicine service management: Application of DFSS (Design for Six Sigma) and SERVQUAL). *Nursing Economics*, *26*(6), 384–388. PMID:19330973

Zadeh, P. E., & Tremblay, M. C. (2016). A review of the literature and proposed classification on e-prescribing: Functions, assimilation stages, benefits, concerns, and risks. *Research in Social & Administrative Pharmacy*, *12*(1), 1–19. doi:10.1016/j.sapharm.2015.03.001 PMID:25847858

Zeng, R., Wang, W., & Wang, Z. (2013). National survey on critical values notification of 599 institutions in China. *Clinical Chemistry and Laboratory Medicine*, *51*(11), 2099–2107. doi:10.1515/cclm-2013-0183 PMID:23839815

Zerth, J., Besser, J., & Reichert, A. (2012). Effectiveness and efficiency for ambulatory care assisted by mobile technological devices. *Biomedizinische Technik. Biomedical Engineering*, *57*(Suppl 1.). doi:10.1515/bmt-2012-4062 PMID:23096280

Zimmerman, B. J., Lindberg, C., & Plsek, P. E. (1998). *Edgeware: insights from complexity science for health care leaders*. Irving, TX: VHA Publishing.

Zygouris, D., Pouliakis, A., Margari, N., Chrelias, C., Terzakis, E., Koureas, N., ... Karakitsos, P. (2014). Classification of endometrial lesions by nuclear morphometry features extracted from liquid-based cytology samples: A system based on logistic regression model. *Analytical and Quantitative Cytopathology and Histopathology*, *36*(4), 189–198. PMID:25291856

About the Contributors

Anastasius Moumtzoglou is a Former Executive Board Member of the European Society for Quality in Health Care, President of the Hellenic Society for Quality & Safety in Health Care, holds B.A in Economics, MA in Health Services Management, MA in Macroeconomics, Ph.D. in Economics. He teaches the module of quality at the graduate and postgraduate level. He has also written three Greek books, which are the only ones in the Greek references. The first deals with "Marketing in Health Care", the following with "Quality in Health Care" and the third with "Quality and Patient Safety in Health Care." He has edited the books "E-Health Systems Quality and Reliability: Models and Standards", "E-health Technologies & Improving Patient Safety: Exploring Organizational Factors", "Cloud Computing Applications for Quality Health Care Delivery", "Laboratory Management Information Systems: Current Requirements and Future Perspectives", " M-Health Innovations for Patient-Centered Care", "Design Development and Integration of Reliable Electronic Healthcare Platforms", and "Mobile Health Applications for Quality Healthcare Delivery". He is the Editor-in-Chief of the "Advances in Healthcare Information Systems and Administration" book series and the International Journal of Reliable & Quality in Healthcare (IJRQEH). He has also served as the scientific coordinator of research programs in Greece and participated as a researcher in European research programs. In 2004, he was declared "Person of Quality," with respect to Greece.

* * *

George Boskou is Assistant Professor in Food Service Management and Organisation at the Department of Nutrition and Dietetics, School of Health Sciences and Education, Harokopio University Athens. His research interests are food safety, total quality management, food service management, food legislation, gastronomy and culinology.

Charalambos Chrelias was born in St Andreas Mesolonghi, Greece in 1951. In 1980 completed the Medical School of Bolognia Italy with a grade of "Very good" and his doctoral dissertation "Rare forms of hyperthyroidism". From 1985-1988 he served as an intern doctor in the 2nd Department of Obstetrics and Gynecology, University of Athens in "Areteion" University Hospital to gain the title of specialist in Obstetrics and Gynecology. In 1989 obtained a PhD from the School of Medicine, University of Athens with a degree of "Excellent" with subject "Study of the levels of FSH and LH in the serum of the mother, the umbilical cord blood and the amniotic fluid during labor". From 1987 until today has served in various Hospital and University positions. Today is associate professor in the Third Department of Obstetrics and Gynecology, National and Kapodistrian University of Athens, University General Hospital "Attikon".

George Chrelias was born in 1979 in Italy. In 2003, he received a degree (Diploma de Licenta) in Medicine from the University of Medicine and Pharmacy "CAROL DAVILA" Bucharest, Romania. In 2014 completed his specialty Training in Gynaecology (ST2/ST3 level) at the GENERAL HOSPITAL LAIKO, Gynecology clinic and today is specialty training in Obstetrics (ST4/ST5 level) at the University Hospital Attikon, Obs & Gynae clinic. He served as clinical attachment at Obstetrics and Gynaecology at South London Healthcare NHS Trust, he has a Master of Science: "Maternal Medicine" from the 3rd department of Obstetrics and Gynaecology, University of Athens. PhD in "Study of the action of the biochemical indicators inhibin, activin and leptin in preeclampsia." At the National and Kapodistrian University of Athens. Today he is a consultant at the 3rd department of Obstetrics and Gynaecology, University of Athens.

Vasileia Damaskou graduated from the School of Medicine Carol Davila in the University of Bucharest, Rumania. This was followed by training in Pathology at the Pathology Department at the General Hospital of Korinthos, Greece. Further specialized training followed in Oncological Pathology at the St Savvas Oncological Hospital in Athens, Greece. After this, she continued training in Cytology at the Alexandra's General Hospital in Athens, Greece. In 2005 The Prefecture of Eastern Attica in Athens Greece awarded Dr Damaskou with a Board Certification in Pathology. To complement her training for a year between 2010 – 2011, she was a visiting Fellow in Dermatopathology under Dr Eduardo Calonje at St John's Institute of Dermatology at St Thomas' Hospital in London, United Kingdom.She was working as a consultant Pathologist with a special interest in Dermatopathology and Oncology, at the Department of Anatomical Pathology at the General Hospital of Patras Greece for 10 years. Currently, she is appointed to the 2nd Department of Pathology of National and Kapodistrian University of Athens. She is a member of the Pan Hellenic Society of Pathologists and the European Society of Pathologists. She is a coordinator of the Hellenic Dermatopathology Working Group. She is a member of the European Dermatopathology, Working Group and of the European task-force for structured reporting. She is a slide manager in 'London Diagnostic Dermatopathology Course". Up to date, she has published more than 15 articles in peer-reviewed journals, with 297 citations (h-index: 7.) and more than 35 poster presentations in international conferences. She is an author of the "Connective tissue tumors" chapter in "McKee's Pathology of the skin" and the "Non- neoplastic skin disorders" chapter in the Hippon e-learning platform.

Katerina Giazitzi is a research fellow at the Department of Nutrition and Dietetics, School of Health Sciences and Education, Harokopio University Athens. She is a dietitian and she has also an MSc in Nutrition and Public Health. Her research interests are nutrition, dietetics, public health and food service management.

Alina Roxani Gouloumi is a pathologist working at Attikon University Hospital in Athens, Greece and a PhD student at Athens Medical School. She graduated from Transilvania University of Brasov (Medical Doctor degree and Master of Science degree). She completed a residency at the Pathology Department of Attikon University hospital and at the Cytology Department of "Alexandra" Hospital.

Sophia Kalantaridou is a Professor of Obstetrics, Gynecology and Infertility. National and Kapodistrian University of Athens, School of Medicine. Chair, 3rd Department of Obstetrics and Gynecology, Special Interest: Reproductive Endocrinology.

Effrosyni Karakitsou has graduated from the School of Applied Mathematical and Physical Sciences of the National Technical University of Athens, Greece in 2014. She obtained a Master's degree in Systems Biology from the University of Surrey, UK in 2015 and she then started her doctorate studies in Computational Biology at the University of Barcelona under HaemMetabolome, a Marie Sklodowska-Curie actions project. She is experienced in information and data processing as well as in software development for the creation of support systems related to cytopathology practice. She has contributed three chapters in honorary books, and numerous publications in international and national conferences as well as in scientific journals. She has also participated in the writing of one book chapter. Her research interests include bioinformatics technologies, information and data processing for knowledge discovery, neural networks, genetic algorithms and distributed computing systems.

Vaios Karathanos is a Professor in Food Engineering at the Department of Nutrition and Dietetics, School of Health Sciences and Education, Harokopio University Athens. His research interests are food chemistry, quality of food and food engineering.

Dimitrios Katehakis holds an Electrical Engineering Diploma from the Technical University of Patras, Greece, and an MS in Electrical Engineering, from the University of Maryland at College Park. He heads the Center for eHealth Applications and Services at FORTH-ICS since 2010. He is also the Secretary General of HL7 Hellas (since 2014), and the Hellenic Health Informatics Association (since 2018). He has participated in the implementation of a large number of eHealth projects, in both Europe and the US. His work focuses on data integration analysis and the design of information systems and distributed architectures for forward-looking, integrated EHR services. Products of his work operate in a large number of health units in Greece. Areas of expertise: Health Information Networks, Health Information Infrastructure, Electronic Health, Health IT Solutions, EHR Standards, EHR Systems, Integrated Care Solutions, Interoperability, eHealth.

Nektarios Koufopoulos graduated from "Grigore T. Popa" Medical University English Faculty, Iasi Romania in 2001. He became a state-certified pathologist in 2014. He was a consultant pathologist in Saint Savvas Cancer hospital of Athens, Greece from 18/08/2014 to 31/12/2018. He currently is a consultant pathologist in the 2nd Department of Pathology, National and Kapodistrian University of Athens. His main research interests are breast, gynecological and urological pathology. He is a member of the Hellenic Society of Pathology, Hellenic Society of Oncology, European Society of Pathology and European Society of Gynaecological Oncology.

Yiannis Koumpouros is an Ass. Professor in the University of West Attica, Department of Informatics and Computer Engineering. Specialized in health informatics, e-health, m-health, telemedicine, subjective satisfaction assessment and strategic management. Expert for the European Commission in the e-health sector and evaluator of numerous research and development projects. Senior manager in business operations with wide expertise in design and implementation of strategic, conceptual and complex changes in an international framework. Significant experience in introducing organizational, process and IT solutions for business performance improvement. Top-level managerial experience in private and public healthcare sector (as chairman of hospitals). Teaching in several universities for almost 15 years. Project and R&D manager in IT fields with European experience. Chairman of several Permanent Committee of Experts (Ministry of Development, General Secretariat of Trade), for issues related to Electronic Scientific Equipments and Medical Equipments. Regular member of the Consultative Technical Council (Ministry of Internal Public Administration and Decentralisation) for subjects on new technologies and IT in the wider public administration, etc.

Angelina Kouroubali is a Collaborating Researcher at Computational BioMedicine Laboratory (CBML) of the Institute of Computer Science at the Foundation for Research and Technology-Hellas (FORTH). She holds a Ph.D. in Management of Medical Informatics from the University of Cambridge Judge Business School, a Masters in Medical Informatics from Columbia University in New York and a BA in Biology from Bard College, USA. Dr. Kouroubali has more than 20 years of professional experience in the field of eHealth and Medical Informatics. She has several peer reviewed scientific publications in international and national journals and conferences. She has been a speaker in highly visible Health IT events such as MEDINFO. Her activities include research, consulting and entrepreneurship. Her interests include health information networks, regional and national information infrastructures, electronic health records, coordinated and integrated care, interoperability, prehospital emergency care, evaluation, certification and quality assurance, complexity, innovation and change in health care. She has been a principle investigator for FORTH in European and National projects. She has won several awards in international competitions such as SlideWiki, Haching Health Athens, Athens Datathon and Smart Cities Datathon.

Niki Margari is a private consultant Cytopathologist. She was lecturer in graduate and post graduate courses related to cytopathology. She is member of the Hellenic Society of Clinical Cytology. She has participations in numerous Greek research programs having yielded 18 publications in international peer reviewed medical journals, more than 30 presentations and lectures in Greek and international scientific congresses, with one scientific award and was in the organisation committee of two Greek conferences. She has participated in the development of a specialized for Cytopathology eLearning platform and contributed to one medical book related to endometrial cytopathology. She is fluent Greek, English, French and Hungarian speaker.

Georgios Michail graduated from Athens University Medical School in 1996. He received the title of Obstetrician-Gynaecologist in 2005, and presented his Thesis, in 2007. After a research fellowship in Ireland (RCSI) and clinical work he acquired the British Society of Colposcopy & Cervical Pathology (B.S.C.C.P.) Diagnosis & Treatment Diploma in 2006. From 2007 onwards he has worked privately, and then served as an Obs/Gynae Consultant. Since 2013 he serves as a Senior Clinical Lecturer in Obstetrics and Gynecology in Patras University Hospital contributing in the clinical and surgical curriculum of the ward. He is Head Colposcopist of the Outpatient Clinic, and a member of the multidisciplinary Oncological Board. He has contributed in scientific protocols under the auspices of the Hellenic Society of Colposcopy and Cervical Pathology (H.S.C.C.P.) and the Hellenic Cervical Pathology Academic (HeCPA) Group. His current research interests are focused in Gynecologic Oncology and Colposcopy, the epidemiology and the molecular mechanisms of HPV infection, HPV vaccination, cervical screening and Gynae Oncology. His teaching experience has been built in Patras University Medical School. He has published in several journals as well as chapters in books. He has membership in several Journal's Editorial Boards, membership of academic bodies and has reviewed numerous articles.

Antonia Mourtzikou obtained a MSc in Biochemistry, a MSc in Health Services Management, a MSc in Public Health (MPH) and a MSc in Clinical Chemistry. She is a PhD (Athens Medical School, Ethnikon kai Kapodistriako Panepistimio Athinon-EKPA).She is also a EurSpecLabMed and has worked as a staff Clinical Biochemist since 1987 in “Asclepeion” Voulas General Hospital. From 2010-present she works in the Department of Cytopathology in University General Hospital “Attikon”. She has attended many scientific seminars, workshops, symposiums, international and Hellenic congresses and conferences. She has published 23 papers at international peer-reviewed scientific journals and 26 papers at greek peer-reviewed scientific journals. She has participated at more than 80 seminars, 24 workshops and at 52 Hellenic and International Congresses with 10 oral presentations and 63 posters, of which 2 oral presentations have been awarded as “the best oral presentation of the congress” and 1 price award of 5000 euros in 2006 for the excellence of the “original work”. She is co-author of 1book chapter. She speaks Greek, English, French and Bulgarian. Her research concerns novel biomarkers, biochemistry and molecular diagnostic methods, flow cytometry, laboratory quality and laboratory management, hospital management and public health. She is reviewer in several international peer-reviewed scientific journals.

Martha Nifora graduated from the University of Patras School of Medicine in 2011 and became a state-certified Pathologist in 2018. She has attended a three-month training program in Forensic Pathology at the University of Athens 1st Pathology Department. Her special interests include Forensic Pathology, Neuropathology, Skin and Soft tissue Pathology. She currently is a consultant pathologist at the 2nd Department of Pathology at the University of Athens Medical School.

Ioannis Panayiotides graduated summa cum laude in 1988 from the University of Ioannina Medical School; he became a state-certified pathologist in 1993 and PhD in 1995 (University of Crete Medical School). He obtained scholarships of the European Society of Pathology and of the European Cancer Centre (Amsterdam) and was further trained in Amsterdam (Vrije Universiteit) and Reims (Université de Reims Champagne-Ardenne). He is a university staff member since 1997 and Head of the 2nd Department of Pathology at the University of Athens Medical School ("Attikon" University Hospital) since 2006. His main research interests (pathology of the skin, cervix uteri, head and neck and CNS, history of pathology) have so far yielded 177 papers in peer-reviewed journals, with 2151 citations (self-citations excluded), amongst which 148 in books. h-index: 28.

George Pangalos of Aristotle University of Thessaloniki, Greece, Dept. of Electrical and Computer Engineering, Information Security laboratory. His research and scientific interests include: Health IT systems design and implementation, Information Systems Security, and e-Gov applications. He has published over 200 articles in international scientific journals and conferences. He has also been author or co-author in several (more than 20) International and Greek books on IT and IT security subjects. He has been involved as project leader - expert in many (more than 50) major international (mostly EU funded) research and development projects in the above areas, most of them in the area of e-Health (epSOS, EXPAND, CEF, e-Helth ID, e-Health Action, NETCARDS, New4EESSI, eHGI, SOHealth, etc.). He has also been the president and member of the board in several national and international scientific and professional bodies and also president and CEO in several Health IT related organizations and departments (President of the Greek Centre for e-government Applications in Social Security and Health (IDIKA), President and CEO of the Regional Health System (PESY) of Thessaly, Director ELKEPA, etc.).

Vasilios Pergialiotis is an Obstetrician and Gynaecologist. He undertook his medical training in the National and Kapodistrian University of Athens, Greece. He graduated from the Athens Medical School at 2004. He completed his specialty training in Laikon General Hospital and Alexandra Maternity Hospital. At 2011 he received the Master of Science Diploma with distinction in "Minimally Invasive Surgery, Robotic Surgery and Telesurgery" from the National and Kapodistrian University of Athens. At 2013 he completed his thesis and received his PhD with distinction in the field of breast cancer. Since February 2014 he is working as a research fellow of the National and Kapodistrian University of Athens at the Laboratory of Experimental Surgery and Surgical Research N.S. Christeas. He is the scientific supervisor of a research team of pre-graduate medical students and post-graduate doctors that is involved in clinical and experimental research. During the last 5 years he has actively participated in more than 100 research projects and for his scientific activity he has been awarded in an international and national level. Since February 2016 he is an Academic Clinical Fellow (Panepistimiakos Ypotrofos) of the 3rd dpt of Obstetrics and Gynecology at Attikon University Hospital. In this position he has participated in all activities of the section of Gynecologic Oncology. At 2016 he received the diploma of Diagnostic Colposcopy from the Hellenic Society of Cervical Pathology and Colposcopy. At 2017 he received the European Certificate of Bachelor in Endoscopy from the European Academy of Gynaecological Surgery after successfully completing the theoretical and practical session. He is a Lecturer in the postgraduate medical programs "Minimally Invasive Surgery, Robotic Surgery and Telesurgery" and "High Risk Pregnancy" of the Athens Medical School of the National and Kapodistrian University of Athens.

Stavros Pitoglou is currently the Chief Technical Officer (CTO) and Head of the Research & Development (R&D) Department of Computer Solutions SA and has been working for the company since 2003. He has graduated from the Physics Department of the University of Patras. Since 2004, participating as Project Director or Senior Project Manager, he successfully administered several large-scale projects in the fields of Health IT and Medical Informatics as well as Public Institutions Enterprise Resource Management. He has coordinated and planned large and diverse working groups, especially for the implementation of European projects under the Third European Community Support Framework and the NSRF -National Strategic Reference Framework (Regions of Attica, Thessaly, Ionian Islands, Eastern Macedonia, and Thrace, Greek Court of Auditors, Therapy Center for Dependent Individuals). He is certified as HL7 Control Specialist by HL7 International Organization. As responsible executive, he laid the groundwork for the company's transformation to a highly respected research and cutting edge technology entity by establishing its R&D Department, in 2013. Leading this department ever since, he currently oversees several internal research projects in the fields of Machine Learning & Artificial Intelligence, Chronic Disease Monitoring, Biosignals and Computer Vision & Image Processing. His personal research interests are focused on issues of Machine Learning and Artificial Intelligence applications, Distributed Networks, and Data Security-Privacy. In addition, he is a Ph.D. candidate in the Biomedical Engineering Laboratory, School of Electrical and Computer Engineering of the National Technical University of Athens. His specific field of study is the combination of system dynamics and artificial neural networks (deep learning) towards the development of a novel model of glucose homeostasis regarding physical exercise with the aim of self-management of diabetes mellitus via cloud and mobile computing.

Abraham Pouliakis is physicist, holds an M.Sc. in electronics and radio-communications, and a Ph.D. degree from the Medical School (University of Athens) related to the application of neural networks in cytopathology. Since 1993 has participated in numerous National, European and European Space Agency Research projects related to information and communication technology, artificial intelligence applied in medicine, collaborative systems, e-learning, e-health, and GIS. Currently is senior researcher in the Second Department of Pathology, National and Kapodistrian University of Athens, School of Medicine, as well as responsible for quality control and assurance of the laboratory. He has more than 80 publications in international peer peer-reviewed scientific magazines, more than 200 presentations in international and Greek conferences and is the co-author of 13 books chapters. His research interests are related to information and communication technology, image/signal processing and artificial intelligence including their applications in the fields of industry and health. Dr. Pouliakis is an active peer reviewer in more than 10 scientific journals and associate editor for the International Journal of Reliable and Quality eHealth care (IJRQEH).

Andriana Prentza is full-time Professor of Software Engineering at the Department of Digital Systems of the University of Piraeus, Greece. She received her Diploma in Computer Engineering and Information Sciences and her M.Sc. in Biomedical Engineering from the University of Patras, Greece, and her Ph.D. degree from the Eindhoven University of Technology, Eindhoven, the Netherlands. She has been very actively involved in a number of European and National R&D programs focusing on Information Communication Technologies (ICT) projects and she serves as expert evaluator and reviewer for the European Commission and national R&D programmes. She has published more than 80 scientific papers in peer-reviewed international journals, book chapters and conference proceedings. Her current research interests include Software Engineering techniques and methodologies for the development and evaluation of software systems and services in the areas of eGovernment and eHealth. She is a Senior Member of IEEE and a member of the Technical Chamber of Greece.

Pranil. V. Sawalakhe has completed his BE from Nagpur University, Nagpur. He received his post graduation M.S. (Advanced Manufacturing Systems) from TEESSIDE University, UK. He had achieved submitted his PhD titled "Model for Evaluating Testing Laboratory performance on Quality Indicators with Six Sigma Scales " in 2019. He had worked as an Assistant professor in the department of Mechanical Engineering at Priyadarshini College of Engineering, Nagpur.

Vasileios Sioulas is a practicing OBGYN and Gynecologic Oncologist, and is affiliated with the National and Kapodistrian University of Athens in Athens, Greece.

Marilena Stamouli received their Diploma in Biology (1986) from the University of Athens, Greece, the MSc degree in Health Management (2010) from the University of Pireus, Greece, and the MSc degree in TQM (2016) from the Hellenic Open University. From 1987 until today she works at the Biopathology Laboratory of the Naval Hospital of Athens, as tenured civilian scientific personnel, and she is supervisor of the Biochemistry Laboratory since 2012. Her main research interests include biochemistry, autoimmunity, thalassaemia and haemoglobinopathies, molecular diagnostic methods and laboratory quality control. She has published 40 related articles in scientific journals and 90 articles in proceedings of peer-reviewed scientific conferences. She has also attended many scientific seminars and workshops. She is a member of the Greek Society of Clinical Chemistry- Clinical Biochemistry, of the Hellenic Society of Immunology and of the European Register of Specialists in Clinical Chemistry and Laboratory Medicine.

George Valasoulis is a consultant Obstetrician & Gynaecologist in IASO Thessaly Hospital, since 2018. He was graduated from the Medical School of the University of Ioannina, Greece in 2004. Dr. Valasoulis has completed his doctorate (PhD) in Gynecology Oncology - Cervical pathology in Medicine with Honours, at the Medical School of the University of Ioannina in 2014. In February 2018 received with Honours, the Postgraduate Diploma of Specialization (MSc) in "Prenatal Diagnosis - Contraception - Childbearing" at the Department of Medicine of the Democritus University of Thrace, Greece. Dr. Valasoulis is author of more than 30 publications in peer reviewed journals, book chapters and reviews, and has more than 320 citations with h-index 11 in SCOPUS. He has more than 180 presentations (invited-oral/poster) at national & international conferences, more than 20 first prize awards (including RCOG, BSCCP, HSCCP, European Congresses of Cytology), scholarships and academic distinctions. He has participated as Sub-researcher - Participation in the HPV Research European Program and a phase 3 clinical trial. Dr. Valasoulis is reviewer in several distinguished gynaecology journals including Gynecologic Oncology, BMJ, BJOG, etc.

Andriani Zacharatou graduated from the University of Crete Medical School in 2013. She currently is a resident at the 2nd Department of Pathology at the University of Athens Medical School. She participates in the Department's training activities including scientific publications in various congresses. Her special interests include Lung and Female Genital Tract Pathology.

Index

G

H

I

J

L

M

N

P

Q

R

S

T

U

V

W

Printed in the USA
CPSIA information can be obtained
at www.ICGtesting.com
LVHW080208230923
759047LV00007B/114

9 781799 823902